G. E. Cold · N. Juul (Eds.)

Monitoring of Cerebral and Spinal Haemodynamics During Neurosurgery

Georg E. Cold · Niels Juul (Eds.)

Monitoring of Cerebral and Spinal Haemodynamics During Neurosurgery

With collaboration of Mads Rasmussen, Alp Tankisi, Helle Bundgaard, Lise Schlünzen, Birgitte Duch, Etienne Karatasi, Lisbeth Krogh, Jens-Aage Kølsen-Petersen, Karsten Skovgaard Olsen, Claus Mosdal and Bent Lob Dahl

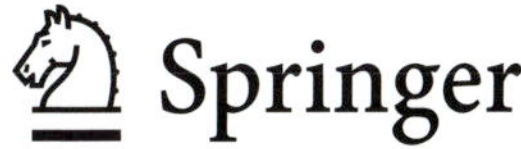

Springer

Georg E. Cold
Hojkolvej 2
8210 Aarhus V
Denmark

Niels Juul
Department of Neuroanaesthesia
Aarhus University Hospital
Norrebrogade 44
8000 Aarhus C
Denmark

ISBN 978-3-540-77872-1   e-ISBN 978-3-540-77873-8

DOI 10.1007/978-3-540-77873-8

Library of Congress Control Number: 2008920954

Cover design: Frido Steinen-Broo, eStudio, Calamar, Spain
Typesetting and Production: le-tex publishing services oHG, Leipzig, Germany

Printed on acid-free paper

9 8 7 6 5 4 3 2 1

springer.com

Preface

Make the best of it (Samuel Pepys)

Everyone interested in neuroanaesthesia talks about intracranial pressure (ICP), but in daily clinical practice nobody measures it during craniotomy. This was our view ten years ago, when Dr. Cold was asked by an international congress to make a speech with the title: Is hyperventilation mandatory during craniotomy? Panic triggered our intellectual resources and, thanks to our good friends the neurosurgeons, we soon performed the first measurement of subdural ICP. Very soon we were convinced that perioperative subdural ICP measurement not only gave important information concerning the occurrence of brain swelling after opening of dura, but also it was possible to follow the effects of ICP-reducing procedures such as hyperventilation, indomethacin, mannitol treatment and surgical decompression by drainage of ventricular fluid or cystic tumours. Moreover, we were convinced that perioperative ICP measurement combined with gas analysis from arterial and jugular venous blood would provide us with important neurophysiological information, instead of the prevailing feeling that the intracranial content is a black box until the exposure of dura. As a consequence, we introduced subdural ICP measurement and insertion of a jugular bulb catheter as routine procedures, provided resources were available, and we soon found that a database containing relevant information for interpretation of ICP data was needed.

Our database contains information from about 1,830 predominantly elective patients undergoing craniotomy. Our first publication concerning the method was published in the *British Journal of Neurosurgery* (1996), and was followed by other publications. Data from these publications are presented in this book and we acknowledge the editors for giving permission to extract data from these publications.

The studies presented in this book are prospectively collected and 8 studies were designed as controlled studies, but the majority of the comparative studies were based on data from the database. In total 16 published and 27 unpublished studies are included in this book. We are well aware that uncontrolled studies, based on collection from a database, can be criticized. Nevertheless, we argue that results from uncontrolled studies may give a hint, and stimulate the repetition of such studies in a controlled design.

As the methods of monitoring, measurement of subdural ICP and data concerning cerebral haemodynamics, and anaesthetic practice are the same, we have chosen to collect these data in a separate chapter (Chapter 2). Moreover, we have preferred the "old fashioned" way of presenting references in the text by name and year of publication, and consequently the reference lists are alphabetical.

Georg E. Cold
Niels Juul

Published papers concerning subdural ICP include the following:

Bundgaard H, Cold GE (2000) Studies of regional subdural pressure gradients during craniotomy. Br J Neurosurg 14:229–234

Bundgaard H, Jensen K, Cold GE et al (1996) Effects of perioperative indomethacin in intracranial pressure, cerebral blood flow, and cerebral metabolism in patients subjected to craniotomy for cerebral tumors. J Neurosurg Anesthesiol 8:273–279

Bundgaard H, Landsfeldt U, Cold GE (1997) Subdural monitoring of ICP during craniotomy: thresholds of cerebral swelling/herniation. Acta Neurochir Suppl 71:276–279

Bundgaard H, von Oettingen G, Larsen KM et al (1998) Effects of sevoflurane on intracranial pressure, cerebral blood flow and cerebral metabolism. Acta Anaesthesiol Scand 42:621–627

Bundgaard H, von Oettingen G, Jørgensen H et al (2001) Effects of dihydroergotamine on intracranial pressure, cerebral blood flow, and cerebral metabolism in patients undergoing craniotomy for brain tumors. J Neurosurg Anesthesiol 3:195–201

Cold GE, Tange M, Jensen TM et al (1996) Subdural pressure measurement during craniotomy. Correlation with tactile estimation of dural tension and brain herniation after opening of dura. Br J Neurosurg 10: 69-75

Cold GE, Bundgaard H, von Oettingen G et al (1998) ICP during anaesthesia with sevoflurane: a dose-response study. Effect of hypocapnia. Acta Neurochir Suppl 71:279–281

Haure P, Cold GE, Hansen TM et al (2003) The ICP-lowering effect of 10° reverse Trendelenburg position during craniotomy is stable during a 10-minute period. J Neurosurg Anesthesiol 15:297–301

Jørgensen HA, Bundgaard H, Cold GE (1999) Subdural pressure measurement during posterior fossa surgery. Correlation studies of brain swelling/herniation after dural incision with measurement of subdural pressure and tactile estimation of dural tension. Br J Neurosurg 13:449–453

Olsen KS, Juul N, Cold GE (2005) Effect of alfentanil on intracranial pressure during propofol-fentanyl anesthesia for craniotomy. A randomized prospective dose-response study. Acta Anaesthesiol Scand 49:445–452

Petersen KD, Landsfeldt U, Cold GE et al (2003) Intracranial pressure and cerebral hemodynamic in patients with cerebral tumors. Anesthesiology 98:329–336

Rasmussen M, Tankisi A, Cold GE (2004) The effects of indomethacin on intracranial pressure and cerebral haemodynamics in patients undergoing craniotomy: a randomized prospective study. Anaesthesia 59:1–8

Rasmussen M, Bundgaard H, Cold GE (2004) Craniotomy for supratentorial brain tumors: risk factors for brain swelling after opening of dura mater. J Neurosurg 101:621–626

Rolighed Larsen JK, Haure P, Cold GE (2002) Reverse Trendelenburg position reduces intracranial pressure during craniotomy. J Neurosurg Anesthesiol 14:16–21

Stilling M, Karatasi E, Rasmussen M et al (2005) Subdural intracranial pressure, cerebral perfusion pressure, and degree of cerebral swelling in supra- and infratentorial space-occupying lesions in children. Acta Neurochir Suppl 95:133–136

Tankisi A, Cold GE (2007) Optimal reverse Trendelenburg position in patients undergoing craniotomy for cerebral tumors. J Neurosurg 106:239–244

Tankisi A, Rolighed Larsen J, Rasmussen M et al (2002) The effects of 10 degrees reverse Trendelenburg position on ICP and CPP in prone positioned patients subjected to craniotomy for occipital or cerebellar tumours. Acta Neurochir (Wien) 144:665–670

Tankisi A, Rasmussen M, Juul N et al (2006) The effects of 10° reverse Trendelenburg position (rTp) on subdural intracranial pressure and cerebral perfusion pressure in patients subjected to craniotomy for cerebral aneurysm. J Neurosurg Anesthsiol 18:11–17

Content

List of Contributors

Helle Bundgaard
Department of Neuroanaesthesia
Aarhus University Hospital
Noorebrogade 44
8000 Aarhus C
Denmark

Georg E. Cold
Hojkolvej 2
8210 Aarhus V
Denmark

Bent Lob Dahl
Department of Neuroanaesthesia
Aarhus University Hospital
Noorebrogade 44
8000 Aarhus C
Denmark

Birgitte Duch
Department of Neuroanaesthesia
Aarhus University Hospital
Noorebrogade 44
8000 Aarhus C
Denmark

Niels Juul
Department of Neuroanaesthesia
Aarhus University Hospital
Norrebrogade 44
8000 Aarhus C
Denmark

Etienne Karatasi
Department of Neuroanaesthesia
Aarhus University Hospital
Noorebrogade 44
8000 Aarhus C
Denmark

Jens Aage Kolsen-Petersen
Department of Neuroanaesthesia
Aarhus University Hospital
Noorebrogade 44
8000 Aarhus C
Denmark

Lisbeth Krogh
Department of Neuroanaesthesia
Aarhus University Hospital
Noorebrogade 44
8000 Aarhus C
Denmark

Claus Mosdal
Department of Neurosurgery
Aarhus University Hospital
Noorebrogade 44
8000 Aarhus C
Denmark

Mads Rasmussen
Department of Neuroanaesthesia
Aarhus University Hospital
Noorebrogade 44
8000 Aarhus C
Denmark

Lise Schlünzen
Department of Neuroanaesthesia
Aarhus University Hospital
Noorebrogade 44
8000 Aarhus C
Denmark

Karsten Skovgaard Olsen
Department of Anesthesia
and Intensive Care
Glostrup University Hospital
University of Copenhagen
2600 Glostrup
Denmark

Alp Tankisi
Department of Neuroanaesthesia
Aarhus University Hospital
Noorebrogade 44
8000 Aarhus C
Denmark

Abbreviations

ARDS	Acute respiratory distress syndrome
AVD	Arteriovenous difference
$AVDO_2$	Arteriovenous oxygen difference
BIS	Bispectral index
BMI	Body mass index
CBF	Cerebral blood flow
CBV	Cerebral blood volume
CI	Confidence interval
$CMRO_2$	Cerebral metabolic rate of oxygen
CPAP	Continuous positive airway pressure
CPP	Cerebral perfusion pressure
CSF	Cerebrospinal fluid
CT	Computed tomography
CVP	Central venous pressure
CVR	Cerebrovascular resistance
DHE	Dihydroergotamine
DPG	2,3-Dephosphoglycerate
DWI	Diffusion-weighted magnetic resonance imaging
EC_{50}	Half maximal effective concentration
EEG	Electroencephalogram
FiO_2	Fraction of inspired oxygen
GCS	Glasgow Coma Scale
GOS	Glasgow Outcome Scale
HES	Hydroxyethyl starch
ICP	Intracranial pressure
IVP	Intraventricular pressure
JBP	Jugular bulb pressure
JP	Jugular pressure
MABP	Mean arterial blood pressure
MAC	Minimal alveolar concentration
MCAO	Middle cerebral artery occlusion
MRI	Magnetic resonance imaging
NIBP	Non-invasive blood pressure

O_2Ct	Venous oxygen content
OR	Odds ratio
$PaCO_2$	Partial pressure of carbon dioxide
PaO_2	Partial pressure of oxygen
$PbrO_2$	Brain tissue oxygen tension
PEEP	Positive end-expiratory pressure
PET	Positron emission tomography
$PtiO_2$	Partial tissue oxygen tension
PVI	Pressure/volume index
PvO_2	Jugular venous oxygen tension
PVR	Peripheral vascular resistance
r	Correlation coefficient
rCBF	Regional cerebral blood flow
rCBV	Regional cerebral blood volume
rTp	Reverse Trendelenburg position
SAH	Subarachnoid haemorrhage
SATv	Jugular venous saturation
SBF	Spinal cord blood flow
SD	Standard deviation
SE	Standard error of mean
SjO_2	Jugular venous/bulb oxygen saturation
SPP	Spinal perfusion pressure
SSP	Spinal subdural pressure
TBI	Traumatic brain injury

Chapter 1
Monitoring of Intracranial Pressure (ICP): A Review

Jens Aage Kolsen-Petersen, Bent Lob Dahl and Georg Emil Cold

Abstract

Everyone interested in neuroanaesthesia talks about intracranial pressure (ICP), but in daily clinical practice nobody measures it during craniotomy. This was the thesis that started this work more than ten years ago. A method for easy monitoring of ICP during surgery, but before opening of dura, was devised and the method was introduced in our daily clinical practice.

In this chapter indications for ICP measurement, critical levels of ICP and regional differences in ICP are described. Medical approaches to ICP control are considered, including body position, hyperventilation, hypothermia and administration of barbiturate. The effect of suctioning, positive end-expiratory pressure, sedatives and analgetics are discussed as well as the use of mannitol and hypertonic saline.

In this chapter, indication for intracranial pressure (ICP) measurement, critical levels of ICP and regional differences in ICP are described. Medical approaches to ICP control are considered, including body position, hyperventilation, hypothermia and administration of barbiturate. The effect of suctioning, positive end-expiratory pressure (PEEP), sedatives and analgesics are discussed as well as mannitol and hypertonic saline.

Lundberg (1960) introduced continuous intraventricular pressure (IVP) monitoring in the neurointensive clinic. This method, based on an intraventricular catheter connected to a pressure transducer at the level of the external auditory meatus, has remained the gold standard ever since. The main limitation of this method is the risk of infection that increases over time and is in the range 6–11% (Mayhall et al. 1984; Aucoin et al. 1986). Owing to the traumatic nature of the method, difficulties concerning the surgical procedure, especially when the cerebral ventricles are compressed, and the relatively high infection rate, other methods have been introduced. These include: epidural transducer; subdural bolt via a burr hole; subdural catheter; peroperative placement of a subdural needle; intraparenchymal transducer; lumbar spinal fluid pressure; and lumbar epidural pressure.

1.1
Normal Intracranial Pressure Values

Cerebrospinal fluid (CSF) pressure data of spinal origin are numerous. Normal pressure is generally defined as pressures below 200 mmH$_2$O, corresponding to 15 mmHg. In supine subjects without cerebral disorders ICP averages 11 mmHg (SD 2 mmHg, range 7–15 mmHg) (Albeck et al. 1998). In the vertical position, the ICP is approximately 10 mmHg, and does not exceed 15 mmHg (Czosnyka and Pickard 2004). Full Term infants have an ICP ranging between 2 and 6 mmHg (Dunn 2002), and during the first days after birth even sub-atmospheric ICP is common (Welch 1980). In children values between 3 and 7 mmHg are within the normal range (Dunn 2002).

1.2
Regional Differences in Intracranial Pressure

1.2.1
Animal Studies

It is generally believed that ICP is the same throughout the CSF spaces within the cranial cavity. Accordingly, in an experimental model of hydrocephalus in dogs, pressure gradients between ventricle, brain and subarachnoid space were not detected (Penn et al. 2005).

Pressure gradients between supra- and infratentorial compartments have been found in a pig model of epidural bleeding during expansion of a supratentorial balloon (Langfitt et al. 1964; Ganz et al. 1995). Pressure gradients within the supratentorial compartment have been studied in monkeys subjected to inflation of a balloon. It was found that pressure forces were not uniformly transmitted from an expanding mass. Even pressure decreases were observed in some brain regions (Kuchiwaki et al. 1992). Miller et al. (1987) showed evidence of temporary interhemispheric ICP gradients, ranging from 5 to 14 mmHg, in animal models of mass lesion. Supratentorial gradients of ICP have also been reported in cats and baboons after middle cerebral artery occlusion (MCAO) (Tulleken et al. 1978), and in mass lesion in the baboon (Symon et al. 1974). In a porcine model of frontal mass lesion, intraparenchymal ICP monitors were placed in the right and left hemispheres. During expansion of the mass, a pressure difference that increased as the size of the mass increased developed between intracranial regions. The regional pressures were found to vary in a consistent fashion. Right and left frontal pressures were equal. The pressure gradients through the brain were as follows: frontal pressures > temporal pressures > midbrain pressures > cerebellar pressures (Wolfla et al. 1996).

1.2.2
Human Studies

Pressure gradients between supra- and infratentorial compartments have been reported during fossa posterior surgery (Rosenwasser et al. 1989; Poon et al. 2002).

Pressure gradients, related to the underlying tumour and/or gravity, have been reported in patients with cerebral tumours (Bundgaard and Cold 2000). Significant and lasting ICP gradients (> 10 mmHg) were found between the frontal hemispheres in all patients with an acute subdural haematoma (Chambers et al. 1998). In patients with mass lesions, supratentorial pressure gradients up to 28 mmHg have been observed (Weaver et al. 1982; Marshall et al. 1986; Broaddus et al. 1989; Chambers et al. 2001), as in patients with intracerebral haematoma (Roux et al. 1984). In clinical studies of head injury, interhemispheric supratentorial pressure gradients have been demonstrated. Mindermann and Gratzl (1998) found that even in patients without space-occupying lesions, pressure difference exists, and argue that simultaneous bilateral ICP measurement may be warranted in the initial posttraumatic phase. Transient gradients that disappear with time are frequently observed, and may indicate an increase in the size of the lesion (Sahuquillo et al. 1999).

Interhemispheric pressure differences were not demonstrated in a clinical study of head injury with bilateral frontal placement of transducers (Yano et al. 1987).

1.3
Pressure/Volume Relationship

Intracranial volume is on average $900\,\mathrm{cm}^3$ in men and $600\,\mathrm{cm}^3$ in women in the first few months of life. By the age of 15 years, it increases up to $1,500\,\mathrm{cm}^3$ in men and $1,300\,\mathrm{cm}^3$ in women. The change in intracranial volume that occurs with age is not linear. Three main periods can be distinguished, each lasting approximately 5 years (0–5, 5–10 and 10–15 years), during which the growth of intracranial volume is linear (Sgouros et al. 1999).

Compliance is defined as the pressure reaction to a change in intracranial volume (DV/DP). The exponential nature of the pressure/volume curve indicates that a similar volume increment at different points of the curve results in a different pressure response. The slope of the pressure/volume curve is dependent on the compensatory mechanisms. Thus, changes in ventricular fluid volume and cerebral blood volume (CBV) influence the pressure increase obtained during volume expansion. Furthermore, the steepness of the pressure/volume curve varies under different pathological circumstances, and is also influenced by therapy with mannitol and steroids. Furthermore, compliance decreases with age and may account for some of the poor outcomes in elderly brain-injured patients (Kiening et al. 2002).

It has been stressed that different compartments exist, not only between supra- and infratentorial regions and interhemispherically, but also between ipsilateral supratentorial regions. Thus, pressure gradients occur between these compartments (see above) and the pressure/volume relationship therefore differs as well (Schaller and Graf 2005).

The pressure/volume index (PVI) is defined as the volume necessary to raise the ICP by a factor of 10 mmHg. By plotting the pressure on a logarithmic axis against volume, the otherwise exponential curve becomes linear. The slope of this curve is the pressure/volume index. In adults the pressure/volume index averages 25 ml, whereas in infants the index averages 10 ml (Shapiro and Marmarou 1989).

Recently, the Spiegelberg intracranial pressure and intracranial compliance monitor system have been tested. Good correlation of compliance was found with the CSF-bolus injection technique in experimental (Yau et al. 2000) and clinical studies (Piper et al. 1999). In a recent study of patients with severe head injury, it was found that at ICP > 20 mmHg, compliance was linearly correlated to cerebral perfusion pressure (CPP) suggesting failure of the autoregulatory mechanism (Protella et al. 2002).

Phase-contrast magnetic resonance imaging (MRI) measurements of systolic CSF peak velocity in the aqueduct of Sylvius is a sensitive method to detect minor changes in cerebral compliance. It has been reported that systolic CSF peak velocity decreases when CSF pressure was experimentally increased by continuous positive airway pressure (CPAP). In anaesthetized patients, hypercapnia increases systolic CSF peak velocity in comparison with normocapnia (Kolbitsch et al. 2002).

1.4
Pressure Waves

Waves occur synchronously with the cardiac cycle and respiration. Waves synchronized with positive pressure ventilation are supposed to be caused by an increase in intrathoracic pressure. Cyclic variation of cerebral pial arteriolar diameter also occurs. The amplitude of these variations is greater during normal arteriolar tone than during vasodilatation caused by hypercapnia (Daley et al. 2002).

Lundberg (1960) described A-waves, B-waves and C-waves. A-waves are characterized as large plateau-like formations recurring at intervals of varying length with duration of 5–20 min and pressure increase of maximally 100 mmHg. A-waves occur in space-occupying lesions. They are associated with an increase in CBV (Risberg et al. 1969), which again may be caused by changes in CPP in patients with intact autoregulation (Rosner and Becker 1984). Experimentally, spontaneous activity of the locus coeruleus complex is suppressed during plateau waves, while the activity of neurons from the cholinoceptive pontine area is increased (Maeda et al. 1989). Other studies indicate that a lesion in the ventral noradrenergic system evoked ICP changes resembling plateau-waves, while activation of the same system by glutamate microinjection produced a decrease in ICP (Maeda et al. 1993). Thus, activity within the cholinergic basal forebrain, as well as the central noradrenergic system, contributes to ICP changes resembling plateau-waves (Maeda and Miyazaki 1998).

B-waves are defined as rhythmic oscillations, with ICP increase above 20 mmHg, occurring more or less regularly at a frequency of 0.5–2 per minute often synchronously with respiration (Lundberg 1960). B-waves are provoked by a decrease in CPP (Rosner and Coley 1986). Concomitance between B-waves and alternating electroencephalogram (EEG) tracings has been documented in patients with traumatic brain injury (Guieu et al. 1979; Munari and Calbucci 1979). Lescot et al. (2005) proposed that a neuropacemaker was the origin of B-waves, which increases the cerebral metabolic rate of oxygen ($CMRO_2$) and CBV, and leads to secondary increases in ICP.

C-waves are defined as rhythmic oscillations occurring with a frequency of 4–8 per minute with amplitude from non-discernable to 20 mmHg. C-waves are related to rhythmic variations of systemic arterial pressure described as Traube-Hering-Mayer waves. The ventrolateral medullary surface is considered as one synaptic relay involved in the generation of arterial blood oscillation (Haxhiu et al. 1989).

1.5
Critical Levels of Intracranial Pressure

Monro (1823) and Kellie (1824) defined the principles of increased ICP. Provided that the fontanels and sutures are closed, the Monro Kellie doctrine states the following: (1) the brain is enclosed in a non-expandable case of bone; (2) the brain parenchyma is nearly incompressible; (3) the volume of the blood in the cranial cavity is therefore nearly constant; and (4) a continuous outflow of venous blood from the cranial cavity is required to make room for continuous incoming arterial blood.

The tolerance to intracranial hypertension depends on the pathophysiology. Thus, high ICP levels are tolerated fairly well as regards neurological status and consciousness, if the pressure increase is developed over months or years and the high pressure is not accompanied by major shifts of the intracranial content. This is observed in obstructive hydrocephalus and slow-growing tumours. On the other hand, if intracranial hypertension is caused by haematomas or cytotoxic oedema, secondary to ischaemia, and is accompanied by a major shift of the intracranial compartments, it is tolerated badly. According to Eide (2003) the actual size or changes in size of the cerebral ventricles are no reliable predictors of ICP or changes in ICP. Thus, great caution should be exercised when predicting ICP on the basis of the size of the cerebral ventricles on cranial CT scanning.

1.5.1
Experimental Studies

In baboons, ischaemic oedema (cytotoxic oedema) is a threshold phenomenon that develops when cerebral blood flow (CBF) is reduced below 20 ml/100 g/min (Symon et al. 1979). However, oedema formation is also dependent on the duration of the ischaemic period and whether ischaemia is complete or incomplete (Ito et al. 1979; Schuier and Hossmann 1980; Todd et al. 1986). Studies in dogs of brain tissue- and CSF oxygen tension indicate that CPP below 80 mmHg is critical. Below this level brain tissue oxygen tension decreases. In the CPP range of 40–60 mmHg a sharp decline in oxygen tensions was found indicating development of cerebral ischaemia (Maas et al. 1993).

In rabbits the critical level at which ICP rises is PaO_2 level of 50 mmHg. Below this level ICP rises steeply (North et al. 1993).

In cats subjected to epidural balloon insufflations CBF increased when ICP began to rise. At ICP levels of 20–30 mmHg CBF and CBV started to decrease. Decompression of the balloon led to an abrupt decrease in ICP and a transient increase in CBF and CBV, after which both CBF and CBV recovered to control values (Kojima et al. 1993).

In cats posttraumatic hypoventilation exacerbates the ICP increase and reduces the pressure/volume index. It is supposed that these events accelerate neuronal damage and produce more extensive brain oedema (Shima and Marmarou 1993).

1.5.2
Human Studies

Cushing (1903) described the haemodynamic response to a high ICP as arterial hypertension accompanied by bradycardia. Tachycardia, however, is also observed and in a recent clinical study arterial hypertension and tachycardia was found to be a better indicator of impaired cerebral perfusion during neuroendoscopy (Kalmar et al. 2005).

During craniotomy, the critical level of ICP for cerebral swelling after opening of dura is 10 mmHg. This threshold has been demonstrated in supratentorial (Bundgaard et al. 1998) and infratentorial tumours (Jørgensen et al. 1999). In a later study it was demonstrated that when ICP exceeds 13 mmHg a 95% risk of cerebral swelling through the opening of dura occurs, whereas at ICP < 5 mmHg only 5% of patients had cerebral swelling (Rasmussen 2004c).

Studies of ICP in patients with severe head injury indicate that pressure levels above 30–40 mmHg for several hours are associated with a poor outcome (Troupp 1967; Vapalahti et al. 1969; Cold et al. 1975; Changaris et al. 1987). In a study of 160 patients with severe head injury Miller et al. (1977) found intracranial hypertension (ICP > 10 mmHg) in 82% of the patients and in 97% of the patients with a mass lesion. Although ICP > 40 mmHg was only observed in 10% of the patients, intracranial hypertension was found to be a primary reason for death in 50% of the patients.

The relationships between ICP, the pulse wave amplitude and CPP indicate a gradual increase in amplitude with CPP decreasing from 75 to 30 mmHg. For CPP below 30 mmHg there is a sharp decrease in amplitude. This change indicates critical disturbance in cerebral circulation (Czosnyka et al. 1994).

In the American Guidelines (2000; http://www.braintrauma.org) the following recommendations are proposed: "There are insufficient data to support a treatment standard for this topic". As an option the American Guidelines propose: that "intracranial pressure (ICP) treatment should be initiated at an upper threshold of 20–25 mmHg". "Interpretation and treatment of ICP based on any threshold should be corroborated by frequent clinical examination and cerebral perfusion pressure data".

1.6
Intracranial Pressure: Impact on Mortality

Although ICP monitoring may guide therapy and is frequently part of the management of patients with severe traumatic brain injury, randomized studies demonstrating improved outcome in patients subjected to ICP monitoring are not available. In a non-randomized study, however, including patients with intracranial haemorrhage, patients subjected to ICP monitoring had an improved outcome (Valentin et al. 2003).

1.7
Intracranial Pressure After Intracranial Surgery

In a retrospective study including 514 consecutive patients with predominantly cerebral tumours ICP was monitored postoperatively. After supratentorial and infratentorial surgery 18.4% and 12.7% had postoperative sustained ICP elevation exceeding 20 mmHg, respectively. Risk factors for postoperative ICP elevation were resection of glioblastoma, repeat surgery and protracted surgery. The most common computed tomography (CT) findings in patients with elevated ICP were brain oedema and bleeding in the tumour bed (Constantini et al. 1988).

1.8
Approaches to Control of Intracranial Hypertension

The operative approach to correction of intracranial hypertension may be restricted if the main reason for intracranial hypertension is cerebral swelling as a consequence of brain oedema or increased CBV. The control of intracranial hypertension under such circumstances is based on the control of intracranial blood volume either via control of cerebral venous distension (central venous pressure, neck compression, dihydroergotamine) or control by neurophysiological mechanisms including the chemical ($PaCO_2$, PaO_2 indomethacin, theophyllamine), neurogenic or hormonal (catecholamine), metabolic (hypnotics, analgesics, hypothermia) and autoregulatory control of cerebral circulation. Finally, control of cerebral tissue water content is possible by osmotic-acting drugs such as mannitol, diuretics and hypertonic saline.

In this chapter, non-surgical principles of control of ICP will be reviewed. New principles of prevention of ischaemic damage of the brain will shortly be commented on with emphasis on their influence on ICP and/or the pressure/volume relationship.

1.9
Control of Cerebral Blood Volume and Intracranial Pressure

In adults the intracranial blood volume is about 60–80 ml with 2/3 in the capillary and venous bed and 1/3 in the arterial vessels. With an average global CBF of 50 ml/100 g/min, about 700–1,000 ml blood (20% of cardiac output) passes through the cerebrum per minute. As CBF, under normal situations, is precisely adjusted to metabolic demand, adjustment of CBV by changes in the cerebral vascular resistance (hypocapnia, indomethacin, theophyllamine) may be potentially detrimental. On the other hand, a decrease in the cerebral venous blood volume does not influence oxygen delivery. As the blood content in venous vessels is double that of the arterial bed, the potentials of manipulation of the venous blood volume theoretically should have a greater impact on ICP.

1.9.1
Head Elevation

In one study, the decrease in ICP during head elevation was smaller than the decline in blood pressure leading to a decrease in CPP. Under these circumstances elevation of the head might precipitate ICP waves of the B-type (Rosner and Coley 1986). In another study, head elevation was not accompanied by a change in CPP because the decrease in ICP corresponded to that of blood pressure (Feldman et al. 1992). Routine nursing of patients with severe head injury at 30 degrees of head elevation within 24 h after trauma leads to a consistent reduction of ICP with preserved CPP (Ng et al. 2004).

A decrease in CBF with patients in the standing position, amounting to approximately 14–21% of flow in recumbence, has been reported (Scheinberg and Stead 1949; Tindall et al. 1967). In comatose patients CBF decreases gradually with head elevation from 0 to 45 degrees, from 46 to 29 ml/100 g/min. During head elevation, the difference between arterial pressure zeroed at the foramen of Monro and jugular pressure was the major determinant of CBF regardless of head position (Moraine et al. 2000). Dynamic cerebral autoregulation is preserved initially after head-up tilt in normal subjects, but deteriorates in patients with vasovagal syncope (Carey et al. 2001). ICP reduction after a change in body position is significantly greater in patients with free CSF flow through the craniospinal junction than in patents with Chiari's malformation, indicating the impairment of CSF displacement into the spinal canal in the latter (Poca et al. 2006).

1.9.2
Reverse Trendelenburg Position

In supine-positioned patients with supratentorial cerebral tumours 10 degrees reverse Trendelenburg position (10° rTp) decreases ICP from 9.5 to 6 mmHg without affecting CPP (Larsen et al. 2002). Similar changes were observed in prone-positioned patients with cerebellar or occipital tumours (Tankisi et al. 2002) and patients with cerebral aneurysm (Tankisi et al. 2006). The ICP-lowering effect of 10° rTp occurs within 1 min after change in position, and mean arterial blood pressure (MABP), CPP and ICP are stable during the following 10 min (Haure et al. 2003).

Repeated measurements of ICP and CPP at neutral position and varying degrees of rTp between 5 and 15 degrees can be obtained within a few minutes, and a decision concerning optimal position, as regards both the level of CPP and ICP, can be drawn. Five degrees rTp reduces ICP without affecting CPP, but a decrease in CPP was observed when further tilting was obtained. The optimal tilting of the operating table, as regards both the fall in ICP and acceptable fall in CPP, was determined to be 15° rTp (Tankisi and Cold 2007).

1.9.3
Head Flexion, Rotation and Tilting

Changes in head position, including maximal flexion and lateral rotation, leads to an increase in ICP, and elevation of the head give rises to a fall in ICP (Nornes and Magnäs 1971; Hulme and Cooper 1976; Kenning et al. 1981; Urlesberger et al. 1991; Yoshida et al. 1991; Williams and Coyne 1993; Meixensberger et al. 1997; Hung et al. 2000). The ICP increase during head rotation is reduced by concomitant head elevation (Hung et al. 2000). The most alarming increase in ICP, however, is observed during head-down position (Hulme and Cooper 1976; Lee 1989; Feldman et al. 1992; Schneider et al. 1993; Yoshida et al. 1993; Mavrocordatos et al. 2000). The mechanisms are intracranial venous distension and an increase in CBV (Mchedlishvili 1988; Schreiber et al. 2002). During bilateral radical neck dissection measurement of ICP indicates a marked increase in ICP immediately after internal jugular vein ligation with a maximum peak at 30 min. Pressure levels of 40 mmHg were observed as well as systemic arterial hypertension in response to the elevated ICP (Weiss et al. 1993).

Some studies indicate that moderate flexion of the head, 15–30 degrees, is associated with a decrease in ICP owing to the improved venous drainage (Kanter et al. 1993). In another study tilting of the head at a steep angle from neutral position (head-tilt position) was compared with the "sniffing position". The sniffing position was found to be superior to the head-tilt position as regards ICP and CPP (Yoshida et al. 1993).

1.9.4
Central Venous Pressure, Intraabdominal Pressure and Body Position

An increase of central venous pressure (CVP), whatever the reason, may contribute to intracranial hypertension and changes in pressure/volume index. Experimental studies indicate that reduction in brain compliance can be secondary to elevation of CVP following resuscitation from haemorrhagic shock (Hariri et al. 1993). Thus, fluid volume replacement in patients with head injury should be done with careful attention to CVP.

In pigs a significant and linear increase in ICP with increased intraabdominal pressure has been demonstrated. This tendency is augmented during head-down position (Josephs et al. 1994; Rosenthal et al. 1997; Halvorson et al. 1998), but is ameliorated when apneumic retractors are applied (Este-McDonald et al. 1995). During prone position the intraabdominal pressure increases (Hering et al. 2001). This effect may lead to an increase in ICP. In one study the prone position resulted in an increase in ICP but improved CPP in patients with subarachnoid haemorrhage (SAH) or traumatic brain injury (Nekludov et al. 2006); in another study turning of the patients from the supine to the prone position did not influence ICP or CPP (Thelandersson et al. 2006).

Acutely increased intraabdominal pressure displaces the diaphragm cranially, narrowing the inferior vena cava, and increasing CVP and thereby ICP and decreasing CPP. The ICP-increasing effect is supposed to be effected by venous stasis and increased pressure in the sagittal sinus with decreased reabsorption of CSF (Bloomfield et al. 1997; Rosenthal et al. 1998).

1.9.5
Endotracheal Suction and Tracheotomy

In patients with acute traumatic head injury the endotracheal suction procedure, in well-sedated subjects, is accompanied by an increase in ICP, CPP and jugular venous saturation. In comparison, in patients who coughed or moved in response to suctioning there was a slight decrease in CPP and venous saturation (Gemma et al. 2002).

In patients with severe brain damage tracheotomy is accompanied by an increase in ICP. Careful monitoring and patient selection is recommended (Stocchetti et al. 2000).

1.10
Positive End-Expiratory Pressure and Continuous Positive Airway Pressure

Coughing, Valsalva manoeuvre, application of PEEP and CPAP, and neck compression are supposed to increase ICP. The mechanisms should be an increase in cerebral venous pressure. Even application of a cervical collar for immobilization might increase ICP (Raphael and Chotai 1994).

In rabbits subjected to elevation of ICP by an epidural balloon, it was demonstrated that the volume needed to reach the deflection point of the volume/pressure course was lower, when PEEP at $10\,cmH_2O$ was applied, compared to the values at PEEP zero. The study suggested that PEEP decreased intracranial compliance (Feldman et al. 1997).

The effect of CPAP on cerebral flow velocity is conflicting. Haring et al. (1994), in volunteers, found that $12\,cmH_2O$ CPAP caused a significant increase in middle cerebral artery velocity. In contrast Bowie et al. (2001) did not find any significant change in velocity during application of 5 and $10\,cmH_2O$ CPAP.

The effect of PEEP on ICP in the clinical setting are conflicting. When patients are maintained in the 30-degree head-up position, PEEP improves arterial oxygenation without increasing ICP (Frost 1977). In another study, including patients with head injury, SAH and hydrocephalus, PEEP at $5\,cmH_2O$ did not alter ICP, and the clinical relevance of ICP increase at PEEP levels of 10 and $15\,cmH_2O$ was questionable, because CPP did not change and remained $> 60\,mmHg$. Furthermore, in patients with stroke (Georgiadis et al. 2001) and patients with increased ICP (McGuire et al. 1997) higher levels of PEEP did not change ICP or CPP. In a recent study application of PEEP at 10 and $15\,cmH_2O$ produced an increase in ICP without significant effect on CPP (Videtta et al. 2002). Generally, PEEP is considered as a valuable form of therapy for the comatose patient with pulmonary disorders such as pneumonia or pulmonary oedema (Frost 1977). The effect of PEEP were studied in patients with severe head injury and acute lung injury. PEEP did not induce any change in CPP and CBF, but ICP was correlated to static elastance of the respiratory system due to alveolar overdistension (Mascia et al. 2000). The same group analysed the effect of PEEP in patients with head injury and acute lung injury, and found that when PEEP induced alveolar hyperinflation leading to an increase in $PaCO_2$, ICP increased, whereas when PEEP caused recruitment ICP was unchanged (Mascia et al. 2005). These findings are in agreement with a study by Kolbitsch et al.

(2000). They found that application of CPAP breathing at $6\,cmH_2O$ had no influence on cerebral compliance. In contrast, CPAP at $12\,cmH_2O$ increased CSF peak velocity measured by phase-contrast MRI. An increase in CBV, which impairs systolic craniocaudal CSF displacement, was considered the most likely underlying mechanism.

Warnings against PEEP are also based on a study in volunteers indicating that CPAP of $12\,cmH_2O$ increased CSF pressure from 7 to 11 mmHg (Hörmann et al. 1994). In the sitting position the combination of head flexion and rotation with institution of PEEP might cause a dangerous increase in ICP (Lodrini et al. 1989).

1.11
Dihydroergotamine (DHE)

Dihydroergotamine (DHE) increases peripheral vascular resistance (PVR), mainly by constriction of the venous capacitance vessels (Mellander and Nordenfelt 1970; Müller-Schweinitzer and Rosenthaler 1987).

In a porcine model of intracranial hypertension DHE administered for 60 min caused a lasting decrease in ICP probably achieved by a decrease in CBV due to constriction of both arterial and venous capacitance vessels (Nilsson et al. 1995).

Dihydroergotamine is a potent constrictor of human basilar arteries in vitro. In normal adults, DHE does not influence CBF (Andersen et al. 1987). Neither does Hydergine, a mixture of three ergot alkaloids, alter CBF even after intraarterial carotid injection (McHenry et al. 1971; Olesen and Skinhøj 1972).

Grände (1989) reported that DHE 0.25 mg intravenously decreased ICP in head-injured patients. The duration of this effect was about one hour and after this period ICP was stabilized at a lower level. Further studies from the same group and others concluded that the decrease in ICP was accompanied by a 30% increase in CBF, a decrease in $AVDO_2$, an increase in CPP and a 6% decrease in CBV (Ryding et al. 1990). In severe head injuries the effect of DHE on ICP is not correlated to CO_2 reactivity. Thus, a decrease in ICP was obtained by DHE in patients with or without impaired CO_2 reactivity (Asgeirsson et al. 1995).

Dihydroergotamine was used at dose of 0.25 mg during craniotomy for cerebral tumours subjected to isoflurane-nitrous oxide anaesthesia. In accordance with the study in head injury patients a significant increase in MABP was observed. ICP, however, increased significantly as well. In several patients, increase in MABP was associated with an increase in CBF, and a fall in $AVDO_2$, suggesting that these patients had impaired cerebral autoregulation. Thus, the increase in ICP was associated with an increase in both CBF and MABP (Bundgaard et al. 2001).

1.12
The Lund Model

The main concept is that opening of the blood-brain barrier upsets the normal regulation of brain volume and aggravetes oedema formation. Dihydroergotamine combined with metoprolol, clonidine and prostaglandin has been introduced in the treatment of severe head injury. Metoprolol and clonidine elicit only a minor effect on cerebral haemodynamics in severely injured patients (Asgeirsson et al. 1995).

The patients were subjected to moderate hyperventilation (30–33 mmHg) and thiopental sedation (0.5–3.0 mg/kg/h). Both metoprolol and clonidine are supposed to decrease hydrostatic capillary pressure and reduce fluid filtration across the damaged blood-brain barrier. DHE in doses declining from 0.8 μg/kg/h to 0.1 μg/kg/h are administered to reduce ICP by precapillary and venous vasoconstriction. Low-dose prostaglandin infusion 0.5–0.8 ng/kg/min is given to improve microcirculation around the contusion, and to heal the disrupted blood-brain barrier (Gründe 1989). This treatment has since been modified with more focus on details in treatment of these patients (Table 1 in Grände 2006).

Preliminary results with this regime seemed promising (Asgeirsson et al. 1994, 1995), however 15 years after its introduction clinical controlled studies have not been performed. Recently data suggested that if pressure autoregulation is intact then Brain Trauma Foundation management is associated with a better outcome than Lund Therapy, but if pressure autoregulation is lost then Lund Therapy is superior at improving outcomes (Howells et al. 2005). It is time to perform rigorous testing of therapeutic strategies for the treatment of severe head trauma (Andrews and Citerio 2006).

1.13
Hyperventilation (HV)

Hypercapnia has been used in the neurosurgical clinic in cases where an increase in CBF is desired, especially during carotid endarterectomy. There is

Table 1.1 Effects of hyperventilation

Beneficial effects	Detrimental effects
Decrease in ICP	Cerebral oligaemia in focal or watershed areas
Respiratory alkalosis neutralizing metabolic acidosis	Decrease in diastolic filling and cardiac output
Normalization of cerebral autoregulation	Decrease in MABP and CPP
Inverse steal phenomenon (Robin Hood)	Water and salt retention
Reduction of CSF formation	Inhibition of oxygen delivery to the tissues Bohr effect
	Lung injury

no doubt, however, that hypercapnia as a general rule is detrimental when intracranial compliance is exhausted. Instead attention will be paid to hypocapnia, which in experimental as well as clinical studies effectively reduces ICP. Hypocapnia, has been used therapeutically in patients with intracranial hypertension (Table 1.1; for review see Laffey and Kavanagh 2002).

1.13.1
Cerebral Blood Flow, Cerebral Blood Volume and Intracranial Pressure

Rosomoff (1963) studied changes in CBV and CSF volume after 30 min of hypocapnia to $PaCO_2$ 20 mmHg in dogs and found a fall in CBV and a compensatory increase in CSF volume. The changes in CBV caused by hypo- and hypercapnia are correlated to changes in CBF. In the monkey regional CBV (rCBV) ranges from 3.8 to 9.2 ml/100 g over the corresponding $PaCO_2$ range of 19 to 92 mmHg. The change in CBV was calculated to be 0.046 ml/mmHg $PaCO_2$ (Phelps et al. 1973). These results were confirmed by Grubb et al. (1974) (0.041 ml/100 g/mmHg $PaCO_2$). Several studies in normal humans and in patients with head injury, cerebral tumours, apoplexy and SAH have shown an increase in cerebrovascular resistance (CVR) and a decrease in CBF during hyperventilation. As a consequence, ICP is reduced. The fall in ICP follows the changes in end-tidal CO_2 and $PaCO_2$, being pronounced during the first 2–3 min. The maximal decrease in ICP is recorded about 15 min after hyperventilation. Following hyperventilation $CMRO_2$ is unchanged.

With MRI technology CBV at normal $PaCO_2$ is 42 µL/g and 29 µL/g for grey and white matter, respectively (Ulatowski et al. 1999). In the normal brain CBV changes by 0.04–0.05 ml/100 g/mmHg $PaCO_2$. In grey and white matter values of 0.053 and 0.043 ml/100 g/mmHg $PaCO_2$ have been found (Greenberg et al. 1978).

In patients with severe head injury a CBV of only 0.5 ml was necessary to produce an ICP change of 1 mmHg (Yoshihara et al. 1995). In another study a change in CBV of 0.72±0.42 ml was found when $PaCO_2$ was changed by 1 mmHg (Stocchetti et al. 1993).

During active hyperventilation cerebral venous drainage is not impaired. During massive passive hyperventilation in dogs a high positive airway pressure impedes cerebral venous drainage, increases cerebral venous pressure and consequently might increase ICP (Kitahata et al. 1971).

1.13.2
Steal and Inverse Steal Phenomenon

Studies of focal ischaemia indicate a decrease in focal pial blood pressure during hypercapnia (Brawley et al. 1967; Symon 1970). This phenomenon is caused by a redistribution of blood flow from regions with a relatively high ICP and low

CO_2 reactivity to regions with a high CO_2 reactivity and relatively low tissue pressure, referred to as a steal phenomenon. In patients with apoplexy and cerebral tumours, hypercapnia might provoke a steal phenomenon by promoting a decrease in CBF in the focal region of incomplete ischaemia (Palvölgyi 1969; Paulson 1970).

The occurrence of the inverse steal phenomenon is of considerable interest and has focused the attention on hypocapnia as a therapeutic tool in experimental brain ischaemia. Although studies in MCAO indicate an increase in lactic acidosis and a decrease in ATP in the focal region (Michenfelder and Sundt 1973), other experimental studies indicate that hypocapnia might redistribute blood flow from healthier regions with low tissue pressure and high CO_2 reactivity to more injured regions with high pressures and relatively low CO_2 reactivity. This reaction is called the inverse steal phenomenon. Preliminary studies in dogs and cats suggested that the size of an infarct was reduced if hypocapnia was applied prior to the insult (Soloway et al. 1968). However, later experimental studies have not corroborated this finding (Soloway et al. 1971). Other studies in isoflurane-anaesthetized rats subjected to MCAO do not provide evidence of a hypocapnia-induced inverse phenomenon (Ruta et al. 1993).

In patients with severe head injury, apoplexy and brain tumours, an inverse steal phenomenon or Robin Hood phenomenon has been observed during hypocapnia (Palvölgyi 1969; Paulson 1970; Pistolese et al. 1972; Fieschi et al. 1974; Cold et al. 1977b; Obrist et al. 1984). However, regions with inverse reactions are scattered over the cerebral hemisphere and sparsely localized to abnormal radiological findings (Cold et al. 1977b). Darby et al. (1988), in a study with enhanced xenon scanning, demonstrated that hypocapnia might provoke a pronounced CBF increase probably resulting in cerebral oedema.

In 1996 Dings et al. introduced measurement of brain tissue oxygen tension in patients with severe head injury. In many cases hypocapnia was associated with an increase in tissue oxygen tension during the first day after trauma.

1.13.3
Bohr Effect

Alkalosis increases the affinity of haemoglobin for oxygen and displaces the dissociation curve to the left (Bohr effect). This mechanism is counteracted by a rapid increase in lactate production (Wasserman 1994), an increase in 2,3-dephosphoglycerate (DPG) mutase and reduced activity of DPG phosphatase (Nunn 1987), which result in an increased activity of 2.3-DPG, resulting in a normalization of the dissociation curve over a period of several hours.

The decrease in oxygen delivery capacity caused by hypocapnia is partly caused by the decrease in CBF (part 75%) and partly by a shift of the dissociation curve of oxyhaemoglobin (part 25%) (Cain 1963; Gotoh et al. 1965; Harp and Wollman 1973).

1.13.4
Risk of Ischaemia

This issue has been debated vigorously during the last decade. The monitored data include regional CBF (rCBF), jugular venous saturation, $AVDO_2$ and brain tissue oxygen tension. A definition of hyperaemia, where CBF outstrips the metabolic demand of the tissue, is used by Bruce et al. (1979) and Obrist et al. (1984). Their studies were primarily based on the $CMRO_2$/CBF relationship ($AVDO_2$) and jugular venous saturation. Real CBF data were used by Cold (1989a) in adult trauma patients, and Skippen et al. (1997) in paediatric head injury patents. Data based on jugular venous saturation are problematic. The two jugular veins have been shown to drain asymmetric parts of the brain, and a significant difference in oxygen saturation in the same patient has been described (Stocchetti et al. 1994). In addition, jugular bulb saturation, by definition, is unable to detect regional areas of ischaemia.

In immature rats hypocapnia increases anaerobic metabolism (Vannucci et al. 1997) and in newborn piglets hypocapnia augments production of cytotoxic excitatory amino acids (Graham et al. 1996). In the pig microdialysis model, hypocapnia decreases brain glucose and increases brain lactate concentration indicating anaerobic metabolism. Hypercapnia has no influence on glucose or lactate (van Hulst et al. 2004). During controlled hyperventilation in non-traumatized pigs no significant change in brain tissue oxygen tension was observed. In contrast, hypercapnia resulted in an increase in brain tissue oxygen tension (van Hulst et al. 2002).

In awake, unsedated patients, active hyperventilation to $PaCO_2$ 20 mmHg induces changes in EEG compatible with cerebral ischaemia (Morgan and Ward 1970). These changes disappeared when hyperbaric oxygenation was provided (Reivich et al. 1966). During hypocapnia EEG slowing is observed when jugular venous oxygen tension is about 22 mmHg (Gotoh et al. 1965). The threshold at which deterioration in consciousness occurs and EEG signs compatible with cerebral hypoxaemia are observed is a jugular venous oxygen tension of about 19–23 mmHg. These low tensions occur at PaO_2 ranging between 26 and 30 mmHg and at a $PaCO_2$ level of 19–23 mmHg. In humans subjected to extreme hypocapnia, a moderate increase in $CMR_{glucose}$ has been found, indicating anaerobic cerebral metabolism (Alexander et al. 1968). This change occurs at CBF levels ranging from 10 to 20 ml/100 g/min, and at jugular venous oxygen tensions of 20 mmHg (Gotoh et al. 1965). In the acute phase of head injury rCBF and global CBF are low (Fieschi et al. 1974; Bouma et al. 1991), and low CBF, in the early phase of head injury, is associated with a poorer outcome (Jaggi et al. 1990; Bouma et al. 1992). Severe cerebral oligaemia accompanying hyperventilation is observed in patients with severe head injury, and in patients with acute brain lesions where hyperventilation decreases rCBF below the ischaemic threshold of 18–20 ml/100 g/min (Cold 1989a; Meixensberger et al. 1993; Stringer et al. 1993). Hyperventilation is also followed by a substantial decrease in jugular bulb saturation (Fortune et al. 1995) and, although normalization of

ICP occurs, it is accompanied by significantly reduced cerebral oxygenation (von Helden et al. 1993; Unterberg et al. 1997). However, in other studies jugular bulb saturation decreases, but not to dangerously low values (Coles et al. 2002; Oertel et al. 2002). In patients with head injury brain tissue oxygen tension might decrease to low values, indicating cerebral ischaemia (van Santbrink et al. 1996; Unterberg et al. 1997; Meixensberger et al. 1998; Fandino et al. 1999; Gopinath et al. 1999; Carmona Suazo et al. 2000; Imberti et al. 2000, 2002). In other studies the fall in brain tissue oxygen tension was not significant (Schneider et al. 1998), and even an increase in oxygen tension has been reported (Gopinath et al. 1999; Imberti et al. 2000, 2002).

It has been proposed that hyperventilation can be optimized on the basis of the level of jugular venous saturation, aiming to normalize ICP and prevent low values of jugular bulb saturation (Cruz 1993, 1998; Cruz et al. 1995). In a recent review the authors concluded that careful use of hyperventilation for the short-term control of ICP remains a useful tool (Stocchetti et al. 2005).

In patients with cerebral contusion the penumbra surrounding the contused region has a high CO_2 reactivity, and the authors hypothesized that hypocapnia may provoke cerebral ischaemia in this vulnerable zone (McLaughlin and Marion 1996). Studies of brain tissue oxygen tension indicate that hyperventilation may reduce oxygen tensions to very low values (Dings et al. 1996). Likewise, manual bagging causes cerebral oligaemia, and precipitates compensatory hypoperfusion with a fall in cerebral venous saturation (Procaccio et al. 1993).

1.13.5
Adaptation to Prolonged Hyperventilation

Hyperventilation causes an increase in arterial pH, but only a small increase in brain pH. The increase in perivascular pH results in vasoconstriction. The stability of brain pH results from processes that counteract changes in intracellular pH. The early processes consist of physiochemical buffering by the CO_2/HCO_3^- system, the imidazole groups of histidine residues of proteins and the free and bound forms of phosphate. Active and passive transport mechanisms such as the Na^+/H^+ exchanger, the Cl^-/HCO_3^- exchanger, the H^+/lactate cotransporter and the H^+ and Na^+/HCO_3^- cotransporters are also included. The latter processes are metabolic pathways that generate or consume H^+ ions, of which increased glycolytic production of lactic acid is the most prominent feature.

In studies in dogs and goats, adaptation to prolonged continuous hypocapnia occurs within 2–3 h (Raichle et al. 1970; Albrecht and Ruttle 1987). Prolonged hypocapnia decreases the rate of formation of CSF. After an initial decrease at 30 and 60 min, however, formation of CSF returns to pre-hypocapnic values (Hochwald et al. 1976; Martins et al. 1976; Artru and Hornbein 1987). In dogs with an intracranial mass-expanding lesion, prolonged hypocapnia initially gives rise to a decrease in CBV. However, the CSF-pressure lowering effect is sustained by a reduction in CSF volume, despite re-expansion of CBV. In the same model brain water content did not contribute to changes in CSF pressure and volume (Artru 1987).

The adaptation to prolonged hypocapnia has been investigated in patients with apoplexy. The half-life of the adaptation mechanism of CSF-pH and CSF bicarbonate averages 6 h, and adaptation is said to be complete within 24–30 h (Christensen 1974). Studies using a non-invasive Doppler ultrasound technique and calculation of the instantaneous mean blood velocity during hypocapnia in normal subjects indicate that blood velocity showed adaptation within 10 min after induction of hypocapnia (Ellingsen et al. 1987).

Cerebral haemodynamic responses to hyperventilation are different in normoxic and hyperoxic conditions. Thus, the CO_2 reactivity is lower with normoxia than hyperoxia, and CBF recovery is more rapid with normoxia than hyperoxia (Johnston et al. 2003). The modulation of the pH control mechanisms is influenced by increased breakdown of hypoxia inducible factor-1 (Minchenko et al. 2002), increased free radical production (Mak et al. 2002) or a direct effect of oxygen on cell membrane proteins (Haddad and Jiang 1997).

In an uncontrolled study of patients with severe head injury no signs of CSF-pH adaptation within periods of 6–24 h were disclosed. It was suggested that ischaemia prevented the CSF-pH adaptation (Cold et al. 1977a). When hyperventilation is used for several days to reduce ICP in the presence of brain oedema, withdrawal of hypocapnia should be cautious as intracranial hypertension very often reappears (Havill 1984). Mechanism of adaptation is supposed to play a role in this rebound intracranial hypertension.

1.13.6
Hyperventilation in Premature, Neonates and Paediatric Patients

In pre-term infants severe hypocapnia, even of relatively short duration, may elicit neurological abnormalities (Greisen et al. 1987). Neurovascular factors that predispose the immature brain include poorly developed cerebral vascular supply to vulnerable regions (De Reuck 1984), antioxidant depletion by excitatory amino acids (Oka et al. 1993) and the effects of lipopolysaccharide (Gilles et al. 1976) and cytokines (Yoon et al. 1997) that potentiate destruction of white matter. Furthermore, abrupt termination of hyperventilation results in cerebral hyperaemia, which may cause intracranial haemorrhage in prematures (Gleason et al. 1989).

In paediatric patients with severe head injury, diffuse brain swelling occurs with high frequency (Bruce et al. 1979). Increase in blood volume attributed to partial or complete impairment of cerebral autoregulation and dysfunction of the blood-brain barrier allowing pathological vasodilatation have been proposed (Bruce et al. 1979). Evidence for this assumption has never emerged. Nevertheless, vasoconstrictory therapy to decrease CBV has been suggested as particularly appropriate in paediatric patients with head injury. Hyperventilation to a $PaCO_2$ level below 25 mmHg has been standard therapy in many paediatric units. In a study by Skippen et al. (1997), 23 paediatric head injury patients were followed with Xe-CT scanning, jugular bulb saturation and ICP monitoring. They found that there is a very little evidence of "absolute" hyperaemia in their patients. Furthermore, they found CBF values < 18 ml/100 g/min even in normocapnic patients. The percentage of areas with oligaemic flow increased during hypocapnia. In children with diabetic ketoacidosis cerebral low $PaCO_2$ and treatment with bicarbonate is associated with the occurrence of cerebral oedema (Glaser et al. 2001).

1.13.7
Hyperventilation as a Lifesaving Procedure

In patients with intracranial hypertension, hypocapnia effectively reduces ICP and CBF. It is accepted that the fall in ICP is caused by vasoconstriction of cerebral arterioles and a secondary decrease in CBV. Although the decrease in CBV is small in comparison with the total brain volume, hypocapnia can be lifesaving in patients with a mass-expanding cerebral lesion. Acute hyperventilation is, therefore, an important tool in the management of acute intracranial hypertension (Lundberg et al. 1959; Bozza et al. 1961; Slocum et al. 1961). On the other hand, hyperventilation must be used cautiously because it might provoke a dangerous decrease in CBF especially in regions with low CBF (Cold 1989b). Ideally the use of prolonged artificial hyperventilation should be guided by measurement of rCBF, $AVDO_2$, venous saturation or tissue oxygen tension.

1.13.8
Guidelines

There are insufficient data to support a level I recommendation for hyperventilation. Level II, prophylactic hyperventilation ($PaCO_2$ of 25 mmHg or less), is not recommended. Level III hyperventilation is recommended as a temporary measure for the reduction of elevated ICP. Hyperventilation should be avoided during the first 24 h after injury when CBF is often critically reduced. If hyperventilation is used, jugular venous oxygen saturation (SjO_2) or brain tissue oxygen tension ($PbrO_2$) measurement is recommended to monitor oxygen delivery.

1.14
Indomethacin

1.14.1
Experimental Studies

Indomethacin is a blocker of cyclooxygenase and thereby prostaglandin synthesis. Indomethacin acts as a cerebral vasoconstrictor and reduces CBF while

CMRO$_2$ remains unchanged (Pichard and MacKenzie 1973; Sakabe and Siesjö 1979; Dahlgren et al. 1981; Wennmalm et al. 1981). In the anaesthetized baboon, PET studies indicate that indomethacin resulted in a marked and homogeneous decrease in CBF in every region analysed and a moderate reduction in CBV. CMRO$_2$ displayed a small increase in thalamus and pons, and oxygen extraction fraction increased greatly in all structures studied (Schumann et al. 1996).

A bolus dose of indomethacin reduces ICP and increases CPP during both propofol and isoflurane anaesthesia in sheep. The ICP-decreasing effect is, however, more pronounced with isoflurane (Rasmussen et al. 2006).

Studies of canine basilar arteries indicate that prostaglandin mediates cerebral oedema (Shohami et al. 1987). In cats subjected to focal ischaemia (Dempsey et al. 1985) and rats subjected to freezing lesions (Yen and Lee 1987) indomethacin reduces cerebral oedema. Also the rapid accumulation of cyclooxygenase degrading products during reperfusion is blocked by indomethacin (Gaudet et al. 1980). In other experimental studies of focal ischaemia (Harris et al. 1982; Awad et al. 1983; Sutherland et al. 1988; Suzuka et al. 1989) and traumatic head injury (Shapira et al. 1988), indomethacin administration was not followed by a decrease in cerebral oedema.

Indomethacin reduces cerebral infarct size in focal ischaemia (Sasaki et al. 1988), enhances post-ischaemic reperfusion after MCAO (Shigeno et al. 1985) and reduces cerebral fluid compression injury (Hallenbeck and Furlow 1979). Furthermore, in rats subjected to fluid percussion trauma pretreatment with indomethacin improves recovery (Kim et al. 1989).

Other experimental studies suggest that the infarct size in focal cerebral ischaemia was not influenced by indomethacin (Harris et al. 1982; Koide et al. 1986).

1.14.2
Human Studies

Studies of non-steroid drugs indicate that ibuprofen (Patel et al. 2000) and diclofenac (Jones and Dinsmore 2002) do not change CBF. In comparison, indomethacin is a strong cerebral vasoconstrictor. In healthy volunteers, the decrease in CBF after a bolus dose of indomethacin followed by continuous infusion is sustained. During hypoxia and during hypercapnia CBF increases indicating normal regulation of CBF (Jensen et al. 1993). In healthy volunteers 0.1, 0.2 and 0.3 mg/kg/h indomethacin decreased CBF to about 45 ml/100 g/min (Jensen et al. 1996). During sensorimotor activation indomethacin reduces the CBF increase otherwise observed, but does not affect the increase in CMRO$_2$ (St Lawrence et al. 2003).

The vasoconstrictor effect of indomethacin has been used in the treatment of intracranial hypertension in patients with head injury. In a preliminary study, indomethacin 30 mg was followed by an immediate decrease in ICP for about one hour. The fall in ICP was accompanied by a decrease in CBF, an increase in $AVDO_2$ and $AVD_{lactate}$, while the $CMRO_2$ was unchanged (Jensen et al. 1991). In another study the effect of a bolus dose (30 mg) of indomethacin on ICP was comparable with the effect of a 1.5-kPa decrease in $PaCO_2$ (Dahl et al. 1991, 1996). Considerable rCBF decrease has been observed after i.v. indomethacin in patients with head injury, also in focal regions where CBF is decreased. However, only a transient increase in $AVD_{lactate}$ has been observed (Jensen et al. 1991).

In patients subjected to craniotomy for cerebral tumours, indomethacin immediately and within seconds after i.v. administration decreased ICP accompanied by a decrease in CBF (Bundgaard et al. 1996). On the other hand prophylactic indomethacin treatment, administered before induction of anaesthesia, does not significantly decrease ICP in patients with cerebral tumours anaesthetized with propofol-fentanyl (Rasmussen et al. 2004a). Administration of indomethacin during propofol anaesthesia is not associated with evidence of ischaemic damage in patients with brain tumours as evaluated by diffusion-weighted imaging (Rasmussen et al. 2004b).

Only one case study of apoplexy is available, indicating a patient with raised ICP where conventional therapies had failed. Indomethacin (50-mg bolus) led to a fall in ICP and an increase in CPP (Schwarz et al. 1999).

In hepatic failure swelling of astrocytes is a common feature and may result in cerebral oedema with intracranial hypertension. There is accumulating evidence that there are high circulating levels of ammonia resulting from the splanchnic vascular bed, and this is a key mediator of these complications (Schenker et al. 1967). Ammonia crosses the blood-brain barrier (Ott and Larsen 2004), influences neurotransmitter trafficking (Filipo and Butterworth 2002) and ammonia concentration correlates to brain water content and ICP in the experimental setting (Takahashi et al. 1990; Olafsson et al. 1995).

In an experimental setting it has been demonstrated that indomethacin prevents the development of ammonia-induced cerebral oedema (Chung et al. 2001). In patients with hepatic failure bolus injection of indomethacin reduces ICP and increases CPP (Clemmensen et al. 1997; Raghavan and Marik 2006) without compromising cerebral perfusion or oxidative metabolism, as indicated by microdialysis values of glutamate and lactate. Indomethacin did not restore cerebral autoregulation (Tofteng and Larsen 2004).

1.15
Metabolic Control of Cerebral Blood Flow

Metabolic control of ICP is based on the concept that CBF is adjusted to the metabolic demand of the brain tissue. If the metabolic demand of the tissue decreases, CBF and volume will decrease, and the ICP will decline. Metabolic regulation of ICP is effected by hypothermia and drugs that reduce the metabolic rate of oxygen in the brain (hypnotics, analgesics). As hypnotic and analgesic treatments depress the respiration, patients subjected to these treatments are intubated and respiration is supported by a ventilator. As this treatment is often supplemented with treatment with muscle relaxants, the effect of muscle relaxants on ICP will also be discussed.

1.15.1
Hypothermia

1.15.1.1
Experimental Studies

Hypothermia decreases $CMRO_2$ and CBF proportionally. In dogs the temperature coefficient Q_{10} (defined as the ratio of metabolic rates at two temperatures differing by 10°C) was 2.2 at temperatures between 37 and 27°C. Below 27°C the Q_{10} was doubled to 4.5 suggesting that the relationship of $CMRO_2$ to brain temperature is variable depending on the functional state of the brain; below 27°C progressive functional depression is supposed to account for the high Q_{10} value (Michenfelder and Milde 1991).

Hypothermia exerts a protective effect on the brain in hypoxic hypoxia (Carlsson et al. 1976), global ischaemia (Chopp et al. 1989), incomplete ischaemia (Hoffman et al. 1991) and in experimental head injury (Clifton et al. 1991). It has been suggested that even a small decrease in temperature of 1–3°C has a protective effect in experimental brain ischaemia (Busto et al. 1989) and an improvement of the blood-brain barrier has been observed (Dietrich et al. 1990). On the other hand, in rats, even small increments in temperature in ischaemic brain tissue seem to accentuate histopathological damage (Kitagawa et al. 1991).

According to Nakamura et al. (2003) rapid increase of brain temperature during re-warming is accompanied by increased extracellular lactate and glutamate. An effect on neuronal cytoskeleton, indicated by an increase of MAP-2 immunoreactivity of the CA1 neurons, was also observed 1 week, but not 1 month after hypothermia.

1.15.1.2
Clinical Studies

A barbiturate in combination with hypothermia might effectively control intracranial hypertension in some patients with severe head injury (Shapiro et al. 1974). Likewise, the combination of barbiturate and hypothermia might accentuate the protective effect in brain ischaemia (Nordström and Rehncrona 1979). On the basis of the experimental studies the use of hypothermia has been discussed and suggested in the intensive care of patients suffering from brain ischaemia (Cohen 1981).

Hypothermia has been used in the treatment of cerebral ischaemia in humans (Connolly et al. 1962) during extracorporeal circulation (duCailar et al.

1964), after circulatory arrest (White 1972), during neurosurgical operations (Uihlein et al. 1966; White et al. 1967) and in the treatment of severe head injury (Sedzimir 1959, Shapiro et al. 1974). Later on, the once common use of hypothermia was abandoned, because studies of hypothermia in the treatment of acute stroke did not prove any beneficial effect. On the contrary, a detrimental effect was observed in primates and dogs (Michenfelder and Milde 1977; Steen et al. 1979).

Mild hypothermia, however, has again been introduced in the treatment of intracranial hypertension in severe head injury. A decrease in ICP accompanied by a decrease in CBF, $AVDO_2$ and $CMRO_2$ have been found (Marion et al. 1993; Shiozaki et al. 1993), and a decrease in $CMR_{lactate}$ has been found (Metz et al. 1996). These changes are accompanied by a moderate decrease in cardiac index, a fall in platelet count and an increased level of serum lipase with signs of pancreatitis (Metz et al. 1996). In an allocated study hypothermia was found to improve outcome (Clifton et al. 1993). In a recent randomized study Marion et al. (1997) found that patients kept at 33°C for 24 h after the injury did not show improved outcome in comparison with normothermic patients.

1.15.1.3
Guidelines

In 2007 American Guidelines there are insufficient data to support level I and level II recommendations for prophylactic hypothermia. The level III recommendation states that pooled data indicate that prophylactic hypothermia is not significantly associated with decreased mortality when compared with normothermic controls. However, preliminary findings suggest that a greater decrease in mortality risk is observed when target temperatures are maintained for more than 48 h.

Prophylactic hypothermia is associated with significantly higher Glasgow Outcome Scale (GOS) scores when compared to scores for normothermic controls.

1.15.2
Hypnotic Agents

In experimental as well as human studies it has been documented that hypnotic agents, including barbiturate, benzodiazepines, etomidate and propofol, increase cerebrovascular resistance and reduce CBF and ICP (Pierce et al. 1962; Michenfelder 1974; Stullken et al. 1977; Larsen et al. 1981; Cold et al. 1986; Stephan et al. 1987). These effects are caused through a metabolic suppression of $CMRO_2$. The metabolic suppression is dose-dependent until the EEG is isoelectric. Beyond this level no further suppression of $CMRO_2$ or CBF occurs (Michenfelder 1974; Kassell et al. 1980; Milde et al. 1985). Hypnotics have been used in the control of intracranial hypertension (Gordon 1970; Hunter 1972; Shapiro et al. 1973).

1.15.3
Vasodilatation

A direct vasodilatory effect of barbiturate has been found on cerebral vessels (Altura and Altura 1975; Edvinsson and McCulloch 1981; Marin et al. 1981). Thus, Edvinsson and McCulloch (1981) in feline middle cerebral arteries found that maximum contractions effected by potassium, noradrenalin and prostaglandin F2a were reduced in the presence of pentobarbital. Gross and Abel (1985) in a rabbit basilar artery model found that concentrations of 3×10^{-5} thiopental caused relaxation of norepinephrine-induced contraction. In the monkey Tsuji and Chiba (1986, 1987) demonstrated a biphasic vascular response, with an initial vasoconstriction followed by a vasodilatation in a dose-dependent manner. It is supposed that this effect modifies the ICP-lowering effect of barbiturate when $CMRO_2$ and electrical and functional capacity are low.

1.15.4
Cerebral Metabolic Rate of Oxygen

In severe head injury (Bruce et al. 1973; Cold 1978; Obrist et al. 1979) and comatose patients with SAH (Grubb et al. 1977; Voldby et al. 1985) $CMRO_2$ is decreased severely, often to values averaging 50% of the values obtained in awake adults. Accordingly, the effect of barbiturate on CBF and $CMRO_2$ is decreased or absent (Messeter et al. 1986; Cold 1989b). Thus, in the acute phase of head injury the barbiturate reactivity, as measured by the decrease in $CMRO_2$ after a bolus dose of 5 mg/kg, seems to be dependent on the $CMRO_2$ level before thiopental injection (Cold 1989a), and in comatose patients with a 50% decrease in $CMRO_2$ the barbiturate reactivity averaged zero (Dahl et al. 1991).

1.15.5
Sedation

Chronic administration of barbiturate has been used in the intensive care management of apoplexy, severe head injury and cerebral aneurysm. As a consequence of respiratory obstruction/failure, risk of aspiration and failure of reflexes combined with unconsciousness, these patients are often intubated and eventually hyperventilated. This regime is supported by sedation with hypnotics/analgesics in order to prevent coughing, stress and anxiety. For sedation pentobarbitone or thiopental are administered at hourly intervals. Alternatively, continuous-infusion thiopental, propofol or midazolam are used. Etomidate is not used for continuous sedation because of its inhibitory effect on adrenal steroid genesis.

Propofol sedation was compared with morphine combined with midazolam sedation in patients with severe head injury. Propofol led to a fall in $AVDO_2$ from 6 to 3 ml O_2/100 ml. However, there was no effect on MABP, ICP or CPP, and outcome was similar in the two groups (Stewart et al. 1994). In a study of head injury, bolus doses of propofol 1.5 mg/kg were compared with thiopental 3 mg/kg. The ICP-reducing effects were comparable. However, the MABP-reducing effect was more pronounced and lasted a longer period when propofol was used (Merlo et al. 1993). Hypnotic drugs (thiopental, propofol or midazolam) for sedation or ICP reduction should be administered by continuous infusion, and continuous monitoring of CPP and cerebral venous saturation are recommended (Andrews et al. 1993).

1.15.6
Intracranial Hypertension

On the basis of the regulatory effect of hypnotic agents on acute intracranial hypertension (Shapiro et al. 1974; Sidi et al. 1983) and the abundance of documentation of a protective effect in acute focal and incomplete ischaemia, prolonged hypnotic sedation has been used prophylactically in severe head injury. In several uncontrolled studies barbiturate-coma treatment has been claimed to prevent or attenuate intracranial hypertension and improve outcome (Rockoff et al. 1979; Saul and Ducker 1982; Eisenberg et al. 1988). In other uncontrolled studies these findings are not supported (Yano et al. 1986). Ward et al. (1985), however, did not find any improvement of outcome in a controlled study where barbiturate was administered in doses sufficient to suppress the EEG to burst suppression level for several days. In the barbiturate-treated group the incidence of arterial hypotension and septicaemia were higher than in the control group. Likewise, Abramson et al. (1983) did not find any beneficial effect of barbiturate in a controlled study of thiopentone administered to patients after cardiac arrest.

1.15.7
Guidelines

In the 2007 American Guidelines, there are insufficient data to support a level I recommendation for the use of anaesthetics, analgesics and sedatives. Level II, prophylactic administration of barbiturates to induce burst suppression EEG, is not recommended. High-dose barbiturate administration is recommended to control elevated ICP refractory to maximum standard medical and surgical treatment. Haemodynamic stability is essential before and during barbiturate therapy. Propofol is recommended for the control of ICP, but not for improvement in mortality or 6-month outcome. High-dose propofol can produce significant morbidity.

1.16
Analgesics

1.16.1
Spontaneous Ventilation

Morphine and analogue drugs should be administered with extreme caution in the spontaneously breathing patient with exhausted intracranial compliance. On the other hand, these drugs are used in SAH and in the postoperative course after craniotomy. Careful monitoring of conscious state, respiration, blood pressure and eventually gas analysis (PaO_2, $PaCO_2$) or capnometry/oximetry is mandatory. Even a small dose of morphine (3 mg i.v.) might provoke a decrease in $AVDO_2$ suggesting a state of hyperaemia (Cold and Felding 1993).

1.16.2
Controlled Ventilation

In the ventilator-treated patient morphine and fentanyl do not increase CBF or ICP. On the contrary, a decrease in ICP is repeatedly observed. This is caused by the sedative effect giving rise to a decrease in CO_2 production, and a decreased level of circulating catecholamine, which otherwise increases cerebral oxygen uptake and CBF when the blood-brain barrier is disrupted (MacKenzie et al. 1976; Berntman et al. 1978; Artru et al. 1981). An additive effect of hypnotics and analgesics on cerebral oxygen uptake may also play a role.

1.16.3
Sufentanil, Alfentanil

Sufentanil and alfentanil should be used with reservation because animal experiments indicate that sufentanil provokes a prolonged period of CBF and CBV increase (Milde et al. 1990). Comparative studies of fentanyl, alfentanil and sufentanil in patients subjected to craniotomy indicate that the use of the two latter drugs was accompanied by a decrease in CPP and an increase in CSF pressure (Marx et al. 1989). Cerebral autoregulation may play a role, because correction of blood pressure normalized ICP. Both sufentanil and alfentanil elicit a decrease in blood pressure. As a consequence, a decrease in CVR and an increase in CBV may occur. Under these circumstances an increase in ICP is observed.

1.17
Muscular Relaxation

In experimental (Cottrell et al. 1983; Lanier et al. 1986) as well as human studies (March et al. 1980) succinylcholine increases ICP. The rise in ICP is caused by activation from peripheral impulses from the muscles (Lanier et al. 1989). Non-depolarizing agents such as pancuronium, atracurium and vecuronium do not increase ICP (Lanier et al. 1985; Giffin et al. 1986; Rosa et al. 1986).

1.18
Osmotic-Acting Drugs, Plasma Expanders and Diuretics

1.18.1
Electrolytes and Proteins and the Blood-Brain Barrier (BBB)

Cerebral tissue is protected by the blood-brain barrier, which allows the passive diffusion of non-electrolytes inclusive of water. The extracellular space in cerebral tissue is negligible under normal circumstances. The electrophysical balance between intra- and extracellular milieu is adjusted with a high intracellular potassium concentration and a high extracellular sodium concentration.

In acute hyperosmolar states there is loss of intracellular water with cell shrinkage followed by gradual restoration of brain volume via the generation of non-electrolyte osmotically active intracellular solute. In the hypo-osmolar state, there is cellular expansion, which is corrected over time by loss of intracellular solute. Low Pl-sodium concentration is accompanied by an increase in cerebral tissue water content. During extreme hyponatraemia brain oedema may develop. If the blood-brain barrier is disrupted an increase in extracellular space with filtration of plasma proteins also occurs.

Patients with severe head injuries might have impaired peripheral circulation, even when normotensive. Volume infusion with crystalloid improves oxygen transport without increasing ICP (Scale et al. 1994).

Changes in protein concentration do not influence the volume of the extracellular space whether the blood-brain barrier is disrupted or not, because the architecture of the extracellular space does not allow any expansion.

1.18.2
Hydroxyethyl Starch and Hyperosmolar/Hyperoncotic Solutions

Following haemorrhagic shock (Kramer et al. 1986; Vollmar et al. 1994) and posttraumatic muscular lesions (Mittlmeier et al. 2003) hyperosmotic and hyperoncotic solutions restore impaired microcirculation related to haemodilution-associated improved rheology, reduced swelling of endothelial cells and increased capillary diameter. Likewise, following traumatic brain injury hyperoncotic/hyperosmolar solutions restore impaired microcirculation and decrease posttraumatic oedema (White and Likavec 1992; Kempski et al. 1996; Qureshi and Suarez 2000) by shifting free water into the intravascular lumen, thereby reducing posttraumatic endothelial swelling (Mazzoni et al. 1988), decreasing capillary resistance and improving the rheological properties of the blood (Mittlmeier et al. 2003), reducing rolling and sticking of white blood cells to the capillary wall in the early phase following experimental brain injury (Nolte et al. 1992; Härtl et al. 1997), and improving pericontusional perfusion and reducing lesion volume following experimental brain injury (Thomale et al. 2004). An early bolus of hyperosmolar/hyperoncotic solution improves long-term outcome after global cerebral ischaemia in rats (Noppens et al. 2006).

In patients with CT signs of blood-brain barrier impairment, penetration of HES into the CSF does not occur (Dieterich et al. 2003).

1.19
Mannitol

1.19.1
Osmotic Gradient

In patients with intracranial hypertension, early studies of intravenous infusion of mannitol showed that this drug effectively reduces ICP (Wise and Chater 1962). After fast intravenous infusion of 0.5–1 g/kg ICP is reduced after 2–5 min. The ICP-reducing effect is of hours duration, depending on the dose and the infusion rate (James 1980).

The osmotic effect of mannitol is dependent on the osmotic gradient in blood (Shenkin et al. 1962). The faster the concentration difference of mannitol occurs between plasma and extracellular fluid, the stronger and the longer the reduction in ICP (Takagi et al. 1993). A difference in osmotic gradient exceeding 10 mOsm always gives rise to a reduction in ICP (Marshall et al. 1978). The decrease in ICP is correlated to the decrease in the water content in brain tissue (Nath and Galbraith 1986).

Long-term administration of mannitol, however, increases spinal fluid osmolarity in patients with SAH or severe head injury. Consequently, it has been advocated to measure CSF osmolarity regularly in patients receiving mannitol for longer than 24 h (Polderman et al. 2003).

1.19.2
Experimental Studies

Following mannitol infusion in cats, blood viscosity decreases immediately. The greatest decrease occurs at 10 min. At 75 min a rebound increase in viscosity occurs. The pial vessel diameter decreased simultaneously, the largest decrease being at 10 min. The changes in pial vessels were interpreted as an autoregulatory process (Muizelaar et al. 1983). Further studies indicate that if cerebral autoregulation is impaired, mannitol infusion is followed by a decrease in ICP, while ICP is unchanged in studies where the autoregulation is intact (Muizelaar et al. 1984). The authors hypothesized that changes in blood viscosity might give rise to compensatory changes in the degree of constriction in cerebral vessels. In studies of vessel diameters with the cranial window technique in cats, it was concluded that mannitol in clinically relevant doses does not exert significant constriction on cerebral vessels. Mannitol therefore exerts its effect on ICP through its osmotic effect, rather than by a direct effect on CBV (Auer and Haselsberger 1987).

Studies of mannitol infusion at normal ICP in baboons (Johnstone and Harper 1973) and dogs (Kassell et al. 1982) have shown an increase in CBF, while CBF is unchanged in animals subjected to intracranial hypertension by an epidural balloon (Johnstone and Harper 1973). In the same study mannitol infusion was followed by an increase in CMRO$_2$.

Studies of cryogenic oedema in the cat indicate that a single dose of mannitol decreases cerebral oedema. However, a repeated dose of mannitol leads to increased water content in oedematous regions (Kaufmann and Cardoso 1992). In rats subjected to cryogenic cortical injury, multiple doses of mannitol did not aggravate total hemispheric swelling or global water content (von Berenberg et al. 1994).

In a rat model of ischaemic cortical infarction, repeated mannitol infusions resulted primarily in a decrease in brain water content of the infarct and in the ipsilateral hemisphere (Paczynski et al. 1997).

Mannitol has a beneficial effect in experimental cerebral ischaemia (Little 1978; Watanabe et al. 1979). In studies of experimental cytotoxic oedema mannitol induces a normalization of EEG (James 1978). Studies in rabbits subjected to MCAO have shown that mannitol administration improves CBF in regions of ischaemia, and that a gradual decline in intercellular pH is prevented (Meyer et al. 1987). Shirane and Weinstein (1992) found that mannitol intensified reperfusion hyperaemia after 30 min temporary ischaemia in rats. Both mannitol and glycerol improve parameters of cerebral energy metabolism during ischaemia and up to 8 h after reperfusion in the gerbil brain (Tsuda et al. 1998). In cats mannitol improves post-ischaemic recovery of blood flow (Tanaka and Tomonaga 1987). In the rats subjected to MCAO the combination of hypothermia plus mannitol have a great neuroprotective effect (Kazan et al. 1999), and in rats subjected to forebrain ischaemia mannitol considerably ameliorated the ischaemic injury (Sutherland et al. 1988). In a swine model of retractor brain ischaemia, mannitol plus nimodipine is superior to either agent alone in maintaining both CBF and evoked potential (Andrews and Muto 1992).

In rats with MCAO mannitol provides neuroprotection by preventing both necrosis and apoptotic components of cell death (Korenkov et al. 2000). Mannitol at clinical concentrations, however, induces apoptosis in endothelial cells (Malek et al. 1998; Famularo 1999), an effect antagonized by adrenomedullin (Kim et al. 2002). One pathway of mannitol-mediated apoptosis is through the degradation of focal adhesion kinase and Akt, and that insulin-like growth factor I protects the cells from apoptosis by blocking the activation of caspases (Kim and Feldman 2002).

Other experimental studies of cerebral ischaemia have failed to demonstrate any enhancement of CBF by mannitol (Seki et al. 1981; Pena et al. 1982).

1.19.3
Human Studies

Studies of central haemodynamics in patients undergoing craniotomy have shown that mannitol infusion is followed by an increase in blood volume, CVP, pulmonary artery wedge pressure and cardiac output and a decrease in the concentration of haemoglobin, plasma sodium and the peripheral resistance (Rudehill et al. 1983; Brown et al. 1986). The concentration of plasma potassium decreases after mannitol 1 g/kg and increases after 2 g/kg (Manninen et al. 1987).

An increase in CBV a few minutes after mannitol infusion has been demonstrated (Ravussin et al. 1986a). Following mannitol infusion blood viscosity decreases for at least 2 h, suggesting an enhancement of cerebral microcirculation (Burke et al. 1981). Accordingly, studies of cerebral circulation indicate an increase in CBF occurring after 10–20 min and lasting for up to 24 h, and a variable increase in $CMRO_2$ (Jafar et al. 1986).

The effect of mannitol on ICP has been studied in patients with cerebral tumours and aneurysms. In patients with normal ICP a transient but significant increase in ICP followed by a steady decrease towards values below control were found. In contrast; in patients with intracranial hypertension ICP decreased immediately after mannitol infusion (Ravussin et al. 1986b). In a clinical trial, patients with acute subdural haematoma had a better outcome and improved control of intracranial hypertension when treated with high doses of mannitol (Cruz et al. 2001).

Other studies suggest that the effect of mannitol is at least partly dependent on other haemodynamic mechanisms. Thus, patients with CPP > 70 mmHg responded relatively poorly to mannitol, while ICP decreased in patients with CPP < 70 mmHg, suggesting that at CPP > 70 mmHg the vasoconstriction is already nearly at maximum. Under this circumstance mannitol is unable to increase resistance further (Rosner and Coley 1987). In general, administration of large doses of mannitol is safe in the presence of intracranial hypertension (Abou-Madi et al. 1993).

In neurointensive patients the volume/pressure relationship improves after mannitol, often without change in ICP (Miller and Leech 1975).

1.19.4
Mannitol in Acute Head Injury

Early administration of mannitol (1.4 g/kg) in the emergency room is associated with improved clinical outcomes for adult comatose patients with acute, non-missile, intraparenchymal temporal lobe haemorrhages and associated abnormal pupillary widening (Cruz et al. 2002). Cruz et al. (2004), in a randomized trial, also demonstrated successful use of mannitol treatment (1.4 g/kg) in patients with Glasgow Coma Scale (GCS) scores of 3 and bilateral abnormal papillary widening.

1.19.5
Mannitol in Cerebral Infarct

Theoretically, mannitol use in large cerebral infarctions may preferentially shrink non-infarcted cerebral tissue, thereby aggravating midline shift and worsening neurological status. That mannitol can accumulate in ischaemic brain tissue has been demonstrated (Maioriello et al. 2002). Acute mannitol used in patients with cerebral oedema after a large hemispheric infarction, however, does not alter midline tissue shifts or worsen neurological outcome (Manno et al. 1999), and improvement of evoked potentials has been demonstrated after mannitol treatment in patients with ischaemic stroke (Onar and Arik 1997). In contrast a Cochrane database review concludes that there is currently no evidence to decide whether the routine use of mannitol in acute stroke would result in any beneficial or harmful effect, and that the routine use of mannitol in patients with acute stroke is not supported by any evidence from randomized trials (Bereczki et al. 2001).

1.19.6
Mannitol and the Blood-Brain Barrier

Osmotic opening of the brain-blood barrier by infusion of hyperosmolar solutions like mannitol has repeatedly been demonstrated. In patients with cerebral tumours hyperosmolar blood-brain barrier disruption with mannitol is used to overcome the relative inaccessibility of infiltrating glioma cells to chemotherapy. It has been argued that opening of tight junctions is the dominant mode of leakage in hyperosmolar opening. The opening of the barrier is independent of energy-producing metabolism. It is supposed that osmotic barrier opening is the result of passive shrinkage of endothelial cells and the surrounding tissue (Greenwood et al. 1988). As a result of the impaired barrier function mannitol diffuses into the cells. In this respect it is of interest that HES macromolecules protect against blood-brain barrier disruption after intracarotid injection of mannitol in rats (Chi et al. 1996).

In patients with space-occupying cerebral processes, the blood-brain barrier may be disrupted. Under these circumstances mannitol may permeate into the cerebral tissue, and even into an ischaemic insult (Maioriello et al. 2002).

1.19.7
Rebound Phenomenon

Cells are able to create osmotically active particles. These particles reduce the transcellular osmotic gradient (Jennett and Teasdale 1981).

After discontinuing the mannitol infusion the osmotic gradient is reversed because mannitol is excreted through the urine, decreasing the concentration in the plasma. Consequently, the concentration of mannitol is found to be higher in the extracellular and intracellular compartments as compared with the concentration in the blood. This rebound phenomenon gives rise to water influx into brain cells, and an increase in ICP (McQueen and Jeanes 1964).

1.19.8
Guidelines

In the Guidelines for the Management of Severe Traumatic Brain Injury (2007), the following recommendations are suggested:

A. Level I: There are insufficient data to support a level I recommendation for hyperosmolar therapy.
B. Level II: Mannitol is effective for control of raised ICP at doses of 0.25–1 g/kg body weight. Arterial hypotension (systolic blood pressure < 90 mmHg should be avoided.
C. Level III: Restrict mannitol use prior to ICP monitoring to patients with signs of transtentorial herniation or progressive neurological deterioration not attributable to extracranial causes. Hypovolaemia, however, should be avoided by fluid replacement. Serum osmolality should be kept below 320 mOsm because of concern for renal failure. Euvolaemia should be maintained by adequate fluid replacement. A Foley catheter is essential in these patients. Intermittent boluses may be more effective than continuous infusion.

In the European guidelines osmotic therapy, preferably mannitol given as repeated infusion, is advocated. Serum osmolality should be maintained < 315 mOsm. Other agents, such as glycerol or sorbitol are not advocated. If osmotherapy has insufficient effect, furosemide can be given additionally (Maas et al. 1997).

In a Cochrane database review Schierhout and Roberts (2000) conclude that there are insufficient data to recommend one form of mannitol infusion over another. Mannitol therapy for raised ICP may have a beneficial effect on mortality when compared to pentobarbital treatment. ICP-directed treatment shows a small beneficial effect compared to treatment directed by neurological signs and physiological indicators. There are insufficient data on the effectiveness of pre-hospital administration of mannitol to preclude either a harmful or a beneficial effect on mortality.

1.20
Glycerol

Glycerol is an alternative to mannitol in the treatment of intracranial hypertension. Glycerol is effective by the oral and i.v. routes. Haemolysis can be provoked but is avoided by reducing the concentration and infusion rate (Quandt and Reyes 1984). In one study equipotent doses of mannitol and glycerol were used in children with intracranial hypertension. Mannitol was found to be superior to glycerol (MacDonald and Uden 1982). In a study of adult patients with intracranial hypertension a greater and longer lasting pressure reduction was found when glycerol was used (Smedema et al. 1993). In another study by Biestro et al. (1997) glycerol and mannitol were compared in patients with head injury. At 1 and 2 h after infusion both agents induced an effective decrease on ICP and increase in CPP. The results suggested that mannitol would be most indicated as a bolus to control sudden rises in ICP, whereas glycerol would be most indicated as a basal treatment.

1.21
Hypertonic Saline

1.21.1
Experimental Studies; Central Haemodynamics

Pigs subjected to haemorrhagic hypotension were resuscitated with hypertonic saline or Ringer's solution. Normalization of blood pressure and oxygen delivery were faster with hypertonic saline (Schmoker et al. 1991). An improved cardiac performance has likewise been observed (Kien et al. 1991a).

In dogs subjected to haemorrhagic hypotension, resuscitation with either 7.2% saline or 20% HES was used. Both fluids restored MABP and cardiac output equally. At 60 min after resuscitation, however, cardiac output decreased in the hypertonic resuscitated group. ICP, CPP and CBF were similar in both groups (Whitley et al. 1991).

In dogs transtentorial herniation was produced by creating a supratentorial intracerebral haemorrhage with autologous blood injection. The state of transtentorial herniation was unresponsive to hyperventilation. Hypertonic saline, however, reversed the transtentorial herniation, normalized ICP and increased CBF as well as $CMRO_2$ (Qureshi et al. 2002).

In a blinded, randomized study in swine hypertonic saline/dextran caused an immediate, transient acidaemia, which primarily was due to hyperchloraemic, hypokalaemic metabolic acidosis with normal anion gap. The acidaemia was transient because of the offsetting alkalotic effects of decreasing serum protein, normalization of electrolytes and the transient nature of an increase in CO_2 tension (Moon and Kramer 1995).

1.21.2
Intracranial Pressure, Cerebral Blood Flow and Blood-Brain Barrier

During resuscitation of animals with acute haemorrhage the ICP level is lower in animals treated with hypertonic saline (Prough et al. 1985, 1991; Ducey et al. 1990; Schmoker et al. 1991). Under this circumstance hypertonic saline also reduces water content in cerebral tissue (Todd et al. 1985), but not in the injured part of the brain (Wisner et al. 1990), CBF improves (Todd et al. 1985; Whitley et al. 1988; Prough et al. 1991; Schmoker et al. 1991; Schürer et al. 1992) and brain tissue oxygen tension normalizes (Schürer et al. 1992).

In cats subjected to fluid percussion injury and mild haemorrhage hypotension, rCBF does not increase sufficiently to restore cerebral oxygen delivery or normalize EEG activity (DeWitt et al. 1996). Studies of rCBF and regional glucose utilization in rats indicate a perfect coupling after resuscitation, although the ratio glucose utilization/rCBF was reset to a higher level (1.5 ml/mmol in the control group, contra 2.7 ml/mmol in the hypertonic saline group) (Waschke et al. 1996). Hypertonic saline injures healthy and glutamate-injured rat hippocampus neurons, but does not affect astrocytes (Himmelseher et al. 2001).

It is supposed that the improvement of CBF and the decrease in ICP are caused by a reduction in the cellular volume of uninjured brain parenchyma, endothelial cells and erythrocytes (Shackford et al. 1992). However, hypertonic saline disrupts the blood-brain barrier (Durwald et al. 1983), and rapid infusion of hypertonic saline might cause acute hypotension by a decrease in total peripheral resistance (Kien et al. 1991b).

1.21.3
Comparative Studies Between Hypertonic Saline and Mannitol

In a canine model of intracranial haemorrhage the effect of 3% and 23.4% hypertonic saline was compared with mannitol (1 g/kg). Hypertonic saline, in both concentrations, is as effective as mannitol in the treatment of intracranial hypertension. Hypertonic saline has a longer duration of action, particularly when used in 3% solution (Qureshi et al. 1999). In rats subjected to cortical cryogenic lesion, hypertonic saline was more effective in reducing ICP than equiosmolar mannitol, and in mannitol-treated animals rebound intracranial hypertension was observed (Mirski et al. 2000). In rabbits subjected to cryogenic lesion, infusion of hypertonic saline induces a decrease in ICP (Härtl et al. 1993). Berger et al. (1995) studied the effect of 7.2% saline/dextran or 20% mannitol in rabbits subjected to focal lesion of vasogenic oedema. They found that hypertonic saline/dextran was as effective as mannitol in reducing ICP.

1.21.4
Human Studies

In a double-blind randomized trial Vassar et al. (1993) used Ringer's solution, 7.5% saline, 7.5% saline combined with dextran 70, and 7.5% saline combined with 12% dextran. Patients with systolic pressure < 90 mmHg were included. They found that hypertonic saline was associated with an increase in blood pressure and an increase in survival at hospital discharge. Patients with low baseline GCS seemed to benefit most from 7.5% NaCl. Hypertonic NaCl without added dextran 70 was as effective as the solution that contained dextran 70. There was, however, no significant effect on neurological outcome after 6 months in hypotensive trauma patients randomized to 250 ml 7.5% NaCl or 250 ml lactated Ringer's solution in addition to conventional fluid therapy (Cooper et al. 2004).

In a randomized trial equipotent rapid infusion of hypertonic saline and mannitol was compared. Hypertonic saline caused a greater ICP decrease than mannitol, and had a longer duration of effect than mannitol (Battison et al. 2005).

Although experimental studies indicate that hypertonic saline is not superior to mannitol in its ability to reduce ICP in cryogenic brain oedema (Scheller et al. 1991), hypertonic saline has been used successfully in children with head injury (Fisher et al. 1992; Khanna et al. 2000), in patients with intractable intracranial hypertension (Worthley et al. 1988) and in patients with brain stem trauma.

Zornow (1996) in an editorial concludes that hypertonic saline reduces ICP and brain volume, and can be used safely in humans with minimal potential for morbidity. On the other hand, Schell et al. (1996) summarize that further studies are needed to measure the functional outcome rather than early parameters of CNS function. In addition hypertonic NaCl has a defined risk including the potential detrimental effects of hypernatraemia (lethargy, seizure and coma), tearing of bridging veins, and development of subdural haematoma, central pontine myelinolysis, cardiac failure and arrhythmia.

1.22
Furosemide

In cats furosemide induces an inhibition of CSF production and a concurrent reduction of ICP. These changes are thought to enhance the clearance of vasogenic oedema (Reulen et al. 1977). In dogs with intracranial hypertension furosemide has no effect on CSF formation rate (Miller et al. 1986). In cats subjected to cold injury furosemide effectively reduces the amount of brain oedema (Long et al. 1976). In dogs subjected to cold injury furosemide decreases brain water content in normal dogs, but not in nephrectomized dogs, indicating that the effect of furosemide is mediated by diuresis (Marshall et al.

1982). In a recent study in rats, however, furosemide alone did not change brain water content at any dose (Thenuwara et al. 2002).

In dogs mannitol and furosemide, when used together, produce a greater and more sustained fall in ICP than mannitol alone (Pollay et al. 1983; Roberts et al. 1987). In the same animal infusion of mannitol followed by furosemide 15 min later resulted in the most profound and sustained ICP reduction (Roberts et al. 1987). In the rats furosemide in doses of 2–8 mg/kg enhances the effect of mannitol on plasma osmolality, resulting in a greater reduction of brain water content. This effect was only observed when mannitol was administered in doses of 4 and 8 g/kg (Thenuwara et al. 2002).

Adding furosemide to hypertonic saline decreases brain water content without causing more increase of osmolality and Na^+ than that caused by hypertonic saline alone (Mayzler et al. 2006).

In clinical studies furosemide does not provoke an initial increase in ICP and does not change serum osmolality or electrolytes to the same degree, as does mannitol (Cottrell et al. 1977). Furosemide decreases CSF formation rate and increases CSF absorption capacity (Sklar et al. 1980).

In patients, with brain tumour or cerebral aneurysm, subjected to a rapid infusion of mannitol (1.4 g/kg) or the same dose combined with furosemide (0.3 mg/kg), brain shrinkage was greater and more consistent with mannitol plus furosemide than with mannitol alone. Rapid electrolyte depletion of sodium was observed with the combination of the two drugs and must be corrected (Schettini et al. 1982).

In patients with intracranial hypertension, the combination of Ringer's solution and furosemide 250 mg resulted in a definite improvement in general condition occurring after 24 h. Forced diuresis with high doses of furosemide is suggested as treatment of choice for acute cerebral oedema (Thilmann and Zeumer 1974).

1.23
Corticosteroids

Glucocorticoids are useful in the resolution of altered vascular permeability in experimental brain oedema. Steroids reduce CSF production (Weiss and Nulsen 1970), attenuate free radical production, and have other beneficial effects in experimental models (Pappius and McCain 1969; Bracken et al. 1985, 1990). The net effect is a reduction of ICP.

In patients with brain tumours steroids result in a marked clinical improvement, also in the perioperative period to patients undergoing craniotomy (French and Galicich 1964; Renaudin et al. 1973). There is evidence in both animals and humans that corticosteroid administration may exacerbate ischaemic brain injury as a result of increases in blood glucose concentration (Norris 1976; Koide et al. 1986; Wass and Lanier 1996). Even a single dose of 10 mg dexamethasone intraoperative in non-diabetic patients undergoing craniotomy produces a significant increase in blood glucose over a 4-h period (Pasternak et al. 2004; Lukins and Manninen 2005). Using Xe-CT scanning an inverse correlation of daily dose, cumulative dose and duration of dexamethasone treatment with rCBF was demonstrated in patients with cerebral tumours (Van Roost et al. 2001).

In patients with severe head injury Gobiet et al. (1976) compared low-dose and high-dose Decadron therapy, and documented a beneficial effect in patients on high-dose therapy. A beneficial effect was also found by Faupel et al. (1976) in a double-blind trial. Subsequently, six major studies were performed. None of these revealed substantial benefits of steroid therapy (Gobiet et al. 1976; Cooper et al. 1979; Gudeman et al. 1979; Braakman et al. 1983; Dearden et al. 1986). In a multicenter study, the CRASH trial, the risk of death from all causes within 2 weeks was higher in patients allocated to corticosteroids (CRASH trial collaboration 2004). The final result of the CRASH study has recently been published. The mortality rate was significantly greater with methylprednisolone (25.7% vs 22.3% for placebo) (Edwards et al. 2005).

In the American Guidelines for the Management of Severe Traumatic Brain Injury (2007) and the European EBIC guidelines (Maas et al. 1997), glucocorticoids are not recommended in the treatment of severe head injury. Level I recommendation of American Guidelines 2007: The use of steroids is not recommended for improving outcome or reducing ICP. In patients with moderate or severe traumatic brain injury (TBI), high-dose methylprednisolone is associated with increased mortality and is contraindicated.

References

Abou-Madi M, Trop D, Ravussin P (1993) The early role of mannitol-induced haemodynamic changes in the control of intracranial hypertension. In: Avezaat CJJ, van Eijndhoven JHM, Maas AIR, Tans JTJ (eds) Intracranial pressure VIII. Springer, Berlin, pp 601–604

Abramson NS, Safar P, Detre K et al (1983) Results of a randomized clinical trial of brain resuscitation with thiopental. Anesthesiology 59:A101

Albeck MJ, Skak C, Nielsen PR et al (1998) Age dependency of resistance to cerebrospinal fluid outflow. J Neurosurg 89:275–278

Albrecht RF, Ruttle M (1987) Cerebral effect of extended hyperventilation in anaesthetized goats. Stroke 18:649–655

Alexander SC, Smith TC, Strobel G et al (1968) Cerebral carbohydrate metabolism of man during respiratory and metabolic alkalosis. J Appl Physiol 24:66–72

Altura BT, Altura BM (1975) Pentobarbital and contraction of vascular smooth muscle. Am J Physiol 229:1635–1640

Andersen AR, Tfelt-Hansen P, Lassen NA (1987) The effect of ergotamine and dihydroergotamine on cerebral blood flow in man. Stroke 18:120–123

Andrews PJD, Citerio G (2006) Lund therapy: pathophysiology-based therapy or contrived over-interpretation of limited data? Intensive Care Med 32:1461–1464

Andrews RJ, Muto RP (1992) Retraction brain ischaemia: mannitol plus nimodipine preserves both cerebral blood flow and evoked potentials during normoventilation and hyperventilation. Neurol Res 14:19–25

Andrews PJD, Dearden NM, Miller JD (1993) Comparison of thiopentone and propofol at two rates of intravenous administration in severely head injured patients. In: Avezaat CJJ, van Eijndhoven JHM, Maas AIR, Tans JTJ (eds) Intracranial pressure VIII. Springer, Berlin, pp 623–628

Artru AA (1987) Reduction of cerebrospinal fluid pressure by hypocapnia: changes in cerebral blood volume, cerebrospinal fluid volume, and brain tissue water and electrolytes. J Cereb Blood Flow Metab 7:471–479

Artru AA, Hornbein TF (1987) Prolonged hypocapnia does not alter the rate of CSF production in dogs during halothane anaesthesia or sedation with nitrous oxide. Anesthesiology 67:66–71

Artru AA, Nugent M, Michenfelder JD (1981) Anesthetics affect the cerebral metabolic response to circulatory catecholamine. J Neurochem 36:1941–1946

Asgeirsson B, Grände PO, Nordström C-H (1994) A new therapy of posttrauma brain oedema based on haemodynamic principles for brain volume regulation. Intensive Care Med 20:260–267

Asgeirsson B, Grände PO, Nordström C-H et al (1995) Cerebral haemodynamic effects of dihydroergotamine in patients with severe traumatic brain lesions. Acta Anesthesiol Scand 39:922–930

Aucoin PJ, Kotilainen HR, Gantz NM et al (1986) Intracranial pressure monitors. Epidemiologic study of risk factors and infections. Am J Med 80:369–376

Auer LM, Haselsberger K (1987) Effect of intravenous mannitol on cat pial arteries and veins during normal and elevated intracranial pressure. Neurosurgery 21:142–146

Awad I, Little JR, Lucas F et al (1983) Modification of focal cerebral ischemia by prostacyclin and indomethacin. J Neurosurg 58:714–719

Battison C, Peter H, Andrews JD et al (2005) Randomized, controlled trial on the effect of 20% mannitol solution and a 7.5% saline/6% dextran solution on increased intracranial pressure after brain injury. Crit Care Med 33:196–202

Bereczki D, Liu M, do Prado GF et al (2001) Mannitol for acute stroke. Cochrane Database Syst Rev 1:CD001153

Berger S, Schürer L, Härtl R et al (1995) Reduction of posttraumatic intracranial hypertension by hypertonic/hyperoncotic saline/dextran and hypertonic mannitol. Neurosurgery 37:98–108

Berntman L, Dahlgren N, Siesjö BK (1978) Influence of intravenously administered catecholamine on cerebral oxygen consumption and blood flow in the rat. Acta Physiol Scand 104:101–108

Biestro A, Alberti R, Galli R et al (1997) Osmotherapy for increased intracranial pressure: comparison between mannitol and glycerol. Acta Neurochir 139:725–733

Bloomfield GL, Ridings PC, Blockers CR et al (1997) A proposed relationship between increased intraabdominal, intrathoracic, and intracranial pressure. Crit Care Med 25:496–503

Bouma GJ, Muizlaar JP, Choi SC et al (1991) Cerebral circulation and metabolism after severe traumatic brain injury: the elusive role of ischemia. J Neurosurg 75:685–693

Bouma GJ, Muizelaar JP, Stringer WA et al (1992) Ultra-early evaluation of regional cerebral blood flow in severely head-injured patients using xenon-enhanced computerized tomography. J Neurosurg 77:360–368

Bowie RA, O'Conner PJ, Hardman JG et al (2001) The effect of continuous positive airway pressure on cerebral blood flow velocity in awake volunteers. Anesth Analg 92:415–417

Bozza MM, Maspes PE, Rossanda M (1961) The control of brain volume and tension during intracranial operations. Br J Anaesth 33:132–147

Braakman R, Schouten HJA et al (1983) Megadose steroids in severe head injury. J Neurosurg 58:326–330

Bracken MB, Shepard MJ, Collins WF et al (1985) A randomized, controlled trial of methylprednisolone or naloxone in the treatment of acute spinal-cord injury. Results of the National Acute Spinal Cord Injury Study. J Neurosurg 63:704–713

Bracken MB, Shepard MJ, Collins WF et al (1990) A randomized, controlled trial of methyl-prednisolone or naloxone in the treatment of acute spinal cord injury. N Engl J Med 322:1405–1411

Brawley BW, Strandness DE, Kelly WA (1967) The physiologic response to therapy in experimental cerebral ischaemia. Arch Neurol 17:180–187

Broaddus WC, Pendleton GA, Delashaw SB et al (1989) Differential intracranial pressure recordings in patients with dual ipsilateral monitors. In: Hoff JH, Betz AL (eds) Intracranial pressure VII. Springer, Berlin, pp 41–44

Brown SC, Lam AM, Manninen PH (1986) Haemodynamic effects of high-dose mannitol in man. Can Anaesth Soc J 33:S92–S93

Bruce DA, Langfitt TW, Miller JD et al (1973) Regional cerebral blood flow, intracranial pressure, and brain metabolism in comatose patients. J Neurosurg 38:131–145

Bruce DA, Raphaely RC, Goldberg AI et al (1979) Pathophysiology, treatment and outcome following severe head injury in children. Childs Brain 5:174–191

Bundgaard H, Cold GE (2000) Studies of regional subdural pressure gradients during craniotomy. Br J Neurosurg 14:229–234

Bundgaard H, Jensen K, Cold GE et al (1996) Effects of perioperative indomethacin on intracranial pressure, cerebral blood flow, and cerebral metabolism in patients subjected to craniotomy for cerebral tumours. J Neurosurg Anesthesiol 8:273–279

Bundgaard H, Landsfeldt U, Cold GE (1998) Subdural monitoring of ICP during craniotomy: thresholds of cerebral swelling/herniation. Acta Neurchir Suppl 71:276–278

Bundgaard H, von Oettingen G, Jørgensen H et al (2001) The effects of dihydroergotamine on intracranial pressure, cerebral blood flow and cerebral metabolism in patients subjected to craniotomy for brain tumours. J Neurosurg Anesthesiol 13:195–201

Burke AM, Quest DO, Chien S et al (1981) The effects of mannitol on blood viscosity. J Neurosurg 55:550–553

Busto R, Globus MYT, Dietrich WD et al (1989) Effect of mild hypothermia on ischemic-induced release of neurotransmitters and free fatty acids in rat brain. Stroke 20:904–910

Cain SM (1963) An attempt to demonstrate cerebral anoxia during hyperventilation of anaesthetized dogs. Am J Physiol 204:323–326

Carey BJ, Manktelow BN, Panerai RB et al (2001) Cerebral autoregulation responses to head-up tilt in normal subjects and patients with recurrent vasovagal syncope. Circulation 21:898–902

Carlsson C, Hägerdal M, Siesjö BK (1976) Protective effect of hypothermia in cerebral oxygen deficiency caused by arterial hypoxia. Anesthesiology 44:27–34

Carmona Suazo JA, Maas AIR, van den Brink WA (2000) CO_2 reactivity and brain oxygen pressure monitoring in severe head injury. Crit Care Med 28:3268–3274

Chambers IR, Kane PJ, Signorini DF et al (1998) Bilateral ICP monitoring: its importance in detecting the severity of secondary insults. Acta Neurochir Suppl 71:42–43

Chambers IR, Banister K, Mendelow AD (2001) Intracranial pressure within a developing intracerebral haemorrhage. Br J Neurosurg 15:140–141

Changaris DG, McGraw CP, Richardson JD et al (1987) Correlation of cerebral perfusion pressure and Glasgow coma scale to outcome. J Trauma 27:1007–1012

Chi OZ, Lu X, Wei HM et al (1996) Hydroxyethyl starch solution attenuates blood-brain barrier disruption caused by intracarotid injection of hyperosmolar mannitol in rats. Anesth Analg 83:226–341

Chopp M, Knight R, Tidwell CD et al (1989) The metabolic effects of mild hypothermia on global cerebral ischemia and recirculation in the cat: comparison to normothermia and hyperthermia. J Cereb Blood Flow Metab 9:141–148

Christensen MS (1974) Acid-base changes in cerebrospinal fluid and blood, and blood volume changes following prolonged hyperventilation in man. Br J Anaesth 46:348–357

Chung C, Gottstein J, Blei AT (2001) Indomethacin prevents the development of experimental ammonia-induced brain edema in rats after portacaval anastomosis. Hepatology 34:249–254

Clemmesen JO, Hansen BA, Larsen FS (1997) Indomethacin normalizes intracranial pressure in acute liver failure: a twenty-three-year-old woman treated with indomethacin. Hepatology 26:1423–1425

Clifton GL, Jiang JY, Lyeth BG et al (1991) Marked protection by moderate hypothermia after experimental traumatic brain injury. J Cereb Blood Flow Metab 11:114–121

Clifton GL, Allen S, Barrodale P et al (1993) A phase II study of moderate hypothermia in severe brain injury. J Neurotrauma 10:263–271

Cohen PJ (1981) To dream the impossible dream (editorial view). Anesthesiology 55:491–493

Cold GE (1978) Cerebral metabolic rate of oxygen (CMR O_2) in the acute phase of brain injury. Acta Anaesthesiol Scand 22:249–256

Cold GE (1989a) Measurement of CO_2 reactivity and barbiturate reactivity in patients with severe head injury. Acta Neurochir 98:153–163

Cold GE (1989b) Does acute hyperventilation provoke cerebral oligaemia in comatose patients after acute head injury? Acta Neurochir (Wien) 96:100–106

Cold GE, Felding M (1993) Even small doses of morphine might provoke "luxury perfusion" in the postoperative period after craniotomy. Neurosurgery 32:327

Cold GE, Enevoldsen EM, Malmros R (1975) The prognostic value of continuous intraventricular pressure recording in unconscious brain-injured patients under controlled ventilation. In: Lundberg N, Pontén U, Brock M (eds) Intracranial pressure II. Springer, Berlin, pp 517–521

Cold GE, Jensen FT, Malmros R (1977a). The cerebrovascular CO_2 reactivity during the acute phase of brain injury. Acta Anaesthesiol Scand 21:222–231

Cold GE, Jensen FT, Malmros R (1977b). The effects of Pa CO_2 reduction on regional cerebral blood flow in the acute phase of brain injury. Acta Anaesth Scand 21:359–367

Cold GE, Eskesen V, Eriksen H et al (1986) Changes in CMR O_2, EEG and concentration of etomidate in serum and brain tissue during craniotomy with continuous etomidate supplemented with N_2O and fentanyl. Acta Anaesthesiol Scand 30:159–163

Cold GE, Tange M, Jensen TM et al (1996) Subdural pressure measurement during craniotomy. Correlation with tactile estimation of dura tension and brain herniation after opening of dura. Br J Neurosurg 10:69–75

Coles JP, Minhas PS, Fryer TD et al (2002) Effect of hyperventilation on cerebral blood flow in traumatic head injury: clinical relevance and monitoring correlates. Crit Care Med 30:1950–1959

Connolly JE, Boyd RJ, Calvin JW (1962) The protective effect of hypothermia in cerebral ischaemia. Experimental and clinical application by selective brain cooling in the human. Surgery 52:15–24

Constantini S, Cotev S, Rappaport H et al (1988) Intracranial pressure monitoring after elective intracranial surgery. J Neurosurg 69:540–544

Cooper PR, Moody S, Clark WK et al (1979) Dexamethasone and severe head injury. A prospective double-blind study. J Neurosurg 51:307–316

Cooper DJ, Myles PS, McDermott FT et al (2004). Prehospital hypertonic saline resuscitation of patients with hypotension and severe traumatic brain injury: a randomized controlled trial. JAMA 291:1350–1357

Cottrell JE, Robustelli A, Post K et al (1977) Furosemide- and mannitol-induced changes in intracranial pressure and serum osmolality and electrolytes. Anesthesiology 47:28–30

Cottrell JE, Hartung J, Giffin JP et al (1983) Intracranial and hemodynamic changes after succinyl administration in cats. Anesth Analg 62:1006–1009

CRASH trial collaboration (2004) Effect of intravenous corticosteroids on death within 14 days in 10008 adults with clinically significant head injury (MRC CRASH trial): randomized placebo-controlled trial. Lancet 364:1321–1328

Cruz J (1993) Combined continuous monitoring of systemic and cerebral oxygenation in acute brain injury: preliminary observations. Crit Care Med 21:1225–1232

Cruz J (1998) The first decade of continuous monitoring of jugular bulb oxyhaemoglobin saturation: management strategies and clinical outcome. Crit Care Med 26:344–351

Cruz J, Jaggi JL, Hoffstad OJ (1995) Cerebral blood flow, vascular resistance, and oxygen metabolism in acute brain trauma: redefining the role of cerebral perfusion pressure? Crit Care Med 23:1412–1417

Cruz J, Minoja G, Okuchi K (2001) Improving clinical outcomes from acute subdural haematomas with the emergency preoperative administration of high doses of mannitol: a randomized trial. Neurosurgery 49:864–871

Cruz J, Minoja G, Okuchi K (2002) Major clinical and physiological benefits of early high doses of mannitol for intraparenchymal temporal hemorrhages with abnormal pupillary widening: a randomized study. Neurosurgery 51:628–637

Cruz J, Minoja G, Okuchi K et al (2004) Successful use of the new high-dose mannitol treatment in patients with Glasgow Coma Scale scores of 3 and bilateral abnormal papillary widening: a randomized trial. J Neurosurg 100:376–383

Cushing H (1903) The blood pressure reaction of acute cerebral compression, illustrated by cases of intracranial hemorrhage. Am J Med Sci 125:1017–1044

Czosnyka M, Pickard JD (2004) Monitoring and interpretation of intracranial pressure. J Neurol Neurosurg Psychiatry 75:813–821

Czosnyka M, Price DJ, Williamson M (1994) Monitoring of cerebrospinal dynamics using continuous analysis of intracranial pressure and cerebral perfusion pressure in head injury. Acta Neurochir (Wien) 126:113–119

Dahl B, Jensen K, Cold GE et al (1991) Studies of barbiturate reactivity in patients with severe head injury. Acta Anaesthesiol Scand Suppl 96:201

Dahl B, Bergholt B, Kjærgaard JO et al (1996) The correlation between CO_2 and indomethacin reactivity in severe head injury. Acta Neurochir 138:265–273

Dahlgren N, Nilsson B, Sakabe T et al (1981) The effect of indomethacin on cerebral blood flow and oxygen consumption in the rat at normal and increased carbon dioxide tensions. Acta Physiol Scand 111:475–485

Daley ML, Han S, Leffler C (2002) Cyclic variation of cerebral pial arteriolar diameter synchronized with positive pressure inhalation. Acta Neurochir Suppl 81:143–145

Darby JM, Yonas H, Marion DW et al (1988) Local inverse steal induced by hyperventilation in head injury. Neurosurgery 23:84–88

Dearden NM, Gibson SJ, McDowall DG et al (1986) Effect of high-dose dexamethasone on outcome from severe head injury. J Neurosurg 64:81–88

Dempsey RJ, Roy MW, Meyer KL et al (1985) Indomethacin-mediated improvement following middle cerebral artery occlusion in cats. Effects of anesthesia. J Neurosurg 62:874–881

De Reuck JL (1984) Cerebral argioarchitecture and perinatal brain lesions in premature and full-term infants. Acta Neurol Scand 70:391–395

DeWitt DS, Prough DS, Deal DD et al (1996) Hypertonic saline does not improve cerebral oxygen delivery after head injury and mild hemorrhage in cats. Crit Care Med 24:109–117

Dieterich H-J, Reutershan J, Felbinger TW et al (2003) Penetration of intravenous hydroxyethyl starch into the cerebrospinal fluid in patients with impaired blood-brain barrier. Anesth Analg 96:1150–1154

Dietrich WD, Busto R, Valdes I et al (1990) Effects of normothermic versus mild hyperthermic forebrain ischemia in rats. Stroke 21:1318–1325

Dings J, Meixenberger J, Amschler J et al (1996) Brain tissue p O_2 in relation to cerebral perfusion pressure, TCD findings and CO_2 reactivity after severe head injury. Acta Neurochir 138:425–434

duCailar J, Rioux J, Groleau D et al (1964) Hypothermie au dessous de 25 par refrigeration externe et sans circulation extra-corporelle. Ann Anesth Franc 4:781–800

Ducey JP, Lamiell JM, Gueller GE (1990) Cerebral electrophysiological effects of resuscitation with hypertonic saline-dextran after hemorrhage. Crit Care Med 18:744–749

Dunn LT (2002) Raised intracranial pressure. J Neurol Neurosurg Psychiatry 73 (suppl 1):i23–i27

Durwald QJ, Del Maestro RF, Amacher AL et al (1983) The influence of systemic arterial pressure and intracranial pressure on the development of cerebral vasogenic edema. J Neurosurg 59:803–809

Edvinsson L, McCulloch J (1981) Effects of pentobarbital on contractile responses of feline cerebral arteries. J Cereb Blood Flow Metab 1:437–440

Edwards P, Arango M, Balica L et al (2005) Final results of MRC CRASH, a randomized placebo-controlled trial of intravenous corticosteroid in adults with head injury: outcomes at 6 months. Lancet 365:1957–1959

Eide PK (2003) The relationship between intracranial pressure and size of cerebral ventricles assessed by computed tomography. Acta Neurochir 145:171–179

Eisenberg HM, Frankowski RF, Contant CF et al (1988) High-dose barbiturate control of elevated intracranial pressure in patients with severe head injury. J Neurosurg 69:15–23

Ellingsen I, Hauge A, Nicolaysen G et al (1987) Changes in human cerebral blood flow due to step changes in PaO_2 and $PaCO_2$. Acta Physiol Scand 129:157–163

Este-McDonald JR, Josephs LG, Birkett DH et al (1995) Changes in intracranial pressure associated with apneumic retractors. Arch Surg 130:362–365

Famularo G (1999) The puzzle of neuronal death and life: is mannitol the right drug for the treatment of brain oedema associated with ischemic stroke? Eur J Emerg Med 6:363–368

Fandino J, Stocker R, Prokop S et al (1999) Correlation between jugular bulb oxygen saturation and partial pressure of brain tissue oxygen during CO_2 and O_2 reactivity tests in severely head-injured patients. Acta Neurochir 141:825–834

Faupel G, Reulen HJ, Muller D et al (1976) Double-blind study on the effects of steroids on severe closed head injury. In: Pappius HM, Feindal W (eds) Dynamics of brain edema. Springer, Berlin, pp 337–343

Feldman Z, Kanter MJ, Robertson CS et al (1992) Effect of head elevation on intracranial pressure, cerebral perfusion pressure, and cerebral blood flow in head-injured patients. J Neurosurg 76:207–211

Feldman Z, Roberson CS, Contant CSF et al (1997) Positive end-expiratory pressure reduces intracranial compliance in the rabbit. J Neurosurg Anesthesiol 9:175–179

Fieschi C, Battistini N, Beduschi A et al (1974) Regional cerebral blood flow and intraventricular pressure in acute head injuries. J Neurol Neurosurg Psychiatry 37:1378–1388

Filipo V, Butterworth RF (2002) Neurobiology of ammonia. Prog Neurobiol 67:259–279

Fisher B, Thomas D, Peterson B (1992) Hypertonic saline lowers raised intracranial pressure in children after head trauma. J Neurosurg Anesthesiol 4:4–10

Fortune JB, Feustel PJ, Graca L et al (1995) Effect of hyperventilation, mannitol, and ventriculostomy drainage on cerebral blood flow after head injury. J Trauma 39:1091–1097

French LA, Galicich JH (1964) The use of steroids for control of cerebral edema. Clin Neurosurg 10:212–223

Frost EA (1977) Effects of positive end-expiratory pressure on intracranial pressure and compliance in brain-injured patients. J Neurosurg 47:195–200

Ganz JC, Hall C, Zwernow NN (1995) Cerebral blood flow during experimental epidural bleeding in swine. Acta Neurochir 103:148–157

Gaudet RJ, Alam I, Levine L (1980) Accumulation of cyclooxygenase products of arachidonic acid metabolism in gerbil brain during reperfusion after bilateral common carotid artery occlusion. J Neurochem 35:653–658

Gemma M, Tommasino C, Cerri M et al (2002) Intracranial effects of endotracheal suctioning in the acute phase of head injury. J Neurosurg Anesthesiol 14:50–54

Georgiadis D, Schwartz S, Baumgartner RW et al (2001) Influence of positive end-expiratory pressure on intracranial pressure and cerebral perfusion pressure in patients with acute stroke. Stroke 32:2088–2092

Giffin JP, Hartung J, Cottrell et al (1986) Effect of vecuronium on intracranial pressure, mean arterial pressure and heart rate in cats. Br J Anesth 58:441–443

Gilles FH, Leviton A, Kerr CS (1976) Endotoxin leucoencephalopathy in the telencephalon of the newborn kitten. J Neurol Sci 27:183–191

Glaser N, Barnett P, McCaslin I et al (2001) Risk factors for cerebral oedema in children with diabetic ketoacidosis. The Pediatric Emergency Medicine Collaborative Research Committee of the American Academy of Pediatrics. N Engl J Med 344:264–269

Gleason CA, Short BL, Jones MD Jr (1989) Cerebral blood flow and metabolism during and after prolonged hypocapnia in newborn lambs. J Pediatr 115:309–314

Gobiet W, Bock WJ, Liesgang J et al (1976) Treatment of acute cerebral edema with high dose of dexamethasone. In: Beks JWF et al (eds) Intracranial pressure III. Springer, Berlin, pp 231–235

Gopinath SP, Valadka AB, Uzura M et al (1999) Comparison of jugular venous oxygen saturation and brain tissue $P O_2$ as monitors of cerebral ischaemia after head injury. Crit Care Med 27:2337–2345

Gordon E (1970) The action of drugs on intracranial contents. In: Boulton TB, Bryce-Smith R et al (eds) Progress in anaesthesiology. Excerpta Medica, Amsterdam, p 60

Gotoh F, Meyer JS, Takagi Y (1965) Cerebral effects of hyperventilation in man. Arch Neurol 12:410–423

Graham EM, Apostolou M, Mishra OP et al (1996) Modification of the N-methyl-D-Aspartate (NMDA) receptor in the brain of newborn piglets following hyperventilation induced ischemia. Neurosci Lett 218:29–32

Grände P-O (1989) The effects of dihydroergotamine in patients with head injury and raised intracranial pressure. Intensive Care Med 15:523–527

Grände P-O (2006) The "Lund Concept" for the treatment of severe head trauma: physiological principles and clinical application. Intensive Care Med 32:1475–1484

Greenberg JH, Alavi A, Reivich M et al (1978) Local cerebral blood volume response to carbon dioxide in man. Circ Res 43:324–331

Greenwood J, Luthert PJ, Pratt OE et al (1988) Hyperosmolar opening of the blood-brain barrier in energy-depleted rat brain. Part I. Permeability studies. J Cereb Blood Flow Metab 8:9–15

Greisen G, Munck H, Lou H (1987) Severe hypocapnia in preterm infants and neurodevelopmental deficit. Acta Paediatr Scand 76:401–404

Gross CE, Abel PW (1985) Contraction and relaxation of rabbit basilar artery by thiopental. Neurosurgery 17:433–435

Grubb RL, Raichle ME, Eichling JO et al (1974) The effects of changes in Pa CO_2 on cerebral blood volume, blood flow, and vascular mean transit time. Stroke 5:630–638

Grubb RL, Raichle ME, Eichling JO et al (1977) Effects of subarachnoid hemorrhage on cerebral blood volume, blood flow and oxygen utilization in humans. J Neurosurg 46:446–453

Gudeman SK, Miller JD, Becker DP (1979) Failure of high-dose steroid therapy to influence intracranial pressure in patients with severe head injury. J Neurosurg 51:301–306

Guieu JD, Lapierre M, Blond S et al (1979) Correlations between intracranial pressure variations and EEG changes in patients with cranial trauma (translated). Rev Electroencephalogr Neurophysiol Clin 9:194–201

Haddad GG, Jiang C (1997) O_2-sensing mechanisms in excitable cells: role of plasma membrane K+ channels. Annu Rev Physiol 59:23–42

Hallenbeck JM, Furlow TW (1979) Prostaglandin I2 and indomethacin prevent impairment of post-ischemic brain reperfusion in the dog. Stroke 10:629–637

Halverson A, Buchanan R, Jacobs L et al (1998) Evaluation of mechanism of increased intracranial pressure with insufflation. Surg Endosc 12:266–269

Haring HP, Hormann C, Schalow S et al (1994) Continuous positive airway pressure breathing increases cerebral blood flow velocity in humans. Anesth Analg 79: 883–885

Hariri RJ, Firlich AD, Shepard SR et al (1993) Traumatic brain injury, hemorrhagic shock, and fluid resuscitation: effects on intracranial pressure and brain compliance. J Neurosurg 79:421–427

Harp JR, Wollman H (1973) Cerebral metabolic effects of hyperventilation and deliberate hypotension. Br J Anaesth 45:256–262

Harris RJ, Bayhan M, Branston NM et al (1982) Modulation of the pathophysiology of primate focal cerebral ischaemia by indomethacin. Stroke 13:17–24

Härtl R, Schürer L, Dautermann C et al (1993) Effect of hypertonic-hyperoncotic solutions (HHS) on increased intracranial pressure after a focal brain lesion and inflation of an epidural balloon. In: Avezaat CJJ, van Eijndhoven JHM, Maas AIR, Tans JTJ (eds) Intracranial pressure VIII. Springer, Berlin, pp 612–614

Härtl R, Medary MB, Ruge M et al (1997) Early white blood cell dynamics after traumatic brain injury: effects on cerebral microcirculation. J Cereb Blood Flow Metab 17:1210–1220

Haure P, Cold GE, Hansen TM et al (2003) The ICP-lowering effect of 10° reverse Trendelenburg position during craniotomy is stable during a 10-minute period. J Neurosurg Anesthesiol 15:297–301

Havill JH (1984) Prolonged hyperventilation and intracranial pressure. Crit Care Med 12:72–74

Haxhiu MA, van Lunteren E, Deal EC et al (1989) Role of the ventral surface of medulla in the generation of Mayer waves. Am J Physiol 257:R804–R809

Hering R, Wrigge H, Vorwerk R et al (2001) The effects of prone positioning in intraabdominal pressure and cardiovascular and renal function in patients with acute lung injury. Anesth Analg 92:1226–1231

Himmelseher S, Pfenninger E, Morin P et al (2001) Hypertonic-hyperoncotic saline differentially affects healthy and glutamate-injured primary rat hippocampus neurons and cerebral astrocytes. J Neurosurg Anesthesiol 13:120–130

Hochwald GM, Wald A, Malhan C (1976) The sink action of cerebrospinal fluid volume flow. Arch Neurol 33:339–344

Hoffman WE, Werner C, Baughman VL et al (1991) Postischemic treatment with hypothermia improves outcome from incomplete cerebral ischemia in rats. J Neurosurg Anesthesiol 3:34–38

Hörmann C, Mohsenipour I, Gottardis M et al (1994) Response of cerebrospinal fluid pressure to continuous positive airway pressure in volunteers. Anesth Analg 78:54–57

Howells T, Elf K, Jones PA et al (2005) Pressure reactivity as a guide in the treatment of cerebral perfusion pressure in patients with brain trauma. J Neurosurg 102:311–317

Hulme A, Cooper R (1976) The effects of head position and jugular vein compression on intracranial pressure. A clinical study. In: Beks JWF, Bosch DA, Brock M (eds) Intracranial pressure III. Springer, Berlin, pp 259–263

Hung OR, Hare GM, Brien S (2000) Head elevation reduces head-rotation associated increased ICP in patients with intracranial tumours. Can J Anaesth 47:415–420

Hunter AR (1972) Thiopentone supplemented anaesthesia for neurosurgery. Br J Anaesth 44:506–510

Imberti R, Ciceri M, Bellinzona G et al (2000) The use of hyperventilation in the treatment of plateau waves in two patients with severe traumatic brain injury: contrasting effects on cerebral oxygenation. J Neurosurg Anesthesiol 12:124–127

Imberti R, Bellinzona G, Langer M (2002) Cerebral tissue $P\,O_2$ and $Sjv\,O_2$ changes during moderate hyperventilation in patients with severe traumatic brain injury. J Neurosurg 96:97–102

Ito U, Ohno K, Nakamura R et al (1979) Brain edema during ischemia after restoration of blood flow. Measurement of water, sodium, potassium content and plasma protein permeability. Stroke 10:542–547

Jafar JJ, Johns LM, Mullan SF (1986) The effect of mannitol on cerebral blood flow. J Neurosurg 64:754–759

Jaggi JL, Obrist WD, Gennarelli TA et al (1990) Relationship of early cerebral blood flow and metabolism to outcome in acute head injury. J Neurosurg 72:176–182

James HE (1978) Cytotoxic edema produced by 6-aminonicotinamide and its response to therapy. Neurosurgery 3:196–200

James HE (1980) Methodology for the control of intracranial pressure with hypertonic mannitol. Acta Neurochir (Wien) 51:161–172

Jennett WB, Teasdale C (1981) Management of head injuries in the acute state. Davis, Philadelphia, pp 240–241

Jensen K, Öhrström J, Cold GE et al (1991) The effects of indomethacin on intracranial pressure, cerebral blood flow, and cerebral metabolism in patients with severe head injury and intracranial hypertension. Acta Neurochir (Wien) 108:116–121

Jensen K, Freundlich M, Bünemann L et al (1993) The effect of indomethacin upon cerebral blood flow in healthy volunteers. The influence of moderate hypoxia and hypercapnia. Acta Neurochir (Wien) 124:114–119

Jensen K, Kjaergaard S, Malte E et al (1996) Effect of graduated intravenous and standard rectal doses of indomethacin on cerebral blood flow in healthy volunteers. J Neurosurg Anesthesiol 8:111–116

Johnston AJ, Steiner LA, Balestreri M et al (2003) Hyperoxia and cerebral haemodynamic responses to moderate hyperventilation. Acta Anaesthesiol Scand 47:391–396

Johnstone IH, Harper AM (1973) The effect of mannitol on cerebral blood flow. An experimental study. J Neurosurg 38:461–471

Jones SJ, Dinsmore J (2002) Effect of diclofenac on cerebral blood flow velocity in patients with supratentorial tumours. Br J Anaesth 89:762–764

Jørgensen HA, Bundgaard H, Cold GE (1999) Subdural pressure measurement during fossa posterior surgery. Br J Neurosurg 13:449–453

Josephs LG, Este-McDonald E, Birkett DH et al (1994) Diagnostic laparoscopy increases intracranial pressure. J Trauma 36:815–818

Kalmar AF, van Aken J, Caemaert J et al (2005) Value of Cushing reflex as warning sign for brain ischaemia during neuroendoscopy. Br J Anaesth 94:791–799

Kanter MJ, Robertson CS, Sheinberg MA et al (1993) Changes in cerebral haemodynamics with head elevated vs. head flat. In: Avezaat CJJ, van Eijndhoven JHM, Maas AIR, Tans JTJ (eds) Intracranial pressure VIII. Springer, Berlin, p 79

Kassell NF, Hitchon PW, Gerk MK et al (1980) Alterations in cerebral blood flow, oxygen metabolism, and electrical activity produced by high dose sodium thiopental. Neurosurgery 7:598–603

Kassell NF, Baumann KW, Hitchon PW et al (1982) The effects of high dose mannitol on cerebral blood flow in dogs with normal intracranial pressure. Stroke 13:59–61

Kaufmann AM, Cardoso ER (1992) Aggravation of vasogenic cerebral edema by multiple-dose mannitol. J Neurosurg 77:584–589

Kazan S, Karasoy M, Baloglu H et al (1999) The effect of mild hypothermia, mannitol and insulin-induced hypoglycaemia on ischemic infarct volume in the early period after permanent middle cerebral artery occlusion in the rat. Acta Neurochir 141:979–987

Kellie G (1824) An account of the appearances observed in the dissection of two of the three individuals presumed to have perished in the storm of the 3rd, and whose bodies were discovered in the vicinity of Leith on the morning of the 4th November 1921 with some reflections on the pathology of the brain. Trans Med Chir Sci, Edinburgh, 1:84–169

Kempski O, Obert C, Mainka T et al (1996) "Small volume resuscitation" as treatment of cerebral blood flow disturbances and increased ICP in trauma and ischemia. Acta Neurochir Suppl 66:114–117

Kenning JA, Toutant SM, Saunders RL (1981) Upright patient positioning in the management of intracranial hypertension. Surg Neurol 15:148–152

Khanna S, Davis D, Peterson B et al (2000) Use of hypertonic saline in the treatment of severe refractory posttraumatic intracranial hypertension in pediatric traumatic brain injury. Crit Care Med 28:4:1144–1151

Kien RD, Reitan JA, White DA et al (1991a) Cardiac contractility and blood flow distribution following resuscitation with 7.5% hypertonic saline in anesthetized dogs. Circ Shock 35:109–116

Kien ND, Kramer GC, White DA (1991b) Acute hypotension caused by rapid hypertonic saline infusion in anesthetized dogs. Anesth Analg 73:597–602

Kiening KL, Schoening WN, Lanksch WR et al (2002) Intracranial compliance as bed-side monitoring technique in severely head-injured patients. Acta Neurochir Suppl 81:177–180

Kim B, Feldman EL (2002) Insulin-like growth factor I prevents mannitol-induced degradation of focal adhesion kinase and Akt. J Biol Chem 26:27393–27400

Kim HJ, Levasseur JE, Patterson JL et al (1989) Effect of indomethacin pretreatment on acute mortality in experimental brain injury. J Neurosurg 71:565–572

Kim W, Moon SO, Sung MJ et al (2002) Protective effect of adrenomedullin in mannitol-induced apoptosis. Apoptosis 7:527–536

Kitagawa K, Matsumoto M, Tagaya M et al (1991) Hyperthermia-induced neuronal protection against ischemic injury in gerbils. J Cereb Blood Flow Metab 11:449–452

Kitahata LM, Galicich JM, Sato I (1971) The effect of passive hyperventilation on intracranial pressure. J Neurosurg 34:185–193

Koide T, Wieloch TW, Siesjö BK (1986) Chronic dexamethasone pretreatment aggravates ischemic neuronal necrosis. J Cereb Blood Flow Metab 6:395–404

Kojima T, Iwat K, Tamai K (1993) Change of cerebral electrophysiological activity, regional cerebral blood flow and regional cerebral blood volume in acute intracranial hypertension. In: Avezaat CJJ, van Eijndhoven JHM, Maas AIR, Tans JTJ (eds) Intracranial pressure VIII. Springer, Berlin, pp 249–252

Kolbitsch C, Lorenz IH, Hoermann C et al (2000) The influence of increased intrathoracic pressure on cerebral compliance in humans. Proc XI ICP Symp, Cambridge P17-8, p 286

Kolbitsch C, Lorenz ICH, Hörmann C et al (2002) The impact of hypercapnia on systolic cerebrospinal fluid peak velocity in the aqueduct of Sylvius. Anesth Analg 95:1049–1051

Korenkov AI, Pahnke J, Frei K et al (2000) Treatment with nimodipine or mannitol reduces programmed cell death and infarct size following cerebral ischemia. Neurosurg Rev 23:145–150

Kramer GC, Perron PR, Lindsey DC et al (1986) Small-volume resuscitation with hypertonic saline dextran solution. Surgery 100:239–247

Kuchiwaki H, Misu N, Takada S et al (1992) Measurement of local directional pressures in the brain with mass. Neurosurgery 31:731–738

Laffey JG, Kavanagh BP (2002) Hypocapnia. N Engl J Med 347:43–53

Langfitt TW, Weinstein JD, Kassell NF et al (1964) Transmission of increased intracranial pressure within the craniospinal axis. J Neurosurg 21:989–997

Lanier WL, Milde JH, Michenfelder JD (1985) The cerebral effects of pancuronium and atracurium in halothane-anesthetized dogs. Anesthesiology 63:589–597

Lanier WL, Milde JH, Michenfelder JD (1986) Cerebral stimulation following succinylcholine in dogs Anesthesiology 64:551–559

Lanier WL, Iaizzo PA, Milde JH (1989) Cerebral function and muscle afferent activity following intravenous succinylcholine in dogs anesthetized with halothane: the effects of pretreatment with a defasciculating dose of pancuronium. Anesthesiology 71:87–95

Larsen R, Hilfiker O, Radle J et al (1981) Midazolam: Wirkung auf allgemeine Hämodynamik, Hirndurchblutung und Cerebralen Sauerstoffverbrauch bei Neurochirurgischen Patienten. Anesthetist 30:18–21

Larsen JR, Haure P, Cold GE (2002) Reverse Trendelenburg position reduces intracranial pressure during craniotomy. J Neurosurg Anesthesiol 14:16–21

Lee ST (1989) Intracranial pressure changes during positioning of patients with severe head injury. Heart Lung 18:411–414

Lescot T, Naccache L, Bonnet MP et al (2005) The relationship of intracranial pressure Lundberg waves to electroencephalograph fluctuations in patients with severe head trauma. Acta Neurochir 147:125–129

Little JR (1978) Modification of acute focal ischaemia by treatment with mannitol. Stroke 9:4–9

Lodrini S, Montolivo M, Pluchino F et al (1989) Positive end-expiratory pressure in supine and sitting positions: its effects on intrathoracic and intracranial pressures. Neurosurgery 24:873–877

Long DM, Maxwell R, Choi KS (1976) A new therapy regimen for brain edema. In: Pappius HM, Feidal W (eds) Dynamics of brain edema. Springer, Berlin, pp 293–300

Lukins MB, Manninen PH (2005) Hyperglycemia in patients administered dexamethasone for craniotomy. Anesth Analg 100:1129–1133

Lundberg N (1960) Continuous recording and control of ventricular fluid pressure in neurosurgical practice. Acta Psychiatr Scand 36(suppl 149):1–193

Lundberg N, Kjällquist A, Bien C (1959) Reduction of increased intracranial pressure by hyperventilation. Acta Psychiatr Neurol Scand 34(suppl 139)

Maas AIR, Fleckenstein W, deJong DA et al (1993) Effect of increased ICP and decreased cerebral perfusion pressure on brain tissue and cerebrospinal fluid oxygen tension. In: Avezaat CJJ, van Eijndhoven JHM, Maas AIR, Tans JTJ (eds) Intracranial pressure VIII. Springer, Berlin, pp 233–237

Maas AIR, Dearden M, Teasdale GM et al (1997) EBIC guidelines for management of severe head injury in adults. Acta Neurochir 139:286–294

MacDonald JT, Uden DL (1982) Intravenous glycerol and mannitol therapy in children with intracranial hypertension. Neurology 32:437–440

MacKenzie ET, McCullock J, O'Keane M et al (1976) Cerebral circulation and norepinephrine: relevance of the blood-brain barrier. Am J Physiol 231:483–488

Maeda M, Miyazaki M (1998) Control of ICP and cerebrovascular bed by the cholinergic basal forebrain. Acta Neurochir Suppl 71:293–296

Maeda M, Miyazaki M, Ishii S (1989) The role of the mutual interaction between the locus coeruleus complex and the cholinoceptive pontine area in the plateau wave. In: Hoff JT, Betz AL (eds) Intracranial pressure VII. Springer, Berlin, pp 228–231

Maeda M, Miyazaki M, Ishii S (1993) Control of ICP by the medullary reticular formation. In: Avezaat CJJ, van Eijndhoven JHM, Maas AIR, Tans JTJ (eds) Intracranial pressure VIII. Springer, Berlin, pp 207–213

Maioriello A, Chaljub G, Nauta HJW et al (2002). Chemical shift imaging of mannitol in acute cerebral ischemia. J Neurosurg 87:687–691

Mak S, Egri Z, Tanna G et al (2002) Vitamin C prevents hyperoxia-mediated vasoconstriction and impairment of endothelium-dependent vasodilatation. Am J Physiol Heart Circ Physiol 282:H2414–H2421

Malek AM, Goss GG, Jiang L et al (1998) Mannitol at clinical concentrations activates multiple signaling pathways and induces apoptosis in endothelial cells. Stroke 29:2631–2640

Manninen PH, Lam AM, Gelb AW et al (1987) The effect of high-dose mannitol on serum and urine electrolytes and osmolality in neurosurgical patients. Can J Anaesth 34:442–446

Manno EM, Adams RE, Derdeyn CP et al (1999) The effects of mannitol on cerebral edema after large hemispheric cerebral infarct. Neurology 52:583–587

March Ml, Dunlop BJ, Shapiro HM et al (1980) Succinylcholine-intracranial pressure effects in neurosurgical patients. Anesth Analg 59:550–551

Marin J, Lobato RD, Rico ML et al (1981) Effect of pentobarbital on the reactivity of isolated human cerebral arteries. J Neurosurg 54:521–524

Marion DW, Obrist WD, Carlien PM et al (1993) The use of moderate therapeutic hypothermia for patients with severe head injuries: a preliminary report. J Neurosurg 79:354–362

Marion DW, Penrod LE, Kelsey SF et al (1997) Treatment of traumatic brain injury with moderate hypothermia. New Engl J Med 336:540–545

Marshall LF, Smith RW, Rauscher LA et al (1978) Mannitol dose requirements in brain-injured patients. J Neurosurg 48:169–172

Marshall WK, Page RB, Milchak MA (1982) Furosemide reduces brain water in cerebral injury in dogs. Anesthesiology 57:A308

Marshall LF, Zovickian J, Ostrup R et al (1986) Multiple simultaneous recordings of ICP in patients with acute mass lesions. In: Miller JD, Teasdale GM, Rowan JO et al (eds) Intracranial pressure VI. Springer, Berlin, pp 184–186

Martins AN, Doyle TF, Newby N (1976) $PaCO_2$ and rate of formation of cerebrospinal fluid in the monkey. Am J Physiol 231:127–131

Marx W, Shah N, Long C et al (1989) Sufentanil, alfentanil, and fentanyl: impact on cerebrospinal fluid pressure in patients with brain tumors. J Neurosurg Anesthesiol 1:3–7

Mascia L, Grasso S, Puntillo F et al (2000) The effects of PEEP on cerebral haemodynamics in severe brain injured patients with acute lung injury. Intensive Care Med 123

Mascia L, Grasso S, Fiore T et al (2005) Cerebro-pulmonary interactions during the application of low levels of positive end-expiratory pressure. Intensive Care Med 31:373–379

Mavrocordatos P, Bissonnette P, Ravussion P (2000) Effects of neck position and head elevation on intracranial pressure in anaesthetized neurosurgical patients: preliminary results. J Neurosurg Anesthesiol 12:10–14

Mayhall CG, Archer NH, Lamb VA et al (1984) Ventriculostomy-related infections. A prospective epidemiological study. N Eng J Med 310:553–559

Mayzler O, Leon A, Eilig I et al (2006) The effect of hypertonic (3%) saline with and without furosemide on plasma osmolality, sodium concentration, and brain water content after closed head trauma in rats. J Neurosurg Anesthesiol 18:24–31

Mazzoni MC, Borgstrom P, Arfors KE et al (1988) Dynamic fluid redistribution in hyperosmotic resuscitation of hypovolemic hemorrhage. Am J Physiol 255:H629–H637

McGuire G, Crossley D, Richards J et al (1997) Effects of varying levels of positive end-expiratory pressure on intracranial pressure and cerebral perfusion pressure. Crit Care Med 25:1059–1062

Mchedlishvili G (1988) Pathogenetic role of circulatory factors in brain oedema development. Neursurg Rev 11:7–13

McHenry LC Jr, Jaffe ME, West JW et al (1972) Regional cerebral blood flow and cardiovascular effects of hexobendine in stroke patients. Neurology (Minneap) 22:217–223

McLaughlin MR, Marion DW (1996) Cerebral blood flow and vasoresponsivity within and around cerebral contusions. J Neurosurg 85:871–876

McQueen JD, Jeanes LD (1964) Dehydration and rehydration of the brain with hypertonic urea and mannitol. J Neurosurg 11:118–128

Meixensberger J, Brawanski A, Danhauser-Leistner I et al (1993) Is there a risk to induce ischemia by hyperventilation therapy? In: Avezaat CJJ, van Eijndhoven JHM, Maas AIR, Tans JTJ (eds) Intracranial pressure VIII. Springer, Berlin, pp 589–591

Meixensberger J, Baunach S, Amschler J et al (1997) Influence of body position on tissue-p O_2, cerebral perfusion pressure and intracranial pressure in patients with acute brain injury. Neurol Res 19:249–253

Meixensberger J, Jager A, Dings J et al (1998) Multimodal haemodynamic neuromonitoring: quality and consequences for therapy of severely head injured patients. Acta Neurochir Suppl 71:260–262

Mellander S, Nordenfelt I (1970) Comparative effects of dihydroergotamine and noradrenalin on resistance exchange and capacitance functions in the peripheral circulation. Clin Sci 39:183–201

Merlo F, Demo P, Moreth T et al (1993) Propofol vs. thiopental for the control of elevated ICP in head injured patients. In: Avezaat CJJ, van Eijndhoven JHM, Maas AIR, Tans JTJ (eds) Intracranial pressure VIII. Springer, Berlin, pp 629–631

Messeter K, Nordström C-H, Sundbärg G et al (1986) Cerebral haemodynamics in patients with severe head trauma. J Neurosurg 64:231–237

Metz C, Holzschuh M, Bein T et al (1996) Moderate hypothermia in patients with severe head injury: Cerebral and extracerebral effects. J Neurosurg 85:533–541

Meyer FB, Anderson RE, Sundt TM et al (1987) Treatment of experimental focal cerebral ischaemia with mannitol. J Neurosurg 66:109–115

Michenfelder JD (1974) The interdependency of cerebral functional and metabolic effects following massive doses of thiopental in the dog. Anesthesiology 41:231–236

Michenfelder JD, Milde JH (1977) Failure of prolonged hypocapnia, hypothermia or hypertension to favourably alter acute stroke in primates. Stroke 8:87–91

Michenfelder JD, Milde JH (1991) The relationship among canine brain temperature, metabolism, and function during hypocapnia. Anesthesiology 75:130–136

Michenfelder JD, Sundt TM (1973) The effect of $Pa\,CO_2$ on the metabolism of ischemic brain in squirrel monkeys. Anesthesiology 38:445–453

Milde LN, Milde JH, Michenfelder JD (1985) Cerebral functional, metabolic, and haemodynamic effects of etomidate in dogs. Anesthesiology 63:371–377

Milde LN, Milde JH, Gallagher W (1990) Effects of sufentanil on cerebral circulation and metabolism in dogs. Anesth Analg 70:138–146

Miller JD, Leech P (1975) Effects of mannitol and steroid therapy on intracranial volume-pressure relationships in patients. J Neurosurg 42:274–281

Miller JD, Becker DP, Ward JD et al (1977) Significance of intracranial hypertension in severe head injury. J Neurosurg 47:503–513

Miller JD, Wilkinson HA, Rosenfeld SA et al (1986) Intracranial hypertension and cerebrospinal fluid production in dogs: effects of furosemide. Exp Neurol 94:66–80

Miller JD, Peeler DF, Pattisapu J et al (1987) Supratentorial pressure. Part 1: differential intracranial pressure. Neurol Res 9:16–26

Minchenko A, Leshchinsky I, Opentanova I et al (2002) Hypoxia inducible factor-1-mediated expression of the 6-phosphofructo-2-kinase/fructose-2,6-biphosphatase-3 (PFKFB3) gene. Its possible role in the Warburg effect. J Biol Chem 277:6183–6187

Mindermann T, Gratzl O (1998) Interhemispheric pressure gradients in severe head trauma in humans. Acta Neurochir Suppl 71:56–58

Mirski AM, Denchev ID, Schnitzer SM et al (2000) Comparison between hypertonic saline and mannitol in the reduction of elevated intracranial pressure in a rodent model of acute cerebral injury. J Neurosurg Anesthesiol 12:334–344

Mittlmeier T, Vollmar B, Menger MD et al (2003) Small volume hypertonic hydroxyethyl starch reduces acute microvascular dysfunction after closed soft-tissue trauma. J Bone Joint Surg Br 85:126–132

Monro A (1823) Observations of the structure and function of the nervous system. Creech and Johnson, Edinburgh, p 5

Moon PF, Kramer GC (1995) Hypertonic saline/dextran resuscitation from hemorrhagic shock induces transient acidosis. Crit Care Med 23:323–331

Moraine J-J, Berré J, Mélot C (2000) Is cerebral perfusion pressure a major determinant of cerebral blood flow during head elevation in comatose patients with severe intracranial lesions? J Neurosurg 92:606–614

Morgan P, Ward B (1970) Hyperventilation and changes in the electroencephalogram and electroretinogram. Neurology 20:1009–1014

Muizelaar JP, Wei EP, Kontos HA et al (1983) Mannitol causes compensatory cerebral vasoconstriction and vasodilatation in response to blood viscosity changes J Neurosurg 59:822–828

Muizelaar JP, Lutz HA, Becker DP (1984) Effect of mannitol on ICP and CBF and correlation with pressure autoregulation in severely head-injured patients. J Neurosurg 61:700–706

Müller-Schweinitzer E, Rosenthaler J (1987) Dihydroergotamine: pharmacodynamics, and mechanism of venoconstrictor action in beagle dogs. J Cardiovasc Pharmacol 9:686–693

Munari C, Calbucci F (1979) Correlations between intracranial pressure (ICP) and EEG changes during traumatic coma. Rev Electroencephalogr Neurophysiol Clin 9:185–193

Nakamura T, Miyamoto O, Sumitani K et al (2003) Do rapid systemic changes of brain temperature have an influence on the brain? Acta Neurochir 145:301–307

Nath F, Galbraith S (1986) The effect of mannitol on cerebral white matter water content. J Neurosurg 65:41–43

Nekludov M, Bellander BM, Mure M (2006) Oxygenation and cerebral perfusion pressure improved in the prone position. Acta Anesthesiol Scand 50:932–936

Ng I, Lim J, Wong HB (2004) Effects of head posture on cerebral haemodynamics: its influence on intracranial pressure, cerebral perfusion pressure, and cerebral oxygenation. Neurosurgery 54:593–598

Nilsson F, Messeter K, Grände PO et al (1995) Effects of dihydroergotamine on cerebral circulation during experimental intracranial hypertension. Acta Anaesthesiol Scand 39:916–921

Nolte D, Bayer M, Lehr HA et al (1992) Attenuation of postischemic microvascular disturbances in striated muscle by hyperosmolar saline dextran. Am J Physiol 263:H1411–H1416

Noppens RR, Christ M, Brambrink AM et al (2006) An early bolus of hypertonic saline hydroxyethyl starch improves long-term outcome after global cerebral ischemia. Crit Care Med 34:2194–2200

Nordström C-H, Rehncrona S (1979) Reduction of cerebral blood flow and oxygen consumption with a combination of barbiturate anesthesia and induced hypothermia in the rat. Acta Anaesthesiol Scand 22:7–12

Nornes H, Magnäs B (1971) Supratentorial epidural pressure recording during posterior fossa surgery. J Neurosurg 35:541–549

Norris JW (1976) Steroid therapy in acute cerebral infarction. Arch Neurol 33:69–71

North JB, Reilly PL, Gorman D et al (1993) The effect of hypoxia on intracranial pressure and cerebral blood flow. In: Avezaat CJJ, van Eijndhoven JHM, Maas AIR, Tans JTJ (eds) Intracranial pressure VIII. Springer, Berlin, pp 238–243

Nunn JF (1987) Applied respiratory physiology, 3rd edn. Butterworth, Cambridge, UK

Obrist WD, Gennarelli TA, Segewa H et al (1979) Relation of cerebral blood flow to neurological status and outcome in head-injured patients. J Neurosurg 51:292–300

Obrist WD, Langfitt TW, Jaggi JL et al (1984) Cerebral blood flow and metabolism in comatose patients with acute head injury. Relationship to intracranial hypertension. J Neurosurg 61:241–253

Oertel M, Kelly DF, Lee JH et al (2002) Is CPP therapy beneficial for all patients with high ICP? Acta Neurochir Suppl 81:67–68

Oka A, Belliveau MJ, Rosenberg PA et al (1993) Vulnerability of oligodendroglia to glutamate: pharmacology, mechanisms, and prevention. J Neurosci 13:1441–1453

Olafsson S, Gottstein J, Blei AT (1995) Brain edema and intracranial hypertension in rats after total hepatectomy. Gastroenterology 108:1097–1103

Olesen J, Skinhøj E (1972) Effects of ergot ankaloids (Hydergine) on cerebral haemodynamics in man. Acta Pharmacol 31:75–85

Onar M, Arik Z (1997) The evaluation of mannitol therapy in acute ischemic stroke patients by serial somatosensory evoked potentials. Electromyogr Clin Neurophysiol 37:213–218

Ott P, Larsen FS (2004) Blood-brain barrier permeability to ammonia in liver failure: a critical reappraisal. Neurochem Int 44:185–198

Paczynski RP, He YY, Diringer MN et al (1997) Multiple-dose mannitol reduces brain water content in a rat model of cortical infarction. Stroke 28:1437–1443

Palvölgyi R (1969) Regional cerebral blood flow in patients with intracranial tumours. J Neurosurg 31:149–163

Pappius HM, McCann WP (1969) Effects of steroids on cerebral edema in cats. Arch Neurol 20:207–216

Pasternak JJ, McGregor DG, Lanier WL (2004) Effect of single-dose dexamethasone on blood glucose concentration in patients undergoing craniotomy. J Neurosurg Anesthesiol 16:122–125

Patel J, Roberts I, Azzopardi D et al (2000) Randomized double-blind controlled trial comparing the effects of ibuprofen with indomethacin on cerebral hemodynamics in preterm infants with patent ductus arteriosus. Pediatr Res 47:36–42

Paulson OB (1970) Regional cerebral blood flow in apoplexy due to occlusion of the middle cerebral artery. Neurology 20:63–77

Pena H, Gaines C, Suess D et al (1982) Effect of mannitol on experimental focal ischaemia in awake monkeys. Neurosurgery 11:477–481

Penn RD, Lee MC, Linninger AA et al (2005) Pressure gradients in the brain in an experimental model of hydrocephalus. J Neurosurg 102:1069–1075

Phelps ME, Grubb RL, Ter-Pogosian MM (1973) Correlation between Pa CO_2 and regional cerebral blood volume by x-ray fluorescence. J Appl Physiol 35:274–280

Pichard JD, MacKenzie ET (1973) Inhibition of prostaglandin synthesis and the response of baboon cerebral circulation to carbon dioxide. Nat New Biol 245:187

Pierce EC, Lambertsen CJ, Deutsch S et al (1962) Cerebral circulation and metabolism during thiopental anesthesia and hyper-ventilation in man. J Clin Invest 41:1664–1671

Piper I, Spiegelberg A, Whittle I et al (1999) A comparative study of the Spiegelberg compliance devices with a manual volume-injection method: a clinical evaluation in patients with hydrocephalus. Br J Neurosurg 13:581–586

Pistolese GR, Faraglia V, Agnoli A et al (1972) Cerebral hemispheric "counter-steal" phenomenon during hyperventilation in cerebrovascular diseases. Stroke 3:456–461

Poca MA, Sahuquillo J, Topczewski T et al (2006) Posture-induced changes in intracranial pressure: a comparative study in patients with and without a cerebrospinal fluid block at the craniovertebral junction. Neurosurgery 58:899–906

Polderman KH, van de Kraats G, Dixon JM et al (2003) Increases in spinal fluid osmolarity induced by mannitol. Crit Care Med 31:584–590

Pollay M, Fullenwider C, Roberts A et al (1983) Effect of mannitol and furosemide on blood-brain osmotic gradient and intracranial pressure. J Neurosurg 59:945–950

Poon WS, Ng SC, Chan MT et al (2002) Neurochemical changes in ventilated head-injured patients with cerebral perfusion pressure treatment failure. Acta Neurochir 81:335–338

Portella G, Cormio M, Cierio G (2002) Continuous cerebral compliance monitoring in severe head injury. Its relationship with intracranial pressure and cerebral perfusion pressure. Acta Neurochir Suppl 81:173–175

Procaccio F, Menasce G, Sacchi L et al (1993) Ischemic insult due to manual ventilation in head injured patients with intracranial hypertension. In: Avezaat CJJ, van Eijndhoven JHM, Maas AIR, Tans JTJ (eds) Intracranial pressure VIII. Springer, Berlin, pp 583–588

Prough DS, Johnson JC, Poole GV et al (1985) Effects on intracranial pressure of resuscitation from hemorrhagic shock with hypertonic saline versus lactated Ringer's solution. Crit Care Med 13:407–410

Prough DS, Withney JM, Taylor CL et al (1991) Regional cerebral blood flow following resuscitation from hemorrhagic shock with hypertonic saline. Anesthesiology 75:319–327

Quandt CM, Reyes RA (1984) Pharmacologic management of acute intracranial hypertension. Drug Intell Clin Pharm 18:105–112

Qureshi AI, Suarez JI (2000) Use of hypertonic saline solutions in treatment of cerebral edema and intracranial hypertension. Crit Care Med 28:3301–3313

Qureshi AI, Wilson DA, Traystman RJ (1999) Treatment of elevated intracranial pressure in experimental intracerebral hemorrhage: Comparison between mannitol and hypertonic saline. Neurosurgery 44:1055–1064

Qureshi AI, Wilson DA, Traystman RJ (2002) Treatment of transtentorial herniation unresponsive to hyperventilation using hypertonic saline in dogs: effect on cerebral blood flow and metabolism. J Neurosurg Anesthesiol 14:22–30

Raghavan M, Marik PE (2006) Therapy of intracranial hypertension in patients with fulminant hepatic failure. Neurocrit Care 4:179–189

Raichle ME, Posner JB, Plum F (1970) Cerebral blood flow during and after hyperventilation. Arch Neurol 23:394–403

Raphael JH, Chotai R (1994) Effects of cervical collar on cerebrospinal fluid pressure. Anaesthesia 49:437–439

Rasmussen M, Tankisi A, Cold GE (2004a) The effects of indomethacin on intracranial pressure and cerebral haemodynamics in patients undergoing craniotomy: a randomized prospective study. Anesthesia 59:229–236

Rasmussen M, Østergaard L, Juul N et al (2004b) Do indomethacin and propofol cause cerebral ischemic damage? Anesthesiology 101:872–878

Rasmussen M, Bundgaard H, Cold GE (2004c) Craniotomy for supratentorial brain tumours: risk factors for brain swelling after opening of dura mater. J Neurosurg 101:621–626

Rasmussen M, Upton RN, Grant C et al (2006) The effects of indomethacin on intracranial pressure and cerebral haemodynamics during isoflurane or propofol anesthesia in sheep with intracranial hypertension. Anesth Analg 102:1823–1829

Ravussin P, Archer DP, Tyler JL et al (1986a) Effects of rapid mannitol infusion on cerebral blood volume. J Neurosurg 64:104–113

Ravussin P, Chiolero R, Buchser E et al (1986b) CSF pressure changes following mannitol in patients undergoing craniotomy. Anesthesiology 65:A303

Reivich M, Cohen PJ, Greenbaum L (1966) Alterations in the electroencephalogram of awake man produced by hyperventilation: effects of 100% oxygen at 3 atmospheres (absolute) pressure. Neurology 16:304

Renaudin J, Fewer D, Wilson CB et al (1973) Dose dependency of Decadron in patients with partially excised brain tumors. J Neurosurg 39:302–305

Reulen HJ, Graham R, Spatz M et al (1977) Role of pressure gradients and bulk flow in dynamics of vasogenic edema. J Neurosurg 46:24–35

Risberg J, Lundberg N, Ingvar D (1969) Regional cerebral blood volume during acute transient rises of the intracranial pressure (plateau waves). J Neurosurg 31:303–310

Roberts PA, Pollay M, Engles C et al (1987) Effect on intracranial pressure of furosemide combined with varying doses and administration rates of mannitol. J Neurosurg 66:440–446

Rockoff MA, Marchall LF, Shapiro HM (1979) High-dose barbiturate therapy in humans: a clinical review of 60 patients. Ann Neurol 6:194–199

Rosa G, Orfie P, Sanfilippo M et al (1986) The effects of atracurium besylate (Tracium) on intracranial pressure and cerebral perfusion pressure. Anesth Analg 65:381–384

Rosenthal RJ, Hiatt JR, Phillips EH et al (1997) Intracranial pressure. Effect of pneumoperitoneum in a large-animal model. Surg Endosc 11:376–380

Rosenthal RJ, Friedman RL, Chidambaram A et al (1998) Effects of hyperventilation and hypoventilation on Pa CO_2 and intracranial pressure during acute elevations of intraabdominal pressure with CO_2 pneumoperitoneum: large animal observations. J Am Coll Surg 187:32–38

Rosenwasser RH, Kleiner LI, Krzeminski JP et al (1989) Intracranial pressure monitoring in the posterior fossa: a preliminary report. J Neurosurg 71:503 505

Rosner MJ, Becker DP (1984) Origin and evolution of plateau waves, experimental observations and a theoretical model. J Neurosurg 60:312–324

Rosner MJ, Coley IB (1986) Cerebral perfusion pressure, intracranial pressure, and head elevation. J Neurosurg 65:636–641

Rosner MJ, Coley I (1987) Cerebral perfusion pressure: a haemodynamic mechanism of mannitol and postmannitol hemogram. Neurosurgery 21:147–156

Rosomoff HL (1963) Distribution of intracranial contents with controlled hyperventilation: implications of neuroanaesthesia. Anesthesiology 24:640–645

Roux FX, Raggueneau JL, Geoerge B et al (1984) Pression epidurale locoregionale et pression intra-cranienne differentielle: interet de leur monitorage chez des patients porters dúe lesion intracerebrale unilaterale. Agressologie 25:559–561

Rudehill A, Lagerkranser M, Lindquist C et al (1983) Effects of mannitol on blood volume and central haemodynamics in patients undergoing cerebral aneurysm surgery. Anesth Analg 62:875–880

Ruta TS, Drummond JC, Cole DJ (1993) The effect of acute hypocapnia on local cerebral blood flow during middle cerebral artery occlusion in isoflurane anesthetized rats. Anesthesiology 78:134–140

Ryding E, Asgeirsson B, Bertman L et al (1990) Dihydroergotamine treatment of increased ICP following severe head injury. 5th Nordic CBF symposium, Lund 27

Sahuquillo J, Poca M-A, Arribas M et al (1999) Interhemispheric supratentorial intracranial pressure gradients in head-injured patients: are they clinically important. J Neurosurg 90:16–26

Sakabe T, Siesjö BK (1979) The effect of indomethacin on blood flow-metabolism couple in the brain under normal, hypercapnic and hypoxic conditions. Acta Physiol Scand 107:283–284

Sasaki T, Nakagomi T, Kirino et al (1988) Indomethacin ameliorates ischemic neuronal damage in the gerbil hippocampal CA 1 sector. Stroke 19:1399–1403

Saul TG, Ducker TB (1982) Effect of intracranial pressure monitoring and aggressive treatment on mortality in severe head injury. J Neurosurg 56:498–503

Scale TM, Meltz S, Yelon J et al (1994) Resuscitation of multiple trauma and head injury: role of crystalloid fluids and inotropes. Crit Care Med 22:1610–1615

Schaller B, Graf R (2005) Different compartments of intracranial pressure and its relationship to cerebral blood flow. J Trauma 59:1521–1531

Scheinberg P, Stead EA Jr (1949) The cerebral blood flow in male subjects as measured by the nitrous oxide technique. Normal values for blood flow, oxygen utilization, glucose utilization, and peripheral resistance, with observations on the effect of tilting and anxiety. J Clin Invest 28:1163–1171

Schell RM, Applegate RL, Cole DJ (1996) Salt, starch and water on the brain. Points of view. J Neurosurg Anesthesiol 8:178–182

Scheller MS, Zornow MH, Oh YS (1991) A comparison of the cerebral and haemodynamic effects of mannitol and hypertonic saline in a rabbit model of acute cryogenic brain injury. J Neurosurg Anesthesiol 3:291–296

Schenker S, McCandless DW, Brophy E et al (1967) Studies on the intracerebral toxicity of ammonia. J Clin Invest 46:838–848

Schettini A, Stahurski B, Young HF (1982) Osmotic and osmotic-loop diuresis in brain surgery. Effects on plasma and CSF electrolytes and ion excretion. J Neurosurg 56:679–684

Schierhout G, Robert I (2000) Mannitol for acute traumatic brain injury. Cochrane Database Syst Rev 2:CD001049

Schmoker JD, Zhuang J, Shackford SR (1991) Hypertonic fluid resuscitation improves cerebral oxygen delivery and reduces intracranial pressure after hemorrhagic shock. J Trauma 31:1607–1613

Schneider GH, von Helden GH, Franke R et al (1993) Influence of body position and cerebral perfusion pressure. Acta Neurochir 59:107–112

Schneider GH, Sarrafzadeh AS, Kiening KL et al (1998) Influence of hyperventilation on brain tissue: PO_2, $PaCO_2$, and pH in patients with intracranial hypertension. Acta Neurochir Suppl 71:62–65

Schreiber SJ, Lambert UKW, Doepp F et al (2002) Effects of prolonged head-down tilt on internal jugular vein cross-sectional area. Br J Anaesth 89:769–771

Schuier FJ, Hossmann KA (1980) Experimental brain infarct in cats. II: Ischemic brain oedema. Stroke 11:593–601

Schumann P, Touzani O, Young AR et al (1996) Effects of indomethacin on cerebral blood flow and oxygen metabolism: a positron emission tomographic investigation in the anaesthetized baboon. Neurosci Lett 220:137–141

Schürer L, Dautermann C, Härtl R et al (1992) Treatment of hemorrhagic hypotension with hypertonic/hyperoncotic solutions: effects on regional cerebral blood flow and brain surface oxygen tension. Eur Surg Res 24:1–12

Schwarz S, Bertram M, Aschoff A et al (1999) Indomethacin for brain edema following stroke. Cardiovasc Dis 9:248–250

Sedzimir CB (1959) Therapeutic hypothermia in cases of head injury. J Neurosurg 16:407–414

Seki H, Ogawa A, Yoshimoto T, Suzuki J (1981) Effect of mannitol on rCBF in canine thalamic ischemia. An experimental study. Brain Nerve (Tokyo) 33:1101–1105

Sgouros S, Goldin JH, Hockley AD et al (1999) Intracranial volume change in childhood. J Neurosurg 91:610–616

Shackford SR, Zhuang J, Schmoker J (1992) Intravenous fluid tonicity: effect on intracranial pressure, cerebral blood flow, and cerebral oxygen delivery in focal brain injury. J Neurosurg 76:91–98

Shapira Y, Davidson E, Weidenfeld Y et al (1988) Dexamethasone and indomethacin do not affect brain edema following head injury in rats. J Cereb Blood Flow Metab 8:395–402

Shapiro K, Marmarou A (1989) Mechanisms of intracranial hypertension in children. In: McLaurin R, Venes J, Schut L et al (eds) Pediatric neurosurgery. Saunders, Philadelphia, p 338

Shapiro HM, Galindo A, Wyte SR et al (1973) Rapid intraoperative reduction of intracranial pressure with thiopental. Br J Anaesth 45:1057–1061

Shapiro HM, Wyte SR, Loeser J (1974) Barbiturate augmented hypothermia for reduction of persistent intracranial hypertension. J Neurosurg 40:90–100

Shenkin HA, Goluboff B, Haft H (1962) The use of mannitol for the reduction of intracranial pressure in intracranial surgery. J Neurosurg 19:897–901

Shigeno S, Fritschka E, Shigeno T et al (1985) Effects of indomethacin on rCBF during and after focal cerebral ischemia in the cat. Stroke 16:235–242

Shima K, Marmarou A (1993) Effect of posttraumatic hypoventilation. In: Avezaat CJJ, van Eijndhoven JHM, Maas AIR, Tans JTJ (eds) Intracranial pressure VIII. Springer, Berlin, pp 476–478

Shiozaki T, Sugimoto H, Taneda M et al (1993) Effect of mild hypothermia on uncontrollable intracranial hypertension after severe head injury. J Neurosurg 79:363–368

Shirane R, Weinstein PR (1992) Effect of mannitol on local cerebral blood flow after temporary complete cerebral ischemia in rats. J Neurosurg 76:486–492

Shohami E, Shapira Y, Sidi A et al (1987) Head injury induces increased prostaglandin synthesis in rat brain. J Cereb Blood Flow Metab 7:58–63

Sidi A, Cotev S, Hadani M et al (1983) Long-term barbiturate infusion to reduce intracranial pressure. Crit Care Med 11:478–481

Skippen P, Sear M, Poskitt K et al (1997) Effect of hyperventilation on regional cerebral blood flow in head-injured children. Crit Care Med 25:1402–1409

Sklar FH, Beyer CW, Ramanathan M et al (1980) The effects of furosemide on CSF dynamics in patients with pseudo tumor cerebri. In: Shulman K, Marmarou A, Miller JD, Becker DP, Hochwald GM, Brock M (eds) Intracranial pressure IV. Springer, Berlin, pp 660–663

Slocum HC, Hayes GW, Laezman BL (1961) Ventilator technique of anesthesia for neuroanaesthesia. Anesthesiology 22:143–145

Smedena RJ, Gaab MR, Hesiler HE (1993) A comparison study between mannitol and glycerol therapy in reducing intracranial pressure. In: Avezaat CJJ, van Eijndhoven JHM, Maas AIR, Tans JTJ (eds) Intracranial pressure VIII. Springer, Berlin, pp 605–608

Soloway M, Nadel W, Albin MS et al (1968) The effect of hyperventilation on subsequent cerebral infarction. Anesthesiology 29:975–980

Soloway M, Moriarty G, Fraser JG et al (1971) Effect of delayed hyperventilation on experimental cerebral infarction. Neurology 21:479–485

Steen PA, Milde JH, Michenfelder JD (1979) No barbiturate protection in a dog model of complete cerebral ischaemia Ann Neurol 5:343–349

Stephan H, Sonntag H, Schenk HD et al (1987) Einfluss von disoprivan (Propofol) auf die Durchblutung und Sauerstoffverbrauch des Gehirns and die CO_2 Reaktivität der Hirngefässe beim Menschen. Anesthetist 36:60–65

Stewart L, Bullock R, Rafferty C et al (1994) Propofol sedation in severe head injury fails to control high ICP but reduces brain metabolism. Acta Neurochir Suppl 60:544–546

St Lawrence KS, Ye FQ, Lewis BK et al (2003) Measuring the effects of indomethacin on changes in cerebral oxidative metabolism and cerebral blood flow during sensorimotor activation. Magn Reson Med 50:99–106

Stocchetti N, Mattioli C, Paparella A et al (1993) Bedside assessment of CO_2 reactivity in head injury: changes in CBF estimated by changes in ICP and cerebral extraction of oxygen (abstract). J Neurotrauma 10(suppl):187

Stocchetti N, Paparella A, Bridelli F et al (1994) Cerebral venous oxygen saturation studied with bilateral samples in the internal jugular veins. Neurosurgery 34:38–43

Stocchetti N, Parma A, Songa V et al (2000) Early translaryngeal tracheostomy in patients with severe brain damage. Intensive Care Med 26:1101–1107

Stocchetti N, Maas AIR, Chieregato A et al (2005) Hyperventilation in head injury. Chest 127:1812–1827

Stringer WA, Hasso AN, Thompson JR et al (1993) Hyperventilation-induced cerebral ischemia in patients with acute brain lesions: demonstrated by xenon-enhanced CT. AJNR Am J Neuroradiol 14:475–484

Stullken AH, Milde JH, Michenfelder JD et al (1977) The nonlinear responses of cerebral metabolism to low concentrations of halothane, enflurane, isoflurane and thiopental. Anesthesiology 46:28–34

Sutherland G, Lesiuk H, Bose R et al (1988) Effect of mannitol, nimodipine, and indomethacin singly or in combination on cerebral ischaemia in rats. Stroke 19:571–578

Suzuka T, Mabe H, Nagai H (1989) Role of arachidonic acid metabolites on development of ischemic cerebral edema in rat middle cerebral artery occlusion. J Cereb Blood Flow Metab 9(suppl 1):S89

Symon L (1970) Regional cerebrovascular responses to acute ischaemia in normocapnia and hypercapnia. J Neurol Neurosurg Psychiatry 33:756–762

Symon L, Pasztor E, Branston NM et al (1974) Effect of supratentorial space-occupying lesions on regional intracranial pressure and local cerebral blood flow: an experimental study in baboons. J Neurol Neurosurg Psychiatry 37:617–626

Symon L, Branston NM, Chikovani O (1979) Ischemic brain oedema following middle cerebral artery occlusion in baboons: relationship between regional cerebral water content and blood flow at 1 and 2 hours. Stroke 10:184–191

Takagi H, Tanaka M, Ohwada T et al (1993) Pharmacokinetic analysis of mannitol in relation to the decrease of ICP. In: Avezaat CJJ, van Eijndhoven JHM, Maas AIR, Tans JTJ (eds) Intracranial pressure VIII. Springer, Berlin, pp 596–600

Takahashi H, Koehler RC, Brusilow SW et al (1990) Glutamine synthetase inhibition prevents cerebral edema during hyperammonemia. Acta Neurochir Suppl 51:346–347

Tanaka A, Tomonaga M (1987) Effect of mannitol on cerebral blood flow and microcirculation during experimental middle cerebral artery occlusion. Surg Neurol 28:189–195

Tankisi A, Cold GE (2007) Optimal reverse Trendelenburg position in patients undergoing craniotomy for cerebral tumors. J Neurosurg 106:239–244

Tankisi A, Rasmussen M, Juul N et al (2002) The effects of 10° reverse Trendelenburg position on ICP and CPP in prone positioned patients subjected to craniotomy for occipital or cerebellar tumours. Acta Neurochir 144:665–670

Tankisi A, Rasmussen M, Juul N et al (2006) The effects of 10° reverse Trendelenburg position on subdural intracranial pressure and cerebral perfusion pressure in patients subjected to craniotomy for cerebral aneurysm. J Neurosurg Anesthesiol 18:11–17

The Brain Trauma Foundation (2000) The American Association of Neurological Surgeons. The Joint Section of Neurotrauma and Critical Care. J Neurotrauma 17

The Brain Trauma Foundation (2007) The American Association of Neurological Surgeons, AANS and CNS the Joint Section of Neurotrauma and Critical Care Guidelines for the management of severe traumatic brain injury. J Neurotrauma 24(suppl 1)

Thelandersson A, Cider Å, Nellgård B (2006) Prone position in mechanically ventilated patients with reduced intracranial compliance. Acta Anaesthesiol Scand 50:937–941

Thenuwara K, Todd MM, Brian JE (2002) Effect of mannitol and furosemide on plasma and brain water. Anesthesiology 96:416–421

Thilmann J, Zeumer H (1974) Untersuchungen zur Behandlung des Hirnödems mit hohen Dosen Furosemid. Dtsch Med Wochenschr 99:932–935

Thomale UW, Griebenow M, Kroppenstedt M et al (2004) Small volume resuscitation with HyperHaes improves pericontusional perfusion and reduces lesion volume following controlled cortical impact injury in rats. J Neurotrauma 21:1737–1746

Tindall GT, Craddock A, Greenfield JC (1967) Effects of the sitting position on blood flow in the internal carotid artery of man during general anaesthesia. J Neurosurg 26:383–389

Todd MM, Tommasino C, Moore S (1985) Cerebral effects of isovolemic hemodilution with a hypertonic solution. J Neurosurg 63:944–948

Todd NV, Picozzi P, Crockard A et al (1986) Reperfusion after cerebral ischemia: influence of duration of ischemia. Stroke 17:460–466

Tofteng F, Larsen FS (2004) The effect of indomethacin on intracranial pressure, cerebral perfusion and extracellular lactate and glutamate concentrations in patients with fulminant hepatic failure. J Cereb Blood Flow Metab 24:798–804

Troup H (1967) Intraventricular pressure in patients with severe brain injuries. J Trauma 7:875–883

Tsuda Y, Kitadai M, Hatanaka Y et al (1998) Effects of mannitol and glycerol on cerebral energy metabolism in gerbils. Acta Neurol Scand 98:36–40

Tsuji T, Chiba S (1986) Responses of isolated canine and simian basilar arteries to thiopentone by a newly designed pharmacological method for measuring vascular responsiveness. Acta Neurochir 80:57–61

Tsuji T, Chiba S (1987) Mechanism of vascular responsiveness to barbiturates in isolated and perfused canine basilar arteries. Neurosurgery 21:161–166

Tulleken CA, von Dieven A, Mollevanger WJ et al (1978) Differential intracranial pressure gradients created by expanding extradural temporal mass lesion. J Neurosurg 86:505–510

Uihlein A, MacCarty CS, Michenfelder JD et al (1966) Deep hypothermia and surgical treatment of intracranial aneurysms. JAMA 195:639–641

Ulatowski JA, Oja JM, Suarez JI et al (1999) In vivo determination of absolute cerebral blood volume using haemoglobin as a natural contrast agent: an MRI study using altered arterial carbon dioxide tension. J Cereb Blood Flow Metab 19:809–817

Unterberg AW, Kiening KL, Hartl R et al (1997) Multimodal monitoring in patients with head injury: evaluation of the effects of treatment on cerebral oxygenation. J Trauma 42:S32–S37

Urlesberger B, Muller W, Ritschi E et al (1991) The influence of head position on the intracranial pressure in preterm infants with post hemorrhagic hydrocephalus. Childs Nerv Syst 7:85–87

Valentin A, Lang T, Karnik R et al (2003) Intracranial pressure monitoring and case mix-adjusted mortality in intracranial haemorrhage. Crit Care Med 31:1539–1542

van Hulst RA, Hassan D, Lachmann B (2002) Intracranial pressure, brain $PaCO_2$, $P O_2$, and pH during hypo- and hyperventilation at constant mean airway pressure in pigs. Intensive Care Med 28:68–73 van Hulst RA, Lameris TW, Haitsma JJ et al (2004) Brain glucose and lactate levels during ventilator-induced hypo- and hypercapnia. Clin Physiol Funct Imaging 24:243–248

Vannucci C, Brucklacher RM, Vannucci SJ (1997) Effect of carbon dioxide on cerebral metabolism during hypoxia-ischemia in the immature rat. Pediatr Res 42:24–29

Van Roost D, Hartmann A, Quade G (2001) Changes of cerebral blood flow following dexamethasone treatment in brain tumour patients. A Xe/CT study. Acta Neurochir 143:37–44

van Santbrink H, Maas AI, Avezaat CJ (1996) Continuous monitoring of partial pressure of brain tissue oxygen in patients with severe head injury. Neurosurgery 38:21–31

Vapalahti M, Troupp H, Heiskanen O (1969) Extremely severe brain injuries treated with hyperventilation and ventricular drainage. In: Brock M, Fieschi C, Ingvar DH, Lassen NA, Schurmann K (eds) Cerebral blood flow. Springer, Berlin, pp 266–267

Vassar MJ, Fischer RP, O'Brien PE (1993) A multicenter trial for resuscitation of injured patients with 7.5% sodium chloride. Arch Surg 128:1003–1013

Videtta W, Villarejo F, Cohen M et al (2002) Effects of positive end-expiratory pressure on intracranial pressure and cerebral perfusion pressure. Acta Neurochir Suppl 81:93–97

Voldby B, Enevoldsen EM, Jensen FT (1985) Regional cerebral blood flow, intraventricular pressure, and cerebral metabolism in patients with ruptured intracranial aneurysms. J Neurosurg 62:48–58

Vollmar B, Lang G, Menger MD et al (1994) Hypertonic hydroxyethyl starch restores hepatic microvascular perfusion in hemorrhagic shock. Am J Physiol 266:H1927–H1934

von Berenberg P, Unterberg A, Schneider GH et al (1994) Treatment of traumatic brain edema by multiple doses of mannitol. Acta Neurochir 60:531–533

von Helden A, Schneider GH, Unterberg A et al (1993) Monitoring of jugular venous saturation in comatose patients with subarachnoid haemorrhage and intracerebral haematomas. Acta Neurochir Suppl 59:102–106

Ward JD, Becker DP, Miller JD et al (1985) Failure of prophylactic barbiturate coma in the treatment of severe head injury. J Neurosurg 62:383–388

Waschke KF, Albrecht DM, van Ackern K et al (1996) Coupling between local cerebral blood flow and metabolism after hypertonic/hyperoncotic fluid resuscitation from hemorrhage in conscious rats. Analg Anesth 82:52–60

Wass CT, Lanier WL (1996) Glucose modulation of ischemic brain injury: review and clinical recommendations. Mayo Clin Proc 71:801–812

Wasserman K (1994) Coupling of external to cellular respiration during exercise: the wisdom of the body revisited. Am J Physiol 266:E519–E539

Watanabe T, Yoshimoto T, Ogawa A et al (1979) The effect of mannitol in preserving the development of cerebral infarction. An electron microscopic investigation. Neurol Surg (Tokyo) 7:859–866

Weaver DD, Winn HR, Jane JA (1982) Differential intracranial pressure in patients with unilateral mass lesions. J Neurosurg 56:660–665

Weiss MH, Nulsen FE (1970) The effect of glucocorticoids on CSF flow in dogs. J Neurosurg 32:452–458

Weiss KL, Wax MK, Haydon RC et al (1993) Intracranial pressure changes during bilateral radical neck dissections. Head Neck 15:546–552

Welch K (1980) Intracranial pressure in infants. J Neurosurg 52:693–699

Wennmalm Å, Eriksson S, Wahren J (1981) Effect of indomethacin on basal and carbon dioxide stimulated cerebral blood flow in man. Clin Phys 1:227–234

White RJ (1972) Preservation of cerebral function during circulatory arrest and resuscitation: hypothermic protective considerations. Resuscitation 1:107–115

White RJ, Likavec MJ (1992) The diagnosis and initial management of head injury. N Engl J Med 327:1507–1511

White RJ, Albin MS, Verdura J et al (1967) Differential extracorporeal hypothermic perfusion of and circulatory arrest to the human brain. Med Res Engineering 6:18–24

Whitley JM, Prough DS, Lamb AK et al (1988) Regional cerebral blood flow following resuscitation from hemorrhagic shock in dogs with a subdural mass. Anesthesiology 69(suppl A):539

Whitley JM. Prough DS, Taylor CL et al (1991) Cerebrovascular effects of small volume resuscitation from hemorrhagic shock: comparison of hypertonic saline and concentrated hydroxyethyl starch in dogs. J Neurosurg Anesthesiol 3:47–55

Williams A, Coyne SM (1993) Effects of neck position on intracranial pressure. Am J Crit Care 2:68–71

Wise BL, Chater N (1962) The value of hypertonic mannitol solution in decreasing brain mass and lowering cerebrospinal-fluid pressure. J Neurosurg 19:1038–1043

Wisner DH, Schuster L, Quinn C (1990) Hypertonic saline resuscitation of head injury: effects on cerebral water content. J Trauma 30:75–78

Wolfla C, Luerssen TG, Bowman RM et al (1996) Brain tissue pressure gradients created by expanding frontal epidural mass lesion. J Neurosurg 84:642–647

Worthley IGL, Cooper DJ, Jones N (1988) Treatment of resistant intracranial hypertension with hypertonic saline. J Neurosurg 68:478–481

Yano M, Nishiyama H, Yokota H et al (1986) Effect of lidocaine on ICP response to endotracheal suctioning. Anesthesiology 64:651–653

Yano M, Ikeda Y, Kobayashi S et al (1987) Intracranial pressure in head-injured patients with various intracranial lesions is identical throughout the supratentorial intracranial compartment. Neurosurgery 21:688–692

Yau YH, Piper IR, Clutton RE et al (2000) Experimental evaluation of the Spiegelberg intracranial pressure and intracranial compliance monitor. Technical note. J Neurosurg 93:1072–1077

Yen MH, Lee SH (1987) Effects of cyclooxygenase and lipoxygenase inhibitors on cerebral edema induced by freezing lesions in rats. Eur J Pharmacol 144:369–373

Yoon BH, Romero R, Kim CJ et al (1997) High expression of tumor necrosis factor-alpha and interleukin-6 in periventricular leukomalacia. Am J Obstet Gynecol 177:406–411

Yoshida A, Shima T, Okada Y et al (1991) Effects of postural changes on epidural pressure in patients with serious intracranial lesions. In: Avezaat CJJ, van Eijndhoven JHM, Maas AIR, Tans JTJ (eds) Intracranial pressure VIII. Springer, Berlin, pp 433–436

Yoshida A, Shima T, Okada Y et al (1993) Effects of postural changes on epidural pressure and cerebral perfusion pressure in patients with serious intracranial lesions. In: Avezaat CJJ, van Eijndhoven JHM, Maas AIR, Tans JTJ (eds) Intracranial pressure VIII. Springer, Berlin, pp 433–436

Yoshihara M, Bandoh K, Marmarou A (1995) Cerebrovascular carbon dioxide reactivity assessed by intracranial pressure dynamics in severely head injured patients. J Neurosurg 82:386–393

Zornow MH (1996) Hypertonic saline as a safe and efficacious treatment of intracranial hypertension. J Neurosurg Anesthesiology 8:175–177

Chapter 2
Material Included in the Database

Georg Emil Cold

Abstract
Since 1994 we have performed perioperative measurement of subdural ICP combined with arterial and jugular blood pressure and gas analysis in primarily elective patients subjected to craniotomy. ICP was measured with a 22G needle connected to a pressure transducer via a polyethylene catheter. Until now (2006), 1,833 patients have been included in our database.

In this chapter the extensive material of the database is disclosed. Patients were entered consecutively over the years, some included as part of controlled trials and some as part of the normal daily routine. The demographics of the patient population are described, likewise the diagnosis, including tumour (if any) localization. The anaesthetics used and ICP-reducing procedures are summarized and the method for ICP monitoring discussed.

Cerebral haemodynamics and the level of ICP are of importance in the surgical management of space-occupying cerebral lesions. At high ICP surgical access to deep cerebral structures is impeded, and pressure by self-retaining specula may decrease cerebral perfusion regionally. Likewise, swelling/herniation of cerebral tissue through the opening of dura may be deleterious by preventing venous outflow from brain tissue, and increases ICP regionally. Thereby, a vicious circle may develop with increasing cerebral oedema and ischaemia, further impeding the surgical access. Preoperative measurement of ICP or other cerebral haemodynamic parameters, however, is rarely a part of the combined surgical or anaesthesiological procedure with the exception when part of a clinical investigation.

Since 1994 we have performed perioperative measurement of subdural ICP combined with arterial and jugular blood pressure and gas analysis in primarily elective patients subjected to craniotomy. ICP was measured with a 22G needle connected to a pressure transducer via a polyethylene catheter. Until May 2006, 1,833 patients have been included in our database. The number of patients per year, and the distribution of men/women are indicated in Table 2.1.

Table 2.1 Number of patients and female/male distribution related to year in 1,833 patients subjected to craniotomy

Year	Number	Women	Men	Percent women
1994	89	48	41	53.9
1995	88	46	42	52.3
1996	131	59	72	45.0
1997	132	57	75	43.2
1998	124	67	57	54.0
1999	143	81	62	56.6
2000	153	77	76	50.3
2001	171	110	61	64.3
2002	157	83	74	52.9
2003	148	66	82	44.6
2004	149	65	84	43.6
2005	207	98	109	47.3
2006	141	68	73	48.2
Total	1,833	925	908	
Percent		50.5	49.5	

Table 2.2 Distribution of age in 1,833 patients subjected to craniotomy

Years	Number	Percent of total
0–10	50	2.7
11–20	53	2.9
21–30	106	5.8
31–40	217	11.8
41–50	377	20.6
51–60	514	28.0
61–70	397	21.7
71–80	111	6.1
81–90	8	0.4
Total	1,833	

In total 1.833 patients were studied, of whom 50.5% were women. The number of patients increased from 89 in 1994 to 207 patients in 2005.

In Table 2.2 the distribution of patients is related to age. Few studies of ICP were performed in children (total 5.6% below the age of 21 years). Between the ages of 51 and 60 years recordings from 514 patients (28.0%) were analysed.

2.1
Diagnosis of Tumour, Localization of Cerebral Aneurysm and Hunt and Hess Gradation

In Table 2.3 the diagnoses of the patients are presented. The three largest groups were supratentorial cerebral tumours (1,326 patients, 72.3%), cerebral aneurysm (225 patients, 12.3%) and infratentorial tumours (150 patients, 8.2%).

Table 2.3 Distribution of patients (number and percent) related to diagnosis in 1,833 patients subjected to craniotomy

	Number	Percent
Supratentorial cerebral tumours	1,326	72.3
Infratentorial cerebral tumours	150	8.2
Cerebral aneurysm	225	12.3
Arteriovenous malformation	28	1.5
Traumatic head injury	15	0.8
Trigeminus neuralgia	26	1.4
Cerebral cyst	14	0.8
Cerebral abscess	10	0.5
Chronic subdural haematoma	7	0.4
Liquorrhea	6	0.3
Cerebral infarct	3	0.2
Parkinson disease	3	0.2
Intracerebral haematoma	11	0.6
Encephalitis	6	0.3
Disseminated sclerosis	3	0.2
Total	1,833	

The localization of cerebral aneurysm related to year is indicated in Table 2.4 (see page 62). After the introduction of coil treatment in 2003 the number of patients subjected to cerebral aneurysm surgery declined. In Table 2.5 (see page 62) patients with cerebral aneurysm are related to Hunt and Hess (H&H) gradation performed immediately before induction of anaesthesia. Sixty-three patients (28.0%) had unruptured aneurysm. In H&H groups I–III the distribution of patients differed from 16.9% to 31.6% of total. Only 4 patients in the H&H group IV were investigated.

2.2
Anaesthesia

In Table 2.6 (see page 63) the number of patients in each diagnostic group is related to choice of anaesthesia. Propofol-fentanyl was used in 1,076 patients (58.7%), propofol-remifentanil was used in 464 patients (25.3%), isoflurane-fentanyl was used in 204 patients (11.1%) and sevoflurane-fentanyl in 76 patients (4.1%). Seven patients were anaesthetized with halothane and 1 with midazolam. In 5 patients ICP was monitored before induction of anaesthesia.

Table 2.4 Number of patients with cerebral aneurysm related to localization of aneurysm and year in 225 patients subjected to craniotomy

	1994	1995	1996	1997	1998	1999	2000	2001	2002	2003	2004	2005	2006	Total
Media	9	5	5	8	5	4	5	4	11	8	10	11	5	90
Arteria communicans anterior	7	2	9	7	7	3	1	1	3	4	4	6	2	56
Carotis	9	9	10	11	3	2	7	4	2			3	2	62
Basilaris	2											5	2	9
Other	1								4	1		1	1	8
Total	28	16	24	26	15	9	13	9	20	13	14	26	12	225

Table 2.5 Patients with cerebral aneurysm related topreoperative Hunt and Hess evaluation

Hunt and Hess gradation	Total	Percent of total
H&H 0	63	28.0
H&H I	49	21.8
H&H II	71	31.6
H&H III	38	16.9
H&H IV	4	1.8
Total	225	100

Table 2.6 The distribution of anaesthesia in patients subjected to craniotomy. The diagnoses are related to anaesthetic technique. Maintenance of anaesthesia during ICP recordings included propofol-fentanyl, propofol-remifentanil, isoflurane-fentanyl, sevoflurane-fentanyl, halothane-fentanyl, midazolam-fentanyl and local anaesthesia (awake)

	Propofol -fentanyl	Propofol -remifentanil	Isoflurane -fentanyl	Sevoflurane -fentanyl	Halothane- fentanyl	Midazolam- fentanyl	Awake	Total
Supratentorial tumours	762	342	142	71	7		2	1,326
Infratentorial tumours	87	50	12	5				150
Cerebral aneurysm	133	51	36			1		225
Arteriovenous malformation	18	4	6					28
Traumatic head injury	15	0	0					15
Trigeminus neuralgia	20	6	0					26
Cerebral cyst	9	3	2					14
Cerebral abscess	8	2	0					10
Chronic subdural haematoma	4	0	3					7
Liquorrhea	4	2	0					6
Cerebral infarct	2	1	0					3
Parkinson's disease	0	0	0				3	3
Intracerebral haematoma	11	0	0					11
Encephalitis	2	2	2					6
Disseminated sclerosis	1	1	1					3
Total	1,076	464	204	76	7	1	5	1,833

2.3
Intracranial Pressure-Reducing Procedures

In Table 2.7 the ICP-reducing procedures are summarized. In total 549 patients underwent ICP-reducing procedures either because ICP exceeded 10 mmHg and/or because the neurosurgeon, by touch of his/her fingers, estimated that dural tension was increased. The ICP-reducing method was decided by the anaesthesiologist in concert with the surgeon. In 188 patients 10° rTp was used and 168 patients were subjected to hyperventilation. In 74 patients decompression by ventricular fluid drainage or puncture of cystic tumour was performed. Mannitol treatment was used in 56 cases, intravenous indomethacin in 51 patients, propofol bolus injection in 8 patients and dihydroergotamine in 4 patients.

Table 2.7　ICP-reducing procedures used in connection with subdural ICP measurements

Procedure	Number of patients	Percent of total (1,833)
Reverse Trendelenburg position	188	10.3
Hyperventilation	168	9.2
Decompression (drainage or puncture of cyst)	74	4.0
Mannitol	56	3.1
Indomethacin	51	2.8
Propofol bolus	8	0.4
Dihydroergotamine	4	0.2
Total	549	30.0

2.4
Discussion

Perioperative ICP monitoring for elective tumour craniotomy is rarely used today, one reason being that preoperative corticosteroids in many cases normalize ICP. Another reason is that electronic monitoring devices used for ICP monitoring are expensive, and the sterilization procedure if possible is time consuming. Furthermore, if the ventricular cavities are compressed, intraventricular catheterization for ICP monitoring, which is considered the "gold standard", may be difficult. Lastly, the application of perioperative ICP monitoring, although of interest for the anaesthesiologist, is dependent on the surgeons attitude and cooperation.

During craniotomy subdural ICP measurement is easily performed. If the surgical team in advance is supplied with a 22G cannula and catheter for connection to a pressure transducer, subdural ICP can be measured within one minute. Furthermore, it is possible to follow changes in ICP during

ICP-reducing therapy such as hyperventilation, indomethacin administration, rTp, mannitol treatment and surgical decompression. Subdural ICP monitoring is a stronger predictor of intraoperative brain swelling than the neuroradiological findings or estimation of dural tension by the neurosurgeon (Rasmussen et al. 2004).

Compared with other ICP-monitoring techniques subdural ICP measurement has limitations. First, a technique that continuously follows ICP during craniotomy would be optimal, because precautions based on both ICP and CPP would secure optimal cerebral perfusion throughout anaesthesia and avoid ischaemic episodes. This is especially relevant at the beginning of the procedure: during intubation, after induction of anaesthesia where blood pressure often fluctuates, during head fixation where an increase in blood pressure might provoke cerebral oedema and in the subsequent period of surgical preparation without surgical stimulation. Finally during incision and galea removal, where the surgical stimulation is very intense, the blood pressure often increases significantly. Nevertheless, preoperative insertion of an epidural transducer or an intraventricular catheter for ICP monitoring is rarely used in elective craniotomy. Large dural lesions limit the use of subdural ICP, but not the use of epidural or intraventricular ICP monitoring. However, small dural lesions (below 2 cm in length) do not limit the use of subdural ICP monitoring.

If dural tension is increased ICP is increased as well, with high probability. At an ICP exceeding 13 mmHg cerebral swelling occurs with 95% probability, and at ICP values greater than 26 mmHg severe brain swelling occurs with 95% probability (Rasmussen et al. 2004). Under this circumstance the use of ICP-reducing therapy might be considered. In the present material, including 1,833 patients, the combination of increased dural tension and ICP exceeding 10 mmHg was registered in 594 patients (32.4%). In this situation ICP-reducing therapy should be considered before opening of dura in order to reduce the risk of cerebral swelling/herniation. Surgical drainage of CSF by an intraventricular catheter, evacuation of cystic processes, change in position from supine to 10° rTp and indomethacin bolus injection might reduce subdural ICP effectively within 1 min, while the maximal effects of hyperventilation and mannitol treatment occur after 10–15 min. The data collected in the present prospective study have clearly given that important information. Besides analysis of the ICP-reducing effects by different techniques, the method provides important information of ICP in tumour patients, where analysis of ICP in relation to anaesthetic technique is one example. Thus, in patients anaesthetized with propofol-fentanyl ICP was significantly lower compared with the ICP in patients anaesthetized with isoflurane-fentanyl or sevoflurane-fentanyl (Petersen et al. 2003). The relationship between pre-anaesthetic Hunt and Hess evaluation and ICP is another example where data collection has provided information. Thus, in patients with unruptured cerebral aneurysms and patients with subarachnoid haemorrhage classified as Hunt and Hess I, the ICP was low and dural tension was normal, while ICP was significantly increased in patients classified as Hunt and Hess II and III (Tankisi et al. 2006). In these patients drainage of ventricular fluid easily controls intracranial hypertension, otherwise early mannitol treatment or 10° rTp adjusted just before opening of dura should be considered.

References

Petersen KD, Landsfeldt U, Cold GE et al (2003) Intracranial pressure and cerebral hemodynamic in patients with cerebral tumours: a randomized prospective study of patients subjected to craniotomy in propofol-fentanyl, isoflurane-fentanyl, or sevoflurane-fentanyl anesthesia. Anesthesiology 98:329–336

Rasmussen M, Bundgaard H, Cold GE (2004) Craniotomy for supratentorial brain tumours: risk factors of brain swelling after opening of the dura. J Neurosurg 101:621–626

Tankisi A, Rasmussen M, Juul N et al (2006) The effects of 10° reverse Trendelenburg position (rTp) on subdural intracranial pressure and cerebral perfusion pressure in patients subjected to craniotomy for cerebral aneurysm. J Neurosurg Anesthesiol 18:11–17

Chapter 3
Method

Niels Juul, Georg Emil Cold

Abstract
Since 1994 we have followed the principles of current neuroanaesthesia, including measurement of subdural ICP and cerebral perfusion pressure, and the data have been prospectively registered. In the first study of the procedure we described the method of subdural ICP monitoring during anaesthesia and found a fairly good correlation in paired subdural ICP measurements and almost identical pressure waves and levels of ICP.

In this chapter the method for subdural ICP monitoring and the monitoring of other physiological parameters that we utilize are described in detail. The anaesthetic techniques used, both inhaled and intravenous, are discussed. The scale for the surgeons' estimation of dural tension is disclosed, and the comparative studies mentioned in subsequent chapters are briefly described. A short summary of the statistical methods used is added.

Since 1994 we have followed the principles of current neuroanaesthesia, including measurement of subdural ICP and CPP, and the data have been prospectively registered. In the first study of the procedure we described the method of subdural ICP monitoring during anaesthesia, and found a fairly good correlation in paired subdural ICP measurements, and almost identical pressure waves and levels of ICP (Cold et al. 1996). In subsequent publications we described the influence of anaesthetic methods, and methods for evaluation of dural tension and degree of cerebral swelling after opening of dura (Bundgaard and Cold 2000; Petersen et al. 2003). Measurements of CBF and $CMRO_2$ were described (Bundgaard et al. 1996, 1998). Methods in connection with subdural ICP monitoring during rTp were published by Tankisi et al. (2002). Measurement of transcranial Doppler sonographics was used and described by Rasmussen et al. (2004). In the following the principles of methods used in studies of subdural ICP and cerebral haemodynamics are summarized.

3.1
Neuroradiological Examination in Patients with Cerebral Tumours

From the latest CT or MR scanning the localization of the tumours and midline shifts were registered. The maximum tumour area was calculated using the formula for area of an ellipse (area = $ab\pi$, where a is half the length and b is half the width of the tumour).

3.2
Localization of Aneurysm and Hunt and Hess Gradation

The localization of the aneurysm was classified with preoperative four-vessel angiography. Classification according to the Hunt and Hess scale was done just before induction of anaesthesia.

3.3
Anaesthesia and Monitoring

If premedication was deemed necessary, diazepam 5–10 mg was administered perorally. If preoperative steroid and/or anticonvulsant treatment were instituted they were given together with diazepam. Any other daily medication was given at the discretion of the attending anaesthesiologist.

Monitoring before induction consisted of automated non-invasive blood pressure (NIBP, oscillometric blood pressure), continuous electrocardiogram and pulse oximetry. After induction of anaesthesia end-tidal CO_2 and concentration of inspired and expired anaesthetic gas were monitored continuously (Datex AS3, Helsinki, Finland). Controlled ventilation (fraction of inspired oxygen (FiO_2) 50–60% by oxygen/air) was applied at a $PaCO_2$ between 30 and 40 mmHg, inspiratory peak pressure < 20 cm H_2O and a respiratory frequency between 10 and 20/min. The level of $PaCO_2$ was achieved by continuous monitoring of pulmonary ventilation and end-tidal CO_2, and verified by arterial blood gas analysis. A Foley catheter was placed in the urinary bladder, and rectal temperature was continuously monitored. A radial artery catheter was inserted for continuous blood pressure monitoring and blood sampling. A catheter was introduced into the bulb of the internal jugular vein for pressure monitoring and blood sampling. The location of the catheter was checked by x-ray. Bupivacaine 2.5 mg/ml with epinephrine or lidocaine with epinephrine were used for infiltration of the scalp. Train-of-four stimulation was used to monitor muscular relaxation, which was achieved by a continuous infusion of atracurium.

The anaesthetic procedures included the following.

Group 1: Propofol-Fentanyl

Anaesthesia was induced with propofol 1–3 mg/kg given over 1 min and fentanyl 3–4 µg/kg. Lidocaine 1 mg/kg was administered over 1 min followed by muscular relaxation by atracurium 0.5 mg/kg. Anaesthesia was maintained with infusions of propofol 6–10 mg/kg/h and fentanyl 2–3 µg/kg/h. Just before incision of the scalp doses of propofol 1 mg/kg and/or fentanyl 1–2 µg/kg/h were supplemented, if necessary. The infusion rates of propofol and fentanyl were unchanged during the ICP measurements and during the estimation of dural swelling.

Group 2: Isoflurane-Fentanyl

Anaesthesia was induced with propofol 1–3 mg/kg given over 1 min and fentanyl 2–3 µg/kg. Lidocaine and atracurium were administered as in group 1. Anaesthesia was maintained with isoflurane (maximally 1.5 minimal alveolar concentration (MAC)) and fentanyl 2–3 µg/kg/h. Just before incision of the scalp fentanyl 1–2 µg/kg/h was supplemented, if necessary. The dose of isoflurane and the infusion rate of fentanyl were unchanged during the ICP measurements and during the estimation of dural swelling.

In Chapter 11, study 1, and in the study in Chapter 12, isoflurane was administered with nitrous oxide 50–67% and fentanyl.

Group 3: Sevoflurane-Fentanyl

Anaesthesia was induced with propofol 1–3 mg/kg given over 1 min and fentanyl 2–3 µg/kg. Lidocaine and atracurium were administered as in group 1. Anaesthesia was maintained with sevoflurane (maximally 1.5 MAC) and fentanyl 2–3 µg/kg/h. Just before incision of the scalp fentanyl 1–2 µg/kg/h was supplemented, if necessary. The dose of sevoflurane and the infusion rate of fentanyl were unchanged during the ICP measurements and during the estimation of dural swelling.

Group 4: Propofol-Remifentanil

Anaesthesia was induced using 1–3 mg/kg propofol supplemented with 0.5–1 µg/kg remifentanil during 1 min followed by 0.1–0.15 mg/kg cisatracurium for muscular relaxation. Anaesthesia was maintained with 0.2–0.5 µg/kg/min remifentanil and 4–8 mg kg/h propofol. The infusion rates of propofol and remifentanil were unchanged during the ICP measurements and during the estimation of dural swelling.

In patients with supratentorial cerebral tumours the effect of anaesthesia on ICP, MABP, CPP and jugular bulb pressure (JBP), and the effect of hyperventilation are indicated in Chapter 10. The same parameters in patients with cerebral aneurysm are indicated in Chapter 19.

3.4
Fluid Administration and Regulation of Blood Pressure

During the first hour of anaesthesia isotonic saline 15 ml/kg was administered, and followed by 2–4 ml/kg/h. If systolic blood pressure decreased > 20 mmHg colloids, in the form of either Haes-Steril 6% (hydroxyethyl starch; Fresenius Kabi, Uppsala, Sweden) or 5% dextran in saline, were administered, if needed, eventually supplemented with ephedrine 5–10 mg intravenously. Packed erythrocytes, albumin or fresh frozen plasma were not given before the ICP measurements.

3.5
Subdural Intracranial Pressure and Cerebral Perfusion Pressure

Subdural ICP was measured during surgery by use of the following method. After removal of the bone flap ICP was measured subdurally by an intravenous needle (22G/0.8 mm), which was connected to a pressure transducer via a polyethylene catheter. The transducer was placed in the same sagittal plane as the dura, and zero point adjustment was performed with the tip of the needle placed at the point of intended insertion of the dura. The needle was introduced through the dura until a continuous recording of ICP with typical cardiac and respiratory waves appeared. After 1 min of stabilization the integrated mean value of subdural pressure was used as an estimate of ICP. The needle was left in situ until the study was finished, and during the measurement no surgical intervention was performed. Simultaneously the integrated value of MABP was recorded via the radial artery catheter. The mid-axillary line was used for zero point adjustment for the arterial blood pressure.

The CPP was calculated as the difference between MABP and ICP. The surgeons were blinded as regards the values of ICP, MABP and JBP. The

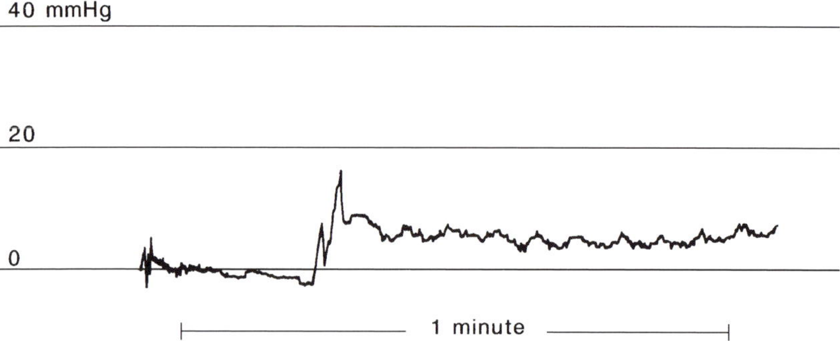

Fig. 3.1 Recording of subdural ICP, with zero-point adjustment, perforation of dura mater and cardiac and respiratory waves

measurement of subdural ICP was normally finished after 1 min. In Figure 3.1 subdural ICP is illustrated with cardiac and respiratory waves.

In Chapter 21 studies of subdural or spinal pressure during spinal surgery are described. In these studies the distance between the skin and the surface of the spinal dura was measured, and the transducer was placed according to this distance.

3.6
Catheterization of the Internal Jugular Vein and Blood Gas Analyses

A jugular bulb catheter was inserted percutaneously at the level of the cricoid. In order to avoid puncture of the carotid artery, catheterization was performed with the head in neutral position (Sulek et al. 1996) and with the patient positioned in 5–10° rTp. This position dilates the jugular vein (Clenaghan et al. 2005). The catheter was introduced 12–14 cm in the cranial direction. Correct cranial position was verified by ascertaining an increase in jugular pressure following neck compression and by unrestrained blood withdrawal. In some cases a lateral x-ray of the neck was exposed to verify correct position of the catheter. The catheter was connected to a transducer and placed in the same sagittal plane as the transducer connected to the needle for subdural ICP measurement.

Blood was withdrawn simultaneously from the arterial and jugular catheters for measurement of PaO_2, $PaCO_2$, pH, glucose lactate, Na^+, K^+ and Ca^{++} (ABL 555 and ABL 700; Radiometer, Copenhagen, Denmark). $AVDO_2$ was calculated as the difference between arterial and jugular venous oxygen content. Furthermore, the arteriovenous difference of $PaCO_2$ ($AVD-CO_2$), pH ($AVD-pH$), lactate (AVD-lactate (mmol/L)), Na^+ ($AVD-Na^+$ (mmol/L)), K^+ ($AVD-K^+$ (mmol/L)) and Ca^{++} ($AVD-Ca^{++}$ (mmol/L)) were calculated.

3.7
Measurement of Cerebral Blood Flow and Cerebral Metabolic Rate of Oxygen

Two angular detectors were placed on each side of the head. As tracer, ^{133}Xe (3–4 mCi i.v.) was used. CBF was measured over a period of 10 min as initial slope index using 10-min clearance curves with a Novo Cerebrograph 10. Correction for rest activity and recirculation was performed. The average of the two CBFs was used. $CMRO_2$ was calculated according to the formula $CMRO_2 = CBF \times AVDO_2$. CBF is measured in Chapter 11, study 1 (indomethacin), Chapter 12 (dihydroergotamine) and Chapter 9 (sevoflurane). In the study of dihydroergotamine (Chapter 12) the CVR was calculated using the formula $CPP = CBF \times CVR$.

3.8
Measurement of Flow Velocity

Transcranial Doppler ultrasonography was used in study 2 in Chapter 11 (indomethacin). In this study middle cerebral artery flow velocity was measured bilaterally. The artery was identified at a depth varying between 45 and 55 mm. The flow velocity was monitored beat-to-beat using a 2-MHz pulsed Doppler probe (TC 2000S; EME Überlingen, Germany). Transcranial Doppler frequency spectra, converted into flow velocity (cm/s), were calculated automatically over 4–5 consecutive cardiac cycles. The mean middle cerebral artery blood flow velocity was recorded and, because flow velocity fluctuates with respiration, the value during end-expiration was used.

3.9
Effect of Hyperventilation and Indomethacin

After the initial ICP measurement the pulmonary ventilation was increased by 30% for 10 min. The measurements were repeated 11 min after the first measurements. CO_2 reactivity was calculated as % change $AVDO_2/\Delta PaCO_2$ mmHg (Chapter 10) or % change $AVDO_2/\Delta PaCO_2$ kPa (Chapter 13).

In some comparable studies the effect of indomethacin and hyperventilation was analysed by comparing the changes in ICP or changes in $AVDO_2$.

3.10
Estimation of Dural Tension and Cerebral Swelling

Before subdural ICP measurement the surgeon made a tactile evaluation of the dural tension. The neurosurgeons were blinded as regards choice of anaesthesia and the ICP value obtained. The tensions were categorized as follows: (1) very slack, (2) normal, (3) increased tension and (4) pronounced increased tension.

The degree of brain swelling during hyperventilation was evaluated by the neurosurgeon after opening of dura. Swelling was estimated as: (1) no swelling, (2) moderate swelling of the brain and (3) pronounced swelling of the brain.

3.11
Measurement of Intracranial Pressure During Tilting
of the Operating Table

The arterial and jugular pressure (JP) transducers were placed on the same horizontal plane as the ICP transducer to eliminate the influence of hydrostatic pressure difference during tilting of the operating table. CPP was calculated as the difference between MABP and subdural ICP. After reference measurements of ICP, MABP and JP in neutral position, the operating table was tilted 5° head-down (5° rTp), with whole-body trunk tilting without flexion of the hips. In this position all pressure transducers were readjusted to the same horizontal level of the dural perforation. The degree of tilting was adjusted using a spirit level fixed to the operating table. A laser pointer fixed to the transducer table was used to place the transducers in the same horizontal plane as the subdural needle. The measurement procedure was repeated after readjustment of the table to 10° and 15° rTp. In accordance with previous investigations performed in our clinic, in which MABP, ICP, CPP and JBP were stable within 1 min after tilting to 10° rTp, the pressure measurements were performed 1 min after a change in position. The effect of rTp on ICP, MABP, CPP and JBP are summarized in Chapter 15.

3.12
Comparative Studies of Intracranial Pressure-Reducing Methods

Data from patients with supratentorial tumours were extracted from our database for the period 1997–2006. The following criteria were used as inclusion in the study: The neurosurgeon estimated that the dura tension was increased and/or ICP exceeded 10 mm Hg at the initial measurement. The following ICP-reducing techniques were used.

3.12.1
Hyperventilation

The minute ventilation of the ventilator was increased by 20–50% for 5 min. In order to keep the peak respiratory pressure below 20 cmH$_2$O, the respiratory rate was eventually increased. Before and 5 min after the increase in minute ventilation subdural ICP and MABP were recorded, and arterial gas tensions were monitored. Thirty patients were included.

3.12.2
Ten Degrees Reverse Trendelenburg Position

After reference measurements of ICP, CPP and MABP in neutral position, the table was adjusted to 10° rTp (whole body trunk tilting without flexion at the hips) and all pressure transducers were re-adjusted to the same level of dural perforation. As a result of a recent study, indicating stable CPP and ICP within 1 min after tilting to 10° rTp, the measurements were performed 1 min after change in position. Sixteen patients were included.

3.12.3
Mannitol Treatment

Over about 5 min, 0.5–1.0 g/kg mannitol was administered intravenously. ICP and CPP were recorded before and 5 min after conclusion of mannitol infusion. Nineteen patients were included.

3.12.4
Indomethacin

Indomethacin 0.5 mg/kg was administered i.v. as a bolus dose. ICP and CPP were recorded for 5 min, and arterial gas analysis was performed before and 5 min after indomethacin. Fifteen patients were included.

3.12.5
Surgical Decompression

Surgical decompression was performed either by drainage via a ventricular catheter inserted during the operation (n=3) or by evacuation of fluid from cystic tumours (n=10). ICP and CPP were recorded before and after decompression, and the volume of fluid from drainage was recorded. Thirteen patients were included.

3.13
Studies of the Effect of Central Analgetics in Patients with Cerebral Tumours

During propofol-fentanyl anaesthesia patients subjected to craniotomy for supratentorial cerebral tumours were subjected to a bolus dose of alfentanil in the following doses: 10, 20 and 30 µg/kg alfentanil followed by an infusion of 10, 20 and 30 µg/kg/h. ICP and CPP were measured continuously before and after administration (Chapter 13). In the same chapter the effects of i.v. fentanyl bolus dose, and remifentanil bolus dose were investigated.

3.14
Studies of Propofol Bolus Dose

In Chapter 14 the effect of an i.v. bolus dose of propofol was studied during propofol-fentanyl and during propofol-remifentanil anaesthesia.

3.15
Patients Subjected to Controlled Studies

After informed consent and before premedication, a sealed numbered envelope indicating anaesthetic procedure or test drug/placebo was opened.

3.16
Statistical Analysis

In intra- and intergroup studies the statistical analyses were as follows: Data within groups were tested for normal distribution. The normality test and equal variance test were applied and one-way ANOVA was used for analysis if these tests were passed. The Tukey test was used for pair-wise multiple comparison procedures. The Kruskal-Wallis one-way analysis of variance on ranks and multiple comparisons versus control groups (Dunn's method) were used for statistical analysis when the normality test or equal variance showed that the data were not normally distributed. These data included subdural ICP, MABP and $AVDO_2$. Bonferroni's test was applied for statistical analysis. In other studies where only two groups were compared the t-test was used if the normality test was passed; if not Mann-Whitney's test was used for intergroup differences and Wilcoxon's test for intragroup changes. The chi-square test was used for statistical analysis of demographic data, localization, size and histopathological diagnosis of the tumours, preoperative steroid administration and position of the head. Difference in tension of dura and the degree of cerebral swelling were tested by the chi-square test in 2×4 or 2×3 tables. For correlation studies Pearson's product moment correlation and linear regression were performed. Means and standard deviation (SD) were calculated in some studies and median and range in others, according to the distribution of the data. $P<0.05$ was considered statistically significant.

References

Bundgaard H, Cold GE (2000) Studies of regional subdural pressure gradients during craniotomy. Br J Neurosurg 14:229–234

Bundgaard H, Jensen K, Cold GE et al (1996) Effects of perioperative indomethacin on intracranial pressure, cerebral blood flow, and cerebral metabolism in patients subjected to craniotomy for cerebral tumours. J Neurosurg Anesthesiol 8:273–279

Bundgaard H, von Oettingen G, Larsen KM et al (1998) Effects of sevoflurane on intracranial pressure, cerebral blood flow, and cerebral metabolism. A dose-response study in patients subjected to craniotomy for cerebral tumours. Acta Anaesthesiol Scand 42:621–627

Clenaghan S, McLaughlin RE, Martyn C et al (2005) Relationship between Trendelenburg tilt and internal jugular vein diameter. Emerg Med J 23:661

Cold GE, Tange M, Jensen TM et al (1996) Subdural pressure measurement during craniotomy. Correlation with tactile estimation of dural tension and brain herniation after opening of dura. Br J Neurosurg 10:69–75

Petersen KD, Landsfeldt U, Cold GE et al (2003) Intracranial pressure and cerebral hemodynamic in patients with cerebral tumours. A randomized prospective study of patients subjected to craniotomy in propofol-fentanyl, isoflurane-fentanyl, or sevoflurane-fentanyl. Anesthesiology 98:329–336

Rasmussen M, Tankisi A, Cold GE (2004) The effects of indomethacin on intracranial pressure and cerebral hemodynamics in patients undergoing craniotomy: a randomized prospective study. Anaesthesia 59:1–8

Sulek CA, Gravenstein N, Blackshear RH et al (1996) Head rotation during internal jugular vein cannulation and the risk of carotid artery puncture. Anesth Analg 82:125–128

Tankisi A, Rolighed Larsen J, Rasmussen M et al (2002) The effects of 10 degrees reverse Trendelenburg position on ICP and CPP in prone positioned patients subjected to craniotomy for occipital or cerebellar tumours. Acta Neurochir 144:655–670

Chapter 4
Comparative Studies of Intracranial Pressure in Patients With and Without Space-Occupying Lesions

Lisbeth Krogh and Georg Emil Cold

Abstract

Anaesthesia for craniotomy has to be carried out with emphasis on haemodynamic stability, a sufficient cerebral perfusion pressure and avoidance of agents or procedures that increase ICP. The patients presented to a current neuroanaesthesiological practice come with a multitude of intracranial pathologies, ranging from discrete unruptured aneurisms to significantly sized tumours that create a midline shift. It is important to relate the ICP measured in patients with space-occupying lesions to the ICP in patients without lesions. Studies of ICP during craniotomy in patients without space-occupying intracerebral lesions, however, are few.

In this chapter data on two populations, one with supratentorial glioblastomas and the other without space-occupying lesions, are presented. Differences between the groups, in ICP and other relevant data obtained, are discussed and the relationship between neuroradiological data and measured ICP correlated.

Anaesthesia for craniotomy has to be carried out with emphasis on haemodynamic stability, a sufficient CPP and avoidance of agents or procedures that increase the ICP. In a randomized study in patients undergoing craniotomy for supratentorial tumours it was concluded that anaesthesia with propofol-fentanyl is to be preferred from anaesthesia with either isoflurane-fentanyl or sevoflurane-fentanyl, because subdural ICP and the degree of cerebral swelling after opening of dura were significantly lower and CPP significantly higher during propofol-fentanyl compared with isoflurane-fentanyl or sevoflurane-fentanyl (Petersen et al. 2003).

Other studies indicate that in patients with space-occupying lesions undergoing supratentorial craniotomy, the degree of cerebral swelling after opening of dura is highly correlated to subdural ICP monitored immediately before opening of dura (Cold et al. 1996; Bundgaard et al. 1998; Rasmussen et al. 2004).

It is important to relate the ICP measured in patients with space-occupying lesions with ICP in patients without lesions. Studies of ICP during craniotomy in patients without space-occupying intracerebral lesions, however, are few. In patients with unruptured cerebral aneurysm, anaesthetized with either propofol-fentanyl or propofol-remifentanil, ICP averaged 2.9 mmHg with the operating table in neutral position; a fall to 0.4 mmHg was found when the table was turned to 10° rTp (Tankisi et al. 2006).

In the present study two populations (one without space-occupying lesion, the other patients with supratentorial glioblastoma) were anaesthetized with either propofol-fentanyl or propofol-remifentanil. Subdural ICP, CPP and jugular pressure were monitored.

Study Outline

Aims 1: To study ICP, CPP and JBP in patients with or without space-occupying lesions. 2: To study the relationship between neuroradiological data (maximal area of tumour, volume of tumour and midline shift) as presented in patients subjected to craniotomy, and to correlate these data with subdural ICP obtained during craniotomy.

Patients The data were collected during the period between 1997 and 2005. Subdural ICP was monitored in 107 patients subjected to propofol-fentanyl and 65 patients subjected to propofol-remifentanil. Of these patients, 132 patients had supratentorial glioblastoma and 40 patients had either unruptured cerebral aneurysm (30 patients) or were operated on for trigeminus neuralgia (10 patients).

Method Concerning neuroradiological findings, histopathology, anaesthetic maintenance dose and monitoring (MABP, ICP, CPP, jugular pressure, arterial gas analysis), degree of dural tension and swelling after opening of dura, see Chapter 3.

Statistical analysis Data within groups were tested for normal distribution. The t-test was used if the normality test was passed; if not Mann-Whitney's test was used for intergroup differences and Wilcoxon's test for intragroup changes. The chi-square test was used for statistical analysis of demographic data, localization, size and histopathological diagnosis of the tumours, preoperative steroid administration and position of the head. Difference in tension of dura and the degree of cerebral swelling were tested by the chi-square test in 2×4 or 2×3 tables. $P<0.05$ was considered statistically significant.

Results In patients with glioblastoma anaesthetized with either propofol-fentanyl or propofol-remifentanil no significant differences were found as regards male/female distribution, age, weight, height, rectal temperature,

PaO_2, jugular venous saturation, $AVDO_2$, neuroradiological findings (maximal area of the tumour, volume of the tumour and midline shift) and $PaCO_2$. The same applies to patients without space-occupying lesions anaesthetized with propofol-fentanyl or propofol-remifentanil (Tables 4.1 and 4.2). The maintenance dose of propofol was significantly higher in propofol-fentanyl-compared with propofol-remifentanil-anaesthetized patients (Table 4.1). In patients with glioblastoma ICP averaged 9.7 mmHg (median 9.0 mmHg) when anaesthetized with propofol-fentanyl, while ICP in propofol-remifentanil-anaesthetized patients averaged 6.7 mmHg (median 6.0 mmHg) ($P<0.05$). In patients without space-occupying lesions ICP averaged 4.3 mmHg (median 5.0 mmHg) when anaesthetized with propofol-fentanyl. This value was significantly lower compared with ICP in patients with glioblastoma ($P<0.05$). In patients without space-occupying lesions ICP averaged 4.4 mmHg (median 4.0 mmHg) when anaesthetized with propofol-remifentanil. This value was not significantly different from patients with glioblastoma subjected to the same anaesthesia (Table 4.3).

In patients with glioblastoma as well as patients without space-occupying lesions both MABP and CPP were significantly lower during anaesthesia with propofol-remifentanil- compared with propofol-fentanyl-anaesthetized patients (Table 4.3). In patients with glioblastoma anaesthetized with propofol-fentanyl jugular pressure was significantly higher (mean 5.4 mmHg) compared with propofol-remifentanil-anaesthetized patients with glioblastoma (mean 2.6 mmHg). No significant difference was found in patients without space-occupying lesions, where mean jugular pressure averaged 3.7 and 3.4 mmHg, respectively (Table 4.2). In patients with glioblastoma the degree of dural tension and swelling after opening of dura were more pronounced in propofol-fentanyl- compared with propofol-remifentanil-anaesthetized patients, with $P=0.042$ (dural tension) and 0.037 (degree of swelling), respectively. In propofol-fentanyl-anaesthetized patients with glioblastoma dural tension and degree of cerebral swelling were significantly different from patients without space-occupying lesions, with P values of 0.001 and <0.001, respectively. In propofol-remifentanil-anaesthetized patients with glioblastoma the degree of dural tension did not differ significantly from patients without space-occupying lesion ($P=0.254$), but the degree of swelling differed significantly ($P<0.001$) (Table 4.4). In patients with glioblastoma as well as patients without space-occupying lesions, whether anaesthetized with propofol-fentanyl or propofol-remifentanil, significant correlations were disclosed between jugular pressure and ICP (correlation coefficients varied from 0.3064 to 0.5800) (Table 4.5). In patients anaesthetized with propofol-fentanyl significant positive correlations were found when neuroradiological data (maximal area of tumour, volume of tumour and midline shift) were correlated to subdural ICP. The corresponding correlations in patients anaesthetized with propofol-remifentanil were also positive but insignificant (Table 4.6).

Table 4.1 Data include patients with supratentorial glioblastoma and patients without space-occupying lesions (unruptured cerebral aneurysm or trigeminus neuralgia). Patients were anaesthetized with propofol-fentanyl or propofol-remifentanil

	Number	Men/ women		Age (year)	Weight (kg)	Height (cm)	Propofol dose (mg//h)
Patients with glioblastoma							
Propofol -fentanyl	89	54/35	Mean±SD	55±11	75±14	174±9	670±186
			Median	56	73	174	700
			Range	17–76	42–120	154–193	250–1,400
Propofol -remifentanil	43	24/19	Mean±SD	52±11	79±15	174±8	400±101*
			Median	55	83	175	400
			Range	52–107	65–119	156–190	250–700
Patients without tumour							
Propofol -fentanyl	18	7/11	Mean±SD	57±11	73±18	175±9	719±199
			Median	57	74	178	700
			Range	37–75	50–124	157–186	300–1,250
Propofol -remifentanil	22	3/19	Mean±SD	53±10	73±14	174±8	425±111*
			Median	53	72	166	400
			Range	27–66	50–98	158–188	200–700

*$P<0.05$ within groups (glioblastoma or patients without space-occupying lesions)

Table 4.2 Data include patients with supratentorial glioblastoma, and patients without space-occupying lesions (unruptured cerebral aneurysm or trigeminus neuralgia). Patients were anaesthetized with propofol-fentanyl or propofol-remifentanil

		Temperature (°C)	PaO_2 (kPa)	Venous saturation (%)	$AVDO_2$ (mmol/L)	Jugular pressure (mmHg)
Patients with glioblastoma						
Propofol -fentanyl	Mean±SD	35.9±0.6	27±10	57±11	3.2±0.9	5.4±4.0
	Median	36.0	26	56.4	3.2	5.0
	Range	34.1–37	10–66	37.3–91	0.9–5.7	−4 to 17
Propofol -remifentanil	Mean±SD	35.9±0.3	24±6	54±8	3.3±0.7	2.6±3.6*
	Median	35.8	24	52.4	3.5	2.5
	Range	35–36.5	12–38	42.7–72	1.8–4.4	−4 to 10
Patients without tumour						
Propofol -fentanyl	Mean±SD	35.8±0.5	27±10	53±13	3.4±1.1	3.7±3.4
	Median	36	24	52	3.4	4.0
	Range	35–37.1	13–42	37.6–88	0.8–5.3	−2 to 12
Propofol -remifentanil	Mean±SD	35.7±0.4	23±6	52±10	3.2±0.8	3.4±3.4
	Median	35.8	24	53	3.0	3.0
	Range	35–36.3	12–33	33.6–65	2.2–5.1	−3 to 10

*$P<0.05$ within groups (glioblastoma or patients without space-occupying lesions)

Table 4.3 Patients with supratentorial glioblastoma, and patients without space-occupying lesions (unruptured cerebral aneurysm or trigeminus neuralgia. Patients were anaesthetized with propofol-fentanyl or propofol-remifentanil

		Tumour area (cm^2)	Tumour volume (cm^3)	Midline shift (mm)	PaCO, (kPa)	MABP (mmHg)	ICP (mmHg)	CPP (mmHg)
Patients with glioblastoma								
Propofol	Mean±SD	17±8	33±22	8.3±5.9	4.5±0.5	85±13	9.7±6.2	75±14
-fentanyl	Median	15.7	26	9.0	4.5	83	9.0	74
	Range	3–42	3–98	0–25	2.7–5.5	56–119	0–34	36–111
Propofol	Mean±SD	15±7	30±19	7.3±6.3	4.5±0.4	74±14*	6.7±4.7*	67±14*
-remifentanil	Median	14.6	26.7	5.0	4.5	70	6.0	65
	Range	3–28	3–71	0–20	3.9–6.0	52–113	0–21	43–100
Patients without tumour								
Propofol	Mean±SD	0	0	0	4.6±0.4	86±12	4.3±3.3**	82±12
-fentanyl	Median				4.6	85	5.0	80
	Range				3.9–5.3	64–106	−2 to 12	58–101
Propofol	Mean±SD	0	0	0	4.6±0.5	74±9*	4.4±2.9	69±10*
-remifentanil	Median				4.5	74	4.0	69
	Range				3.7–5.7	60–93	0–9	51–91

*P<0.05 within groups (glioblastoma or patients without space-occupying lesions)
**P<0.05 between propofol-fentanyl-anaesthetized patients with and without space-occupying lesions

Table 4.4 Data indicate tension of dura before opening and degree of brain swelling after opening of dura in patients with supratentorial glioblastoma and patients without space-occupying lesions anaesthetized with either propofol-fentanyl or propofol-remifentanil. Number (%) of patients is indicated

	Supratentorial glioblastoma present		No space-occupying lesion	
	Propofol -fentanyl	Propofol -remifentanil	Propofol -fentanyl	Propofol -remifentanil
Tension of dura				
Normal tension	42 (47.2%)	30 (69.8%)	17 (94.4%)	19 (86.3%)
Moderate tension	40 (44.9%)	10 (23.3%)	1 (5.6%)	3 (13.6%)
Pronounced tension	7 (7.9%)	3 (7.0%)	0 (0.0%)	0 (0.0%)
Degree of swelling				
No swelling (group 1)	41 (46.1%)	30 (69.8%)	17 (94.4%)	21 (95.5%)
Moderate swelling (group 2)	32 (36.0%)	9 (20.9%)	1 (5.6%)	1 (4.5%)
Pronounced swelling (group 3)	16 (17.9%)	4 (9.3%)	0 (0.0%)	0 (0.0%)

Table 4.5 ICP related to JBP. Correlation coefficient, significance (P value) and linear regression are indicated

	Correlation coefficient (r)	P value	Linear regression
Glioblastoma			
Propofol-fentanyl	0.3064	0.003	ICP=7.38 + 0.51 × JBP (mmHg)
Propofol-remifentanil	0.3969	0.025	ICP=5.23 + 0.52 × JBP (mmHg)
Without tumour			
Propofol-fentanyl	0.5800	<0.001	ICP=1.19 + 0.86 × JBP (mmHg)
Propofol-remifentanil	0.4714	0.027	ICP=3.03 + 0.40 × JBP (mmHg)

Conclusion In propofol-fentanyl- and propofol-remifentanil-anaesthetized patients no significant differences in ICP and CPP were found in patients without space-occupying tumours. In contrast, in patients with glioblastoma both ICP and jugular pressure were significantly higher in propofol-fentanyl-anaesthetized patients compared with patients anaesthetized with propofol-remifentanil.

Discussion

The significantly higher ICP and CPP found in the propofol-fentanyl-anaesthetized patients, compared with the propofol-remifentanil-anaesthetized patients were not caused by differences in $PaCO_2$, tumour size or midline shift.

Table 4.6 ICP correlated to neurological findings (maximal area of tumour, volume of tumour and midline shift). Correlation coefficient, significance (*P* value) and linear regression are indicated

	Correlation coefficient (r)	P value	Linear regression
Correlation between maximal area of tumour and subdural ICP			
Propofol-fentanyl	0.4240	<0.001	ICP=4.55 + 0.34 × area (cm^2)
Propofol-remifentanil	0.3558	0.019	ICP=3.15 + 0.23 × area (cm^2)
Correlation between volume of tumour and subdural ICP			
Propofol-fentanyl	0.4530	<0.001	ICP=5.71 + 0.14 × volume (cm^3)
Propofol-remifentanil	0.3698	0.015	ICP=4.17 + 0.52 × volume (cm^3)
Correlation between midline shift of tumour and ICP			
Propofol-fentanyl	0.3359	0.003	ICP=7.36 + 0.38 × midline shift (mm)
Propofol-remifentanil	0.0810	0.606	Not significant

Accordingly, both dural tension before opening and the degree of cerebral swelling after opening of dura were less pronounced in patients anaesthetized with propofol-remifentanil. The difference in ICP was surprising because the maintenance dose of propofol was significantly lower in the propofol-remifentanil-anaesthetized patients compared with patients undergoing anaesthesia with propofol-fentanyl. According to experimental and clinical studies, propofol induces a dose-related decrease in $CMRO_2$ and CBF, and consequently a lower ICP level should be expected in the propofol-fentanyl group (Moss and Price 1990; Pinaud et al. 1990; Ramani et al. 1992; Alkire et al. 1995). In a comparative study of fentanyl and remifentanil, ICP and CPP did not differ significantly when administered in equipotent doses together with nitrous oxide to patients with supratentorial space-occupying lesions (Guy et al. 1997). Furthermore, recent studies indicate that the CO_2 reactivity is preserved during remifentanil-nitrous oxide anaesthesia (Baker et al. 1997), and the CO_2 reactivity is similar during remifentanil-nitrous oxide and fentanyl-nitrous oxide anaesthesia (Ostapkovich et al. 1998).

The significant difference in subdural ICP might be explained by the difference in CPP, which, dependent on the status of cerebral autoregulation, might influence ICP. On the one hand, a fall in ICP is a consequence of a low CPP if cerebral autoregulation is abolished. On the other hand, an increase in ICP is suspected if cerebral autoregulation is intact. As cerebral autoregulation was not tested in the present study, it is impossible to answer whether autoregulation-induced changes in ICP, caused by different levels of CPP, can explain the difference in ICP levels between the two groups. The differences in ICP might also be caused by differences in JBP between the two anaesthetic groups. In support of this, we found that JBP was significantly lower during propofol-remifentanil anaesthesia compared with the propofol-fentanyl anaesthesia, and significant correlations between JBP and subdural ICP were observed in patients with glioblastoma as well as in patients without space-occupying lesions. Thus, ICP seems to be dependent on the level of JBP in patients undergoing craniotomy in propofol-fentanyl or propofol-remifentanil anaesthesia. This finding is supported by other studies indicating that 5° or 10° rTp is accompanied by a decrease in both JBP and subdural ICP (Rolighed Larsen et al. 2002; Tankisi et al. 2002, 2006; Haure et al. 2003). The fall in ICP during rTp is thought to be due to a decrease in intracranial blood volume caused by augmented venous outflow (Lovell et al. 2000).

In patients anaesthetized with either propofol-fentanyl or propofol-remifentanil significant positive correlations were also disclosed between maximal area of the tumour or volume of the tumour and subdural ICP. The P values were lower and the powers were higher in patients with glioblastoma anaesthetized with propofol-fentanyl compared with glioblastoma patients anaesthetized with propofol-remifentanil. The difference in number of patients in the two anaesthetic groups did not explain the discrepancy, because the correlation coefficients and powers were still of the same numerical size, even when the number of patients in the propofol-fentanyl group was reduced to the first 43 investigations, a number in correspondence with the number in the propofol-remifentanil group.

In awake patients without cerebral pathology ICP averages 11 mmHg (range 7–15 mmHg) (Albeck et al. 1991). In the present study the level of ICP in patients without space-occupying lesions averaged 4.3 and 4.4 mmHg in patients anaesthetized with propofol-fentanyl and propofol-remifentanil, respectively. The difference in ICP between the awake and anaesthetized state is supposed to be caused by propofol that in experimental (Vandesteene et al. 1988; Ramani et al. 1992; Watts et al. 1998) and clinical studies (Madsen 1991; Stephan et al. 1987) reduces cerebral oxygen uptake, CBF and ICP.

Furthermore, the low ICP may be caused by hypocapnia (Petersen et al. 2003). In the present study, both the estimation of dural tension and the degree of cerebral swelling after opening of dura are semiquantitative as well as subjective. Nevertheless, these estimates were used because the presence of brain swelling increases retractor pressure resulting in low regional perfusion pressure (Hongo et al. 1987; Rosenørn 1987), thereby increasing the risk for development of cerebral ischaemia. Furthermore, brain swelling makes surgical access difficult. Another limitation in the present study is the lack of randomization. Data, however, were collected prospectively and continuously between the years 1997 and 2005. In this period subdural ICP monitoring and jugular bulb catheterization were performed in 132 patients with supratentorial glioblastoma, of which 89 patients were anaesthetized with propofol-fentanyl and 43 patients with propofol-remifentanil. The anaesthetic groups were not of equal size, propofol-fentanyl being the largest group. Propofol-remifentanil was used over the period 2000–2005, while propofol-fentanyl was used over the entire period. The maintenance dose of propofol and CPP differed significantly, which makes interpretation of the results difficult. The staff of neurosurgeons and anaesthesiologists involved in craniotomy, however, was almost the same over the period. The same applies to preoperative care, principles of steroid treatment and the operating and monitoring conditions.

References

Albeck MJ, Børgesen SE, Gjerris F et al (1991) Intracranial pressure and cerebrospinal fluid outflow conductance in healthy subjects. J Neurosurg 74:597–600

Alkire MT, Haier RJ, Barker SJ et al (1995) Cerebral metabolism during propofol anesthesia in humans studied with positron emission tomography. Anesthesiology 82:393–403

Baker KZ, Ostapkovich N, Sisti MB, et al (1997) Intact cerebral blood flow reactivity during remifentanil/nitrous oxide anesthesia. J Neurosurg Anesthesiol 9:134–140

Bundgaard H, Landsfeldt U, Cold GE (1998) Subdural monitoring of ICP during craniotomy: thresholds of cerebral swelling/herniation. Acta Neurochir Suppl (Wien) 71:276–278

Cold GE, Tange M, Jensen TM, Ottesen S (1996) Subdural pressure measurement during craniotomy. Correlation with tactile estimation of dural tension and brain herniation after opening of dura. Br J Neurosurg 10:69–75

Guy J, Hindman BJ, Baker KZ, et al (1997) Comparison of remifentanil and fentanyl in patients undergoing craniotomy for supratentorial space-occupying lesions. Anesthesiology 86:514–524

Haure P, Cold GE, Hansen TM et al (2003) The ICP-lowering effect of 10° reverse Trendelenburg position during craniotomy is stable during a 10-minute period. J Neurosurg Anesthesiol 15:297–301

Hongo K, Kabayashi S, Yokoh A et al (1987) Monitoring retraction pressure in the brain. An experimental and clinical study. J Neurosurg 66:270–275

Lovell AT, Marshall AC, Elwell E, et al (2000) Changes in cerebral blood volume with changes in position in awake and anesthetized subjects. Anesth Analg 90:372–376

Madsen JB (1991) Changes in CBF and CMRO$_2$ in patients undergoing craniotomy with propofol infusion. In: Prys-Roberts C (ed) Focus on infusion. Current Medical Literature, London, pp 162–164

Moss E, Price DJ (1990) Effect of propofol on brain retraction pressure and cerebral perfusion pressure. Br J Anaesth 65:823–825

Ostapkovich ND, Baker KZ, Fogarty-Mack P et al (1998) Cerebral blood flow and CO$_2$ reactivity is similar during remifentanil/N$_2$O and fentanyl/N$_2$O anesthesia. Anesthesiology 89:358–363

Petersen KD, Landsfeldt U, Cold GE et al (2003) Intracranial pressure and cerebral hemodynamic in patients with cerebral tumours. Anesthesiology 98:329–336

Pinaud M, Lelausque JN, Chetanneau A (1990) Effects of propofol on cerebral hemodynamics and metabolism in patients with brain trauma. Anesthesiology 73:404–409

Ramani, R, Todd MM, Warner DS (1992) A dose-response study of the influence of propofol on cerebral blood flow, metabolism and the electroencephalogram in the rabbit. J Neurosurg Anesthesiol 4:110–119

Rasmussen M, Bundgaard H, Cold GE (2004) Craniotomy for supratentorial tumours: risk factors for brain swelling after opening of dura. J Neurosurg 101:621–626

Rolighed Larsen JK, Haure P, Cold GE (2002) Reverse Trendelenburg position reduces intracranial pressure during craniotomy. J Neurosurg Anesthesiol 14:16–21

Rosenørn J (1987) Self-retaining brain retractor pressure during intracranial procedures. Acta Neurochir 85:17–22

Stephan H, Sonntag H, Schenk HD et al (1987) Effect of Disoprivan (propofol) on the circulation and oxygen consumption of the brain and CO_2 reactivity of brain vessels in the human. Anaesthesist 36:60–65

Tankisi A, Rolighed Larsen J, Rasmussen M, Dahl B, Cold GE (2002) The effects of 10 degrees reverse Trendelenburg position on ICP and CPP in prone positioned patients subjected to craniotomy for occipital or cerebellar tumours. Acta Neurochir 144:665–670

Tankisi A, Rasmussen M, Juul N et al (2006) The effects of 10° reverse Trendelenburg position on subdural intracranial pressure and cerebral perfusion pressure in patients subjected to craniotomy for cerebral aneurysm. J Neurosurg Anesthesiol 18:11–17

Vandesteene A, Trempont V, Engelman E et al (1988) Effect of propofol on cerebral blood flow and metabolism in man. Anaesthesia 43(suppl):42–43

Watts AD, Eliasziw M, Gelb AW (1998) Propofol and hyperventilation for the treatment of increased intracranial pressure in rabbits. Anesth Analg 87:564–568

Chapter 5
Studies of Regional Subdural Pressure Gradients During Craniotomy

Helle Bundgaard and Georg Emil Cold

Abstract

Intracranial pressure monitoring is based on the premise that the intracranial space is one compartment without pressure differences between brain regions. To what extent the pressure within the subarachnoid space correlates with pressures in other brain regions and whether an increase in pressure within the brain substance is transmitted to the rest of the brain and to the subarachnoid and ventricular cerebrospinal fluid are debated.

In this chapter we summarize and discuss four studies dealing with regional subdural pressure gradients during craniotomy. The first study refers to studies of pressure gradients between subdural ICP and pressures within the neuroaxis, including intraventricular pressure and lumbar spinal pressure. The second study refers to subdural pressure gradients within the surgical field in patients with supratentorial tumour, the third study to pressure gradients within the surgical field in patients with infratentorial tumour, and the fourth study to changes in subdural ICP during opening of dura.

The existence of intercompartmental pressure gradients in conditions of intracranial hypertension has been reported in experimental (Kaufmann and Clark 1970; Takizawa et al. 1986) and clinical studies (Langfitt et al. 1964a, b; Johnston and Rowan 1974). These pressure gradients occur between supratentorial and infratentorial compartments across the tentorium cerebelli or between infratentorial and spinal compartments across the foramen magnum, and develop because displaced brain tissue obstructs the subarachnoid space. Pressure gradients between supratentorial and infratentorial spaces have also been demonstrated in the absence of transtentorial herniation (Smyth and Henderson 1938) and it has been demonstrated that even with patent CSF flow and without tentorial herniation, pressure gradients as high as 12 mmHg exist (Soni 1974).

Concerning intracompartmental pressure gradients, several experimental studies have indicated that gradients occur within the supratentorial compartment between the two hemispheres after cryogenic damage (Langfitt et al. 1964b; Weinstein et al. 1968; Reulen and Kreysch 1973; Symon et al. 1974; Brock et al. 1975; Reulen et al. 1977; Furuse et al. 1981) or after cerebrovascular occlusion (Brock et al. 1972; Iannotti et al. 1985) in one of the hemispheres. Even pressure gradients within one hemisphere have been reported (Wolfla et al. 1996). Clinical research, however, involving head-injured patients has yielded conflicting results. Weaver et al. (1982) documented markedly asymmetric pressures between hemispheres in patients with unilateral mass lesions, and Park et al. (1989) found significant differences in ICP, where the location of higher pressure predicted the region of major pathology. In contrast, Yano et al. (1987) studied comparative ICPs in head-injured patients and found no differences in comparative ICPs, despite the difference in severity of the lesions between the right and left hemispheres.

Intracranial pressure monitoring is based on the premise that the intracranial space is one compartment without pressure differences between brain regions. To what extent the pressure within the subarachnoid space correlates with pressures in other brain regions, and whether an increase in pressure within the brain substance is transmitted to the rest of the brain and to the subarachnoid and ventricular CSF, are debated.

During craniotomy opening of dura occasionally may be followed by herniation of cerebral tissue. This swelling is secondary to a high ICP, where the pressure difference between the intracranial compartment and the ambient pressure forces cerebral tissue through the opening of dura. In some patients this process is self-limiting, where decompression like suction of CSF balances the development of brain herniation. In patients with fast-developing mass-expansion of tumour tissue, haematoma or oedema, cerebral swelling develops so rapidly that evacuation of cerebral tissue may be necessary to provide access to deeper structures. Furthermore, venous engulfment with development of cerebral oedema and ischaemia may develop in the herniated tissue. We therefore found it of interest to measure changes in subdural ICP in the operating field during opening of dura.

In this chapter we summarize and discuss four studies. The first study refers to studies of pressure gradients between subdural ICP and pressures within the neuroaxis, including intraventricular pressure and lumbar spinal pressure. The second study refers to the subdural pressure gradient within the surgical field in patients with supratentorial tumour, the third study to pressure gradients within the surgical field in patients with infratentorial tumour, and the fourth study to changes in subdural ICP during opening of dura. The second and the third studies have been presented by Bundgaard and Cold in Br J Neurosurg (2000) 14:229–234.

Study 1: Studies of Pressure Gradients Between Subdural Intracranial Pressure and Pressures Within the Neuroaxis, Including Intraventricular Pressure and Lumbar Spinal Pressure

Aim   Toinvestigate pressure gradients within the neuroaxis.

Method   In 13 patients undergoing supratentorial craniotomy in the supine position for SAH ($n=9$), tumour ($n=3$) and intraventricular haematoma ($n=1$). A ventricular catheter was inserted preoperatively. After exposure of the dura, subdural ICP and intraventricular pressure were measured with the transducers placed in the same horizontal plane. In 6 patients subjected to fossa posterior surgery in the prone position for tumour ($n=3$), haematoma ($n=2$) and arteriovenous malformation ($n=1$), intraventricular pressure and subdural ICP in the posterior fossa were measured simultaneously. In 5 patients (4 patients with SAH and 1 patient with trigeminus neuralgia) a lumbar spinal catheter was inserted and subdural ICP and lumbar spinal pressures were measured simultaneously.

Statistical analysis   Median and range were calculated. Non-parametric tests (Wilcoxon and Mann-Whitney) were used for statistical analyses within and between groups. Linear regression and correlation analysis (Spearman's rho) were used.

Results   The results are given in Tables 5.1, 5.2 and 5.3 and Fig. 5.1. The values of subdural ICP were higher compared with intraventricular pressure and spinal pressure. The mean values for difference in pressures were 0.1 mmHg when comparing supratentorial subdural ICP with intraventricular pressure,

Table 5.1   Values of subdural ICP and intraventricular pressure in patients undergoing supra- and infratentorial surgery

Patient number	Supratentorial subdural ICP (mmHg)	Intraventricular pressure (mmHg)	Difference in pressures (mmHg)
1	3	7	−4
2	13	17	−4
3	6	6	0
4	10	10	0
5	5	6	−1
6	22	12	10
7	7	5	2
8	13	13	0
9	5	5	0
10	0	2	−2
11	1	1	0
12	7	7	0
13	0	0	0
Mean±SD	7.1±6.2	7.0±4.9	0.1±3.4

Table 5.2 Values of infratentorial subdural ICP and intraventricular pressure in patients undergoing infratentorial surgery

Patient number	Infratentorial subdural ICP (mmHg)	Intraventricular pressure (mmHg)	Difference in pressure (mmHg)
1	7	5	2
2	10	5	5
3	9	6	3
4	14	10	4
5	19	12	7
6	15	7	8
Mean±SD	12.3±4.5	7.5±2.9	4.8±2.3

Table 5.3 Values of subdural ICP and spinal pressure in patients undergoing supratentorial surgery

Patient number	Subdural ICP (mmHg)	Spinal pressure (mmHg)	Difference in pressure (mmHg)
1	10	7	3
2	11	5	6
3	8	1	7
4	9	2	7
5	10	0	10
Mean±SD	9.6±1.1	3.0±2.9	6.6±2.5

4.8 mmHg when comparing infratentorial subdural ICP with intraventricular pressure, and 6.6 mmHg when comparing supratentorial subdural ICP with spinal pressure.

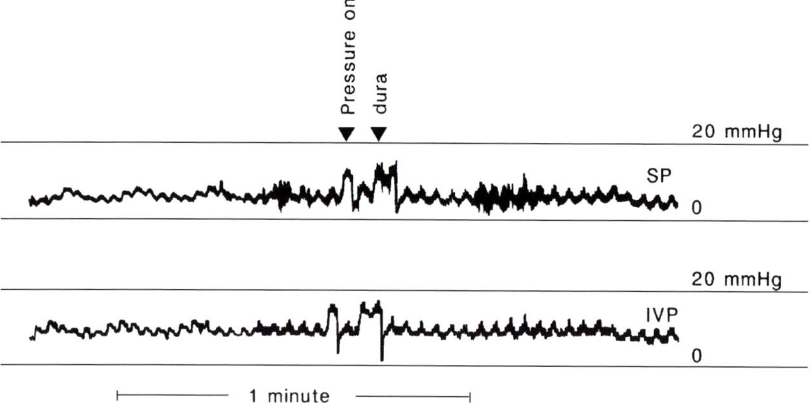

Fig. 5.1 Simultaneous recording of subdural (SP) and intraventricular (IVP) pressures

Conclusion   This study indicates that between compartments of the neuroaxis differences in pressures exist, with the smallest differences within the supratentorial compartment, higher differences between the supra- and infratentorial compartments, and the highest difference between the supratentorial and spinal compartments.

Study 2: Subdural Intracranial Pressure Gradients Within the Supratentorial Surgical Field

Aim   To measure gradients of subdural ICP in the sagittal and horizontal plane within the surgical field during craniotomy.

Method   Thirty-seven patients with supratentorial space-occupying lesions were subjected to craniotomy in the supine position. Twenty-nine patients had

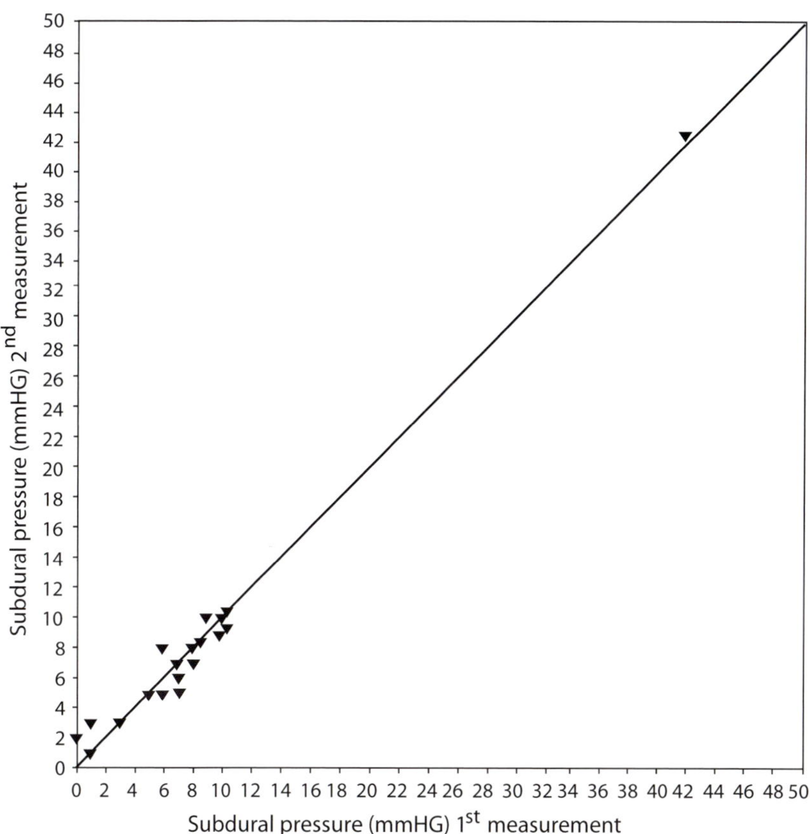

Fig. 5.2   Correlation between paired subdural pressure measurements in the same horizontal plane in 19 patients with supratentorial cerebral tumours

a brain tumour, 5 patients had SAH and were operated on for cerebral aneurysm in the acute phase within 1 week after the haemorrhage and 3 had an arteriovenous malformation. Propofol-fentanyl or isoflurane-nitrous oxide-fentanyl anaesthesia was used for maintenance of anaesthesia. Subdural ICP were measured twice in each patient. In 19 patients the two measurements were performed in the same horizontal plane with a distance of approximately 2–4 cm, and in 18 patients the two measurements were performed in the same vertical plane. The distances between the two vertical measurements of subdural pressure were measured by use of a laser light placed on a ruler. For details concerning induction and maintenance of anaesthesia and monitoring, see Chapter 3.

Statistical analysis   Median and range were calculated. Non-parametric tests (Wilcoxon and Mann-Whitney) were used for statistical analyses within and between groups. Linear regression and correlation analysis (Spearman's rho) were used.

Results   In the study period (5 min) no surgical intervention occurred apart from the subdural pressure measurements. The patients were in steady-state and no changes in mean arterial blood pressure or $PaCO_2$ were observed. In the study of paired subdural pressure measurements in the same horizontal plane, a good correlation between the measurements was found (y=0.976x+0.197, r=0.992, P<0.001) (Fig. 5.2).

In the study of paired subdural pressure measurements in the same vertical plane, the graphical representation of the results indicate that there is a corre-

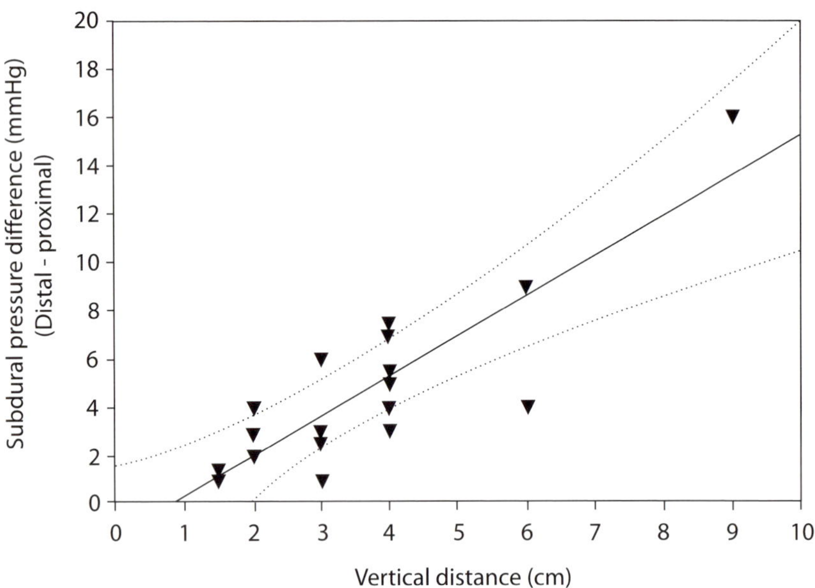

Fig. 5.3   Correlation between the vertical distance (cm), and the difference in subdural ICP in 18 patients with supratentorial space-occupying lesions

lation between the vertical distance of the two measurements and the difference in subdural pressure, with the highest subdural pressure in the most downward portion of the brain ($r=0.85$, $P<0.001$) (Fig. 5.3).

Conclusion   No difference in subdural pressure was observed in the horizontal plane. A correlation between pressure on the vertical axis with the highest pressure in the caudal regions of the brain exists.

Study 3: Subdural Intracranial Pressure Gradients Within the Surgical Field in Infratentorial Surgery

Aim   To measure the difference in subdural ICP in the horizontal plane in patients with midline and unilateral cerebellar tumour.

Method   Sixteen patients with cerebellar tumours were subjected to posterior fossa surgery in the prone position. Ten patients had a tumour in one cerebellar hemisphere (group 1) and 6 patients had a midline cerebellar tumour or tumour in both cerebellar hemispheres (group 2). Propofol-fentanyl or isoflurane-nitrous oxide-fentanyl anaesthesia was used for maintenance of anaesthesia. Subdural pressures were measured bilaterally in the horizontal plane over the right and left cerebellar hemispheres. For details concerning maintenance of anaesthesia and monitoring, see Chapter 3.

Statistical analysis   Median and range were calculated. Non-parametric tests (Wilcoxon and Mann-Whitney) were used for statistical analyses within and between groups. Linear regression and correlation analysis (Spearman's rho) were used.

Table 5.4   Group 1. Paired measurements of subdural ICP on the tumour side and the contralateral side, and differences in pressures are indicated

Patient number	ICP tumour side (mmHg)	ICP contralateral side (mmHg)	Difference in pressure(mmHg)
1	37	28	9
2	16	14	2
3	5	2	3
4	13	7	6
5	22	12	10
6	28	12	16
7	16	13	3
8	36	27	9
9	18	13	5
10	32	27	5
Median	20	13*	5.5
Range	(5–37)	(2–18)	(2–16)

*$P=0.002$ between median subdural pressure on tumour side and the contralateral side

Table 5.5 Group 2. Paired measurements of subdural pressure in 6 patients with midline cerebellar tumour

Patient number	ICP right cerebellar hemisphere (mmHg)	ICP left cerebellar hemisphere (mmHg)	Difference in pressure (mmHg)
1	11	11	0
2	14	15	1
3	14	13	1
4	34	36	2
5	10	11	1
6	23	22	1
Median	14	14	1
Range	(10–34)	(11–36)	(0–2)

No statistical significant difference found

Results In patients with tumour in one cerebellar hemisphere, subdural pressure measured over the cerebellar hemisphere ipsilateral to the tumour side was significantly higher than subdural pressure measured on the contralateral side (median 20 and 13 mmHg, $P=0.002$) (Table 5.4). In contrast, in patients with midline cerebellar tumours no difference was found in the median subdural pressure (14 mmHg) (Table 5.5). A significant difference between median subdural pressure differences in the groups was found ($P=0.002$) (Fig. 5.4).

Conclusion Unilateral cerebellar tumours exert local pressure in the ipsilateral hemisphere.

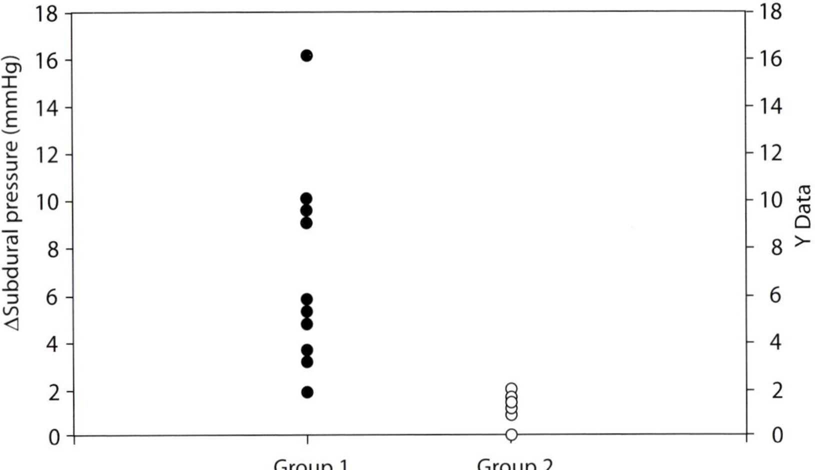

Fig. 5.4 Numerical differences in subdural pressure in 16 patients with cerebellar tumours. Numerical difference in subdural pressure from the left and right cerebellar hemisphere in 10 patients with tumour in one cerebellar hemisphere (group 1; $n=10$). Numerical differences in subdural pressure from the left and right cerebellar hemisphere in 6 patients with midline cerebellar tumour (group 2; $n=6$). $P=0.002$ between median subdural pressure differences in the two groups

Study 4: Changes in Subdural Intracranial Pressure During Opening of Dura

Aim   To measure subdural ICP during opening of dura.

Method   In 21 patients with supratentorial cerebral tumours subdural ICP was measured continuously 2 min before opening of dura, and 3–5 min after opening of dura. Subdural ICP was measured at a distance of about 1 cm from the initial opening of dura close to the bone margin.

Statistical analysis   Median and range were calculated. Non-parametric tests (Wilcoxon and Mann-Whitney) were used for statistical analyses within and between groups.

Results   In 8 patients with median ICP of 6 mmHg (range 2–9 mmHg) herniation never occurred, and opening of dura was followed by a rapid decline of subdural ICP over 2–3 min. In 9 patients with median subdural ICP of 10 mmHg (range 8–17 mmHg) cerebral swelling developed after dural incision, but severe herniation with venous engorgement/oedema was not observed. In these patients subdural ICP decreased slowly but steadily over 3–5 min. In four patients with median subdural ICP of 16 mmHg (range 12–32 mmHg) before opening of dura, severe herniation developed. An initial decrease in subdural ICP was followed by a secondary increase occurring 2–3 min after opening of dura. In these patients cerebral swelling was uncontrolled and evacuation of cerebral tissue was necessary to gain access to deeper structures (Table 5.6).

Conclusion   The risk of cerebral swelling after opening of dura is dependent on ICP. Severe cerebral swelling was only observed at subdural ICP > 12 mmHg before opening of dura.

Discussion

Clinical and diagnostic inferences drawn from ICP-monitoring devices frequently make the assumption that ICP is uniform throughout the subarachnoid space, although the relevant pathology observed on CT or MRI is often found to be asymmetrical, but only few clinical studies are available.

Nearly all the research concerning cerebral pressure gradients has been performed experimentally on the basis of fluid infusion to imitate a rapidly expanding intracranial mass. It is reasonable that differential pressures must exist in relation to a rapidly expanding intracranial mass whose rate of expansion exceeds the rate of the adaptive capacity of the cranial space. Whether slowly expanding lesions are able to create pressure differences or not, is questionable. One problem is related to the methodology of ICP measurements. In slowly expanding lesions, where the capacity of adaptive compliance mechanisms is not exhausted, the pressure gradients are so localized and small that they are almost immeasurable. However, regional pressure gradients are important factors influencing CPP, rCBF and oedema mobilization.

Table 5.6 Changes in subdural ICP 2 min before and 3–5 min after opening of dura

Patient number	ICP, −1 min (mmHg)	ICP, zero (mmHg)	ICP, 1 min (mmHg)	ICP, 2 min (mmHg)	ICP, 3 min (mmHg)	ICP, 4 min (mmHg)	ICP, 5 min (mmHg)
Patients where subdural ICP decreases to zero within 5 min							
1	2	2	1	0			
2	2	2	1	0			
3	5	4	2	1	0		
4	6	6	5	5	4	3	0
5	7	7	6	5	4	3	0
6	8	8	0				
7	8	8	6	2	0		
8	9	9	6	2	0		
Patients where subdural ICP decreases to levels ranging from 3 to 7 mmHg							
1	8	8	7	7	5	5	4
2	9	9	7	7	5	5	4
3	10	10	10	8	3	3	3
4	10	10	7	4	4	4	3
5	10	10	10	8	6	4	3
6	11	11	11	9	8	6	5
7	11	11	11	10	8	6	5

Table 5.6 *(continued)*

Patient number	ICP, −1 min (mmHg)	ICP, zero (mmHg)	ICP, 1 min (mmHg)	ICP, 2 min (mmHg)	ICP, 3 min (mmHg)	ICP, 4 min (mmHg)	ICP, 5 min (mmHg)
Patients where subdural ICP remains higher than 9 mmHg							
1	12	12	12	20	30	28	25
2	16	16	9	9	9	12	15
3	16	16	14	12	20	13	10
4	32	32	30	23	15	17	20

Under normal conditions, there is no evidence of a naturally occurring subdural space (Haines et al. 1993). It is supposed that the pressures measured in the present study originated either from the dural border cell layer or from the subarachnoid space. It is impossible to determine from which space the pressures were measured.

Satisfactory records were obtained in all patients within 1 min. Cardiac and respiratory waves were present immediately after insertion of the needle. The reproducibility of the subdural pressure was high, as evaluated by the studies of subdural pressures performed twice and simultaneously in the same horizontal plane. The pressures never differed more than 2 mmHg, and the regression line ($y=0.976x+0.197$, $r=0.992$, $P<0.001$) was close to the line of identity.

Pressure gradients within the neuroaxis were demonstrated in study 1, where pressure gradients between supratentorial subdural ICP and ventricular pressure were smaller than pressure gradients between the supra- and infratentorial compartments, while pressure gradients between the supratentorial and spinal compartments were greatest. These findings question the use of spinal pressure in studies of intracranial space-occupying lesions.

The pressure gradients originating from a space-occupying process were studied by measuring differences in subdural pressures over the right and the left cerebellar hemispheres in 16 patients operated on in the prone position for cerebellar tumours. We distinguished between patients with tumour in one cerebellar hemisphere and patients with midline cerebellar tumours. Subdural pressure measured over the cerebellar hemisphere ipsilateral to the tumour side was significantly higher than subdural pressure measured on the contralateral side ($P=0.002$). A pressure difference as high as 16 mmHg was seen in one patient. In patients with midline cerebellar tumours subdural pressure gradients never exceeded 2 mmHg. Our results are in accordance with other studies. Cairns expressed the opinion that intracranial pressure produced by a tumour may be greater in the brain adjacent to the tumour (Cairns (1939). Weaver et al. (1982) documented markedly asymmetric pressures between hemispheres in patients with unilateral mass lesions, and Broaddus (1989) found that the location of higher pressure was predicted by the region of major pathology. The influence of a supratentorial tumour on subdural pressure was not evaluated in the present study. However, it is likely that pressure gradients due to a mass-expanding process are also present in the supratentorial compartment within the area of the exposed dura.

The actual pathophysiological mechanisms of pressure gradients in the brain are debated. During expansion of an intracranial mass, vascular compression, ischaemia of brain tissue and oedema adjacent to the lesion may occur. Formation of vasogenic brain oedema is associated with an increase in local brain tissue pressure in the white matter adjacent to the lesion site (Reulen and Kreysch 1973). It has been argued that local differences of brain water content, regional blood flow and brain tissue elastance are responsible for pressure gradients between and within hemispheres, in the presence of an expanding intracranial lesion (Ecker 1955; Lundberg 1960; Miller and Garibi

1972; Leech 1974; Symon et al. 1974; Miller et al. 1975; Piek et al. 1988). Furthermore, the pressures are influenced by obstruction of the venous vascular bed in response to increased ICP (Ecker 1955; Lundberg 1960). In addition, the physical properties of the dura mater and its attachment to the cranium play a role (Langfitt and Elliott 1967).

Other pressure gradients, not originating from an intracranial mass lesion, normally exist within the cranial vault. Tissue pressure is the sum of hydrostatic, osmotic and oncotic pressure gradients. However, it is technically challenging to record each of the components. The hydrostatic pressure measured by current techniques is more analogous to the term total tissue pressure because it also includes osmotic and oncotic forces (Rosner 1996).

The hydrostatic pressure of blood varies normally within the intact skull depending on the size of the vessel and the resistance of the vascular bed. Our results indicate that gravity might influence the regional subdural pressure in the open area of the craniotomy. A vertical pressure gradient was observed with the highest subdural pressure in the most downward portion of the brain (Fig. 5.3). It is probable, however, that the measured subdural pressure in addition to gravity was influenced by the presence of the underlying space-occupying process.

References

Broaddus WC (1989) Differential intracranial pressure recordings in patients with dual ipsilateral monitors. In: Hoff JT, Bentz AL (eds) Intracranial pressure VII. Springer, Berlin

Brock M, Beck J, Markakis E et al (1972) Intracranial pressure gradients associated with experimental cerebral embolism. Stroke 3:123–130

Brock M, Furuse M, Weber R et al (1975) Brain tissue pressure gradients. In: Lundberg N, Ponten U, Brock M (eds) Intracranial pressure II. Springer, Berlin, pp 215–220

Bundgaard H, Cold GE (2000) Studies of regional subdural pressure gradients during craniotomy. Br J Neurosurg 14:229–234

Cairns H (1939) Raised intracranial pressure: hydrocephalic and vascular factors. Br J Surg 27:275–294

Ecker A (1955) Irregular fluctuation of elevated cerebrospinal fluid pressure. Such fluctuations as a measure of dysfunction of cerebrovascular episodes, pseudotumour cerebri, and head injury. Arch Neurol Psychiatry 74:641–649

Furuse M, Brock M, Hasuo M et al (1981) Relationship between brain tissue pressure gradients and cerebral blood flow distribution studied in circumscribed vasogenic cerebral oedema. Neurochirurgia (Stuttg) 24:10–14

Haines DE, Harkey HL, Mefty O (1993) The 'subdural' space: a new look at an outdated concept. Neurosurgery 32:111–120

Iannotti F, Hoff JT, Schielke GP (1985). Brain tissue pressure in focal cerebral ischemia. J Neurosurg 62:83–89

Johnston IH, Rowan JO (1974) Raised intracranial pressure and cerebral blood flow. 4. Intracranial pressure gradients and regional cerebral blood flow. J Neurol Neurosurg Psychiatry 37:585–592

Kaufmann GE, Clark K 1970) Continuous simultaneous monitoring of intraventricular and cervical subarachnoid cerebrospinal fluid pressure to indicate development of cerebral or tonsillar herniation. J Neurosurg 33:145–150

Langfitt TW, Elliott FA (1967) Pain in the back and legs caused by cervical spinal cord compression. JAMA 200:382–5

Langfitt TW, Weinstein JD, Kassell NE et al (1964a) Transmission of increased intracranial pressure I. Within the craniospinal axis. J Neurosurg 21:989–997

Langfitt TW, Weinstein JD, Kassell NF et al (1964b) Transmission of increased intracranial pressure II. Within the supratentorial space. J Neurosurg 21:998–1005

Leech PJ (1974) Intracranial pressure-volume relationships during experimental brain compression in primates. J Neurol Neurosurg Psychiatry 37:1093–1098

Lundberg N (1960) Continuous recording and control of ventricular fluid pressure in neurosurgical practice. Acta Psychiat Scand 36(suppl 149):1–193

Miller JD, Garibi J (1972) Intracranial volume/pressure relationships during continuous monitoring of ventricular fluid pressure. In: Brock M, Dietz H (eds) Intracranial pressure. Experimental and clinical aspects. Springer, Berlin, pp 270–274

Miller JD, Leech PJ, Pickard JD (1975) Volume pressure response in various experimental and clinical conditions. In: Lundberg N, Ponten U, Brock M (eds) Intracranial pressure II. Springer, Berlin, pp 97–100

Park TS, Cail WS, Broaddus et al (1989) Lumboperitoneal shunt combined with myelotomy for treatment of syrengohydromyelia. J Neurosurg 70:721–727

Piek J, Plewe P, Bock WJ (1988) Intrahemispheric gradients of brain tissue pressure in patients with brain tumours. Acta Neurochir (Wien) 93:129–132

Reulen HJ, Kreysch HG (1973) Measurement of brain tissue pressure in cold induced cerebral oedema. Acta Neurochir (Wien) 29:29–40

Reulen HJ, Graham R, Spatz M et al (1977) Role of pressure gradients and bulk flow in dynamics of vasogenic brain edema. J Neurosurg 46:24–35

Rosner M (1996) Techniques for intracranial pressure monitoring. In: Tindall G, Cooper P, Borrow D (eds) The practice of neurosurgery. Williams and Wilkins, Baltimore, pp 95–119

Smyth GE, Henderson WR (1938) Observations on the cerebrospinal fluid pressure on simultaneous ventricular and lumbar punctures. J Neurol Neurosurg Psychiatry 1:226–237

Soni SR (1974) Continuous measurement of differential CSF pressures across the tentorium. J Neurol Neurosurg Psychiatry 37:1283–1284

Symon L, Pasztor E, Branston NM (1974) Effect of supratentorial space-occupying lesions on regional intracranial pressure and local cerebral blood flow: an experimental study in baboons. J Neurol Neurosurg Psychiatry 37:617–626

Takizawa H, Gabra Sanders T et al (1986) Analysis of changes in intracranial pressure and pressure-volume index at different locations in the craniospinal axis during supratentorial epidural balloon inflation. Neurosurgery 19:1–8

Weaver DD, Winn HR, Jane JA (1982) Differential intracranial pressure in patients with unilateral mass lesions. J Neurosurg 56:660–665

Weinstein JD, Langfitt TW, Bruno L et al (1968) Experimental study of patterns of brain distortion and ischemia produced by an intracranial mass. J Neurosurg 28:513–521

Wolfla CE, Luerssen TG, Bowman RM (1996) Brain tissue pressure gradients created by expanding frontal epidural mass lesion. J Neurosurg 84:642–647

Yano M, Ikeda Y, Kobayashi S (1987) Intracranial pressure in head-injured patients with various intracranial lesions is identical throughout the supratentorial intracranial compartment. Neurosurgery 21:688–692

Chapter 6
Subdural Intracranial Pressure and Degree of Swelling After Opening of Dura in Patients with Supratentorial Tumours

Mads Rasmussen and Georg Emil Cold

Abstract

During craniotomy for a mass-expanding cerebral process such as tumour or haematoma, opening of dura mater represents a critical moment. Cerebral swelling through the craniotomy can seriously jeopardize surgical access and increase the risk of cerebral ischaemia with possible worsening of the outcome. Traditionally, preoperative CT data together with the neurological examination and level of consciousness are used to assess the risk of high ICP. As a consequence, the neurosurgeon together with the anaesthesiologist may decide whether ICP-reducing therapy is indicated before opening of the dura and exposing of the brain.

In this chapter two studies of the relationship between subdural ICP and the degree of cerebral swelling after opening of dura mater are presented. The first study examined the relationship between subdural ICP before opening of the dura mater and the dural tension and degree of brain swelling in patients undergoing craniotomy for cerebral tumours or subarachnoid haemorrhage. In the second study we further investigated the relationship between subdural ICP and the degree of brain swelling in a larger population of patients.

During craniotomy for a mass-expanding cerebral process like tumour or haematoma, opening of dura mater represents a critical moment. Cerebral swelling through the craniotomy can seriously jeopardize surgical access and increase the risk of cerebral ischaemia with possible worsening of the outcome. Traditionally, preoperative CT data with estimation of tumour size, midline shift and oedema formation together with the neurological examination and level of consciousness are used to assess the risk of intracranial hypertension. As a consequence, the neurosurgeon together with the anaesthesiologist, may decide whether ICP-reducing therapy is indicated before opening of dura and exposing the brain.

In this chapter two studies of the relationship between subdural ICP and the degree of cerebral swelling after opening of dura will be presented. The first study has been presented by Bundgaard et al. in Acta Neurochir Suppl (1998) 71:276–278 and the second study has been presented by Rasmussen et al. in J Neurosurg (2004) 101:621–626.

Study 1: Subdural Monitoring of ICP During Craniotomy: Thresholds of Cerebral Swelling/Herniation

Aim To correlate ICP immediately before opening of dura mater with the tendency to cerebral swelling/herniation after opening of dura mater, and to define thresholds for cerebral swelling/herniation. Furthermore to correlate the surgeons tactile estimation of dural tension to the degree of cerebral swelling/herniation after opening of dura mater.

Patients One hundred and seventy-eight patients subjected to craniotomy for either supratentorial cerebral tumour ($n=126$) or subarachnoid haemorrhage ($n=52$) were included in the study.

Method Subdural ICP was measured before opening of dura. The degree of dural tension immediately before opening of dura was estimated (for details see Chapter 3). The degree of cerebral swelling after opening of dura was estimated by the surgeon and classified in accordance with Chapter 3: group 1: the brain below the level of dura; group 2: the brain at the level of dura, without swelling; group 3: moderate swelling of the brain; group 4: pronounced swelling of the brain. One hundred and six patients underwent propofol-fentanyl anaesthesia and 72 patients were subjected to isoflurane-nitrous oxide-fentanyl anaesthesia.

Statistical analysis Median, 5% and 95% confidence intervals (CI) of the subdural ICP are indicated. The Mann-Whitney test was used to analyse intergroup data and the Kruskal-Wallis one-way analysis of variance on ranks was used to compare groups. $P<0.05$ was considered significant.

Results Pair-wise multiple comparisons showed a significant difference in subdural ICP between all groups except between group 1 and group 2 and group 3 and group 4. At subdural ICP < 7 mmHg cerebral swelling/herniation rarely occurred after opening of dura. At subdural ICP > 10 mmHg, cerebral swelling/herniation occurred with high probability (Figure 6.1).

The 178 patients were divided into subgroups according to pathology (subarachnoid haemorrhage versus cerebral tumours), anaesthetic agents (isoflurane-nitrous oxide-fentanyl contra propofol-fentanyl) and the level of $PaCO_2$ (< 4.0 kPa, > 4.0 kPa). No significant intergroup difference in the subdural ICP levels were disclosed (Tables 6.1–6.3). Generally, a good correlation between tactile estimation of dural tension and the degree of cerebral swelling after opening of dura was found. However, in 15 patients (8.5%) where swelling/herniation were disclosed the neurosurgeon predicted normal tension of dura,

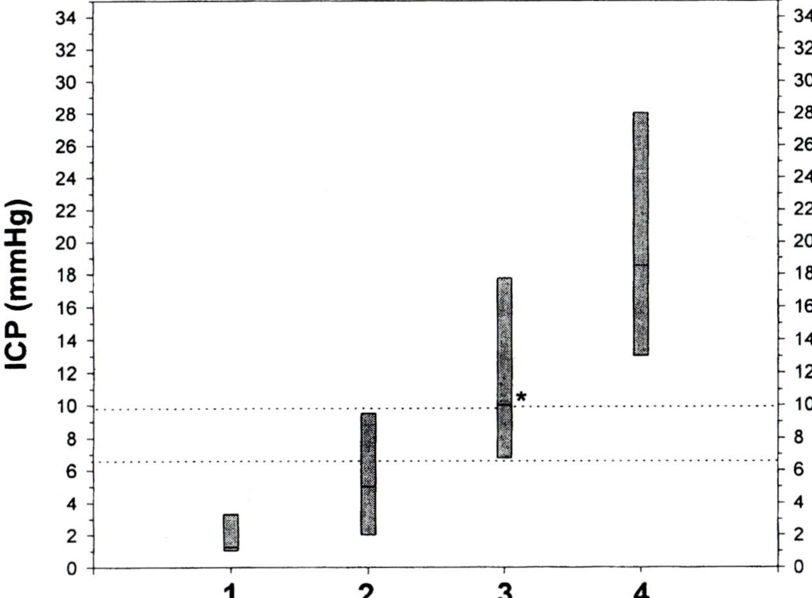

Fig. 6.1 Degree of cerebral swelling/herniation correlated to subdural ICP (N = 178). 1 The brain below the level of dura (n = 10). 2 no swelling or herniation of the brain (n = 107). 3 Swelling or herniation of the brain (n = 43). 4 Pronounced herniation of the brain (n = 18). The dotted lines indicate the thresholds for cerebral swelling/herniation. At ICP below the bottom line cerebral swelling or herniation rarely occur. At ICP above the top line cerebral swelling or herniation occur with high probability. Median and 5% to 95% confidence intervals are indicated. *Indicate $p < 0.05\%$ (comparison between 2 and 3)

Table 6.1 Relationship between level of ICP and degree of cerebral swelling after opening of dura in patients with cerebral tumours and patients with subarachnoid haemorrhage. No significant differences in the levels of ICP in the respective swelling groups were found between patients with cerebral tumour and subarachnoid haemorrhage. Group A: cerebral tumour (n=126), mean $PaCO_2$ 4.5 kPa, MABP 77 mmHg. Group B: subarachnoid haemorrhage (n=52), mean $PaCO_2$ 4.3 kPa, MABP 77 mmHg

	Degree of cerebral swelling			
	Group 1	Group 2	Group 3	Group 4
Group A				
Number	5	78	30	13
Median ICP (mmHg) (5% and 95% CI)	1 (1–4)	5 (1–10)	11 (6–21)	18 (11–31)
Group B				
Number	5	29	13	5
Median ICP (mmHg) (5% and 95% CI)	1 (1–4)	5 (1–13)	10 (6–19)	21 (13–30)

Table 6.2 Relationship between level of ICP and degree of cerebral swelling after opening of dura in patients anaesthetized with isoflurane-nitrous oxide-fentanyl or propofol-fentanyl. No significant differences in the levels of ICP in the respective swelling groups were found between patients with cerebral tumour and subarachnoid haemorrhage. Group A: isoflurane-nitrous oxide anaesthesia (n=72, mean $PaCO_2$ 4.3 kPa, MABP 73 mmHg). Group B: propofol-fentanyl anaesthesia (n=106, mean $PaCO_2$ 4.5 kPa, MABP 80 mmHg)

	Degree of cerebral swelling			
	Group 1	Group 2	Group 3	Group 4
Group A				
Number	4	36	19	13
Median ICP (mmHg) (5% and 95% CI)	2 (1–4)	5 (1–12)	12 (6–19)	17 (11–31)
Group B				
Number	6	71	24	5
Median ICP (mmHg) (5% and 95% CI)	1 (1–4)	5 (1–10)	11 (6–20)	23 (13–30)

Table 6.3 Relationship between level of ICP and degree of cerebral swelling after opening of dura in patients with $PaCO_2$ level of $\leq$ 4.0 kPa and > 4.0 kPa. No significant differences in the levels of ICP in the respective swelling groups were found between patients with cerebral tumour and subarachnoid haemorrhage. Group A: mean $PaCO_2$ $\leq$ 4.0 kPa, MABP 79 mmHg (n=50). Group B: mean $PaCO_2$ > 4.0 kPa, MABP 80 mmHg (n=128)

	Degree of cerebral swelling			
	Group 1	Group 2	Group 3	Group 4
Group A				
Number	5	28	10	7
Median ICP (mmHg) (5% and 95% CI)	1 (1–4)	5 (1–10)	9 (5–15)	20 (17–30)
Group B				
Number	6	79	33	10
Median ICP (mmHg) (5% and 95% CI)	1 (1–4)	5 (1–11)	10 (6–21)	17 (10–32)

and in 13 patients (7.5%) the neurosurgeon estimated increased tension of the dura but no swelling or herniation occurred after opening of dura.

Conclusion Generally a good correlation between the tactile estimation of dural tension and the degree of cerebral swelling after opening of dura was found. In 8.5% of patients, however, the neurosurgeons were unable to predict the occurrence of cerebral swelling. In contrast, at subdural ICP < 7 mmHg cerebral swelling rarely occurred, while at subdural ICP > 10 mmHg cerebral swelling occurred with high probability. The subdural ICP levels at which cerebral swelling occurred were independent of pathology, anaesthetic regime and level of $PaCO_2$.

Study 2: Craniotomy for Supratentorial Brain Tumours: Risk Factors for Brain Swelling After Opening of Dura Mater

Aim The primary aim was to determine risk factors, including subdural ICP, patient characteristics, histopathology, neuroradiology, anaesthetic regimen and perioperative physiological data, predictive for brain swelling through the dural opening. As a secondary aim we wanted to define subdural ICP thresholds of brain swelling.

Method Data were collected prospectively and included demographic, anaesthetic, physiological and radiographic data from patients subjected to elective craniotomy in the supine position for supratentorial brain tumours. Since January 1994 we have routinely performed measurement of subdural ICP for elective craniotomy. Data were collected in the period from March 1994 to January 2003, and included 975 patients. Two hundred and eighty-three records were excluded because data concerning one or more of the independent variables were missing leaving 692 patients for the analysis. Preoperative CT or MR images classified the location of the tumour and extent of the midline shift. The neuroradiological examination was usually performed within 30 days of the operation. To estimate tumour size the maximum cross-sectional area was calculated on the basis of the CT or MR images using the formula for the area of an ellipse (area = abπ, where a is half the length and b is half width of the tumour). Histopathological diagnosis was obtained from the neuropathology report. A radial artery catheter was inserted for continuous blood pressure monitoring and blood sampling. Controlled ventilation (FiO_2 40–50% by oxygen/air) was applied, and the patients were ventilated with $PaCO_2$ and PaO_2 levels attempted to be between 4–5 kPa and >13 kPa, respectively. The level of $PaCO_2$ was achieved by continuous monitoring of pulmonary ventilation and end-tidal CO_2 and verified by arterial blood gas analysis. Four different anaesthetic regimes were used at our Department as "standard" anaesthesia for supratentorial craniotomy (see Chapter 3 for details): isoflurane-fentanyl, sevoflurane-fentanyl, propofol-fentanyl and propofol-remifentanil.

Subdural ICP was measured according to the description in Chapter 3. The integrated mean value of subdural pressure was used as an estimate of ICP. CPP was calculated as the difference between MABP and ICP. Blood was withdrawn simultaneously from the arterial catheter for measurement of arterial oxygen tension and $PaCO_2$. The number of subdural ICP readings with corresponding arterial blood samples ranged from 1 to 3 in each patient, depending on whether ICP-reducing therapy (see below) was instituted. The measurements were performed during a 2- to 15-min time-frame, depending on the number of measurements.

The degree of cerebral swelling was evaluated by the neurosurgeon after opening of dura. Swelling was estimated as follows: (1) the brain below the level of dura; (2) the brain at the level of dura; (3) moderate swelling of the brain; (4) pronounced swelling of the brain.

In study 1 we demonstrated that subdural ICP $\geq 10\,$mmHg is associated with a high probability of cerebral swelling through the dural opening. Consequently, we developed a guideline at our Department to stepwise institute hyperventilation (PaCO$_2$ attempted to be between 3 and 4 kPa), osmotherapy (mannitol 0.5–1 g/kg), 5–15° rTp or indomethacin (bolus dose of 0.2–0.4 mg/kg) to reduce ICP when perioperative recordings of ICP $\geq 10\,$mmHg were obtained. These therapies were instituted in random order in cooperation with the neurosurgeon. None of these therapeutic measures were incorporated in the study. The data selected for analysis from each patient therefore represent the last recording of ICP, haemodynamic and ventilatory values performed immediately before opening of dura and estimation of the degree of brain swelling.

Statistical analysis The outcome variable was dichotomized as the presence (patients classified as having moderate or pronounced brain swelling) or absence (patients classified as having the brain below or at the level of the dura) of cerebral swelling through the dural opening during craniotomy. Several continuous (age, weight, tumour size, midline shift, ICP, MABP, CPP) and categorical (sex, histopathology, tumour localization, anaesthetic regime) independent variables were chosen that potentially contribute to perioperative brain swelling (Table 6.4).

A multivariate logistic regression was performed to determine the predictors of intraoperative brain swelling. The listed independent variables might contribute to the degree of subdural ICP. Consequently the logistic regression analysis was performed with and without adjustment for ICP.

The results of the logistic regression analysis are presented as odds ratios (OR) with confidence intervals and P values. For a continuous variable x, the odds ratio is a measure of the risk change associated with a unit change in x. This estimate is obtained as the logarithm of the slope estimate from the logistic regression analysis. A *P* value <0.05 was considered to be significant. To illustrate the impact of ICP on the risk of brain swelling, a logistic regression curve was computed using the equation $P = P(x_1) = \exp(b_0 + b_1x_1)/[1 + \exp(b_0 + b_1x_1)]$ where *P* is the probability of brain swelling, b_0 and b_1 are the intercept and slope estimates from the logistic regression analysis and x is the ICP. The surgical access during craniotomy often depends on the degree of brain swelling observed. Therefore, the population of patients with brain swelling was selected and divided into two groups: those with moderate brain swelling and those with pronounced brain swelling. Logistic regression analysis was further used to calculate the impact of ICP on the risk of severe brain swelling using the above-mentioned equation.

Table 6.4　Risk factors included in the analysis of perioperative brain swelling

Risk factor	Number	Mean±SD	Percent of total
Age (years)	692	50.0±15.0	
Weight (kg)	692	73.0±16.0	
Men/women	340/352		49.0/51.0
Histopathology			
Glioblastoma	197		28.5
Meningioma	153		22.1
Metastasis	102		14.7
Glioma	182		26.3
Other	58		8.4
Tumour localization			
Frontal	266		38.4
Parietal	136		19.6
Temporal	197		28.5
Occipital	15		2.2
Central	76		11.0
Other	2		0.3
Tumour size (cm^2)	692	13.3±10.0	
Midline shift (mm)	692	5.4±5.8	
Anaesthesia			
Sevoflurane-fentanyl	52		7.5
Isoflurane-fentanyl	120		17.3
Propofol-fentanyl	457		66.0
Propofol-remifentanil	63		9.1
Physiological parameters			
$PaCO_2$ (kPa)	692	4.4±1.0	
MABP (mmHg)	692	81.0±14.0	
Subdural ICP (mmHg)	692	7.0±5.5	
CPP (mmHg)	692	73.0±15.0	

Results　A total of 692 patients were included in this study. Classification of the patients according to the degree of brain swelling is demonstrated in Table 6.5. The logistic regression analysis identified four independent predictors of intraoperative brain swelling (Table 6.6). Subdural ICP was the strongest predictor of intraoperative brain swelling (OR=1.9, 95% CI=1.72–2.10, $P<0.0001$).

Table 6.5 Classification of brain swelling in 692 patients undergoing craniotomy for cerebral tumour

Classification of swelling	Number of patients (% of total)
Brain below the level of dura	59 (8.5%)
Brain at the level of dura	386 (55.8%)
Moderate brain swelling	205 (29.6%)
Pronounced brain swelling	42 (6.1%)

Table 6.6 Risk factors for intraoperative brain swelling after opening of dura in 692 patients with cerebral tumour. Odds ratios are presented without (OR) and with (OR_{adj}) adjustment for subdural ICP. The 95% CI and probability values are listed for each OR_{adj}

Risk factor	OR	OR_{adj}	CI_{adj}	P value$_{adj}$
Age (years)	0.99	1.01	0.99–1.03	0.13
Weight (kg)	1.02	1.01	0.99–1.03	0.16
Men/women	1.08	1.12	0.67–1.83	0.65
Histopathology				
Glioblastoma	1.60	2.10	1.01–4.30	0.047*
Meningioma	1.00	1.00		
Metastasis	2.1	2.9	1.3–6.9	0.011*
Glioma	1.10	1.66	0.77–3.60	0.19
Other	1.10	1.34	0.50–3.60	0.56
Tumour localization				
Frontal	1.00	1.00		
Parietal	1.03	0.74	0.38–1.43	0.37
Temporal	0.97	0.85	0.48–1.52	0.58
Occipital	5.29	3.05	0.49–19.1	0.23
Central	1.90	1.43	0.46–4.51	0.54
Tumour size (cm^2)	1.01	1.01	0.98–1.03	0.68
Midline shift (mm)	1.02	1.06	1.02–1.11	0.008*
Anaesthesia				
Sevoflurane-fentanyl	1.67	1.28	0.50–3.03	0.66
Isoflurane-fentanyl	2.18	1.34	0.72–2.52	0.36
Propofol-fentanyl	1.00	1.00		
Propofol-remifentanil	0.73	1.57	0.63–3.89	0.33
Physiological parameters				
MABP (mmHg)	1.00	1.00	0.98–1.02	0.96
Subdural ICP (mmHg)		1.90	1.72–2.10	0.0001*
CPP (mmHg)	0.973	0.990	0.96–0.98	0.82

*$P<0.05$

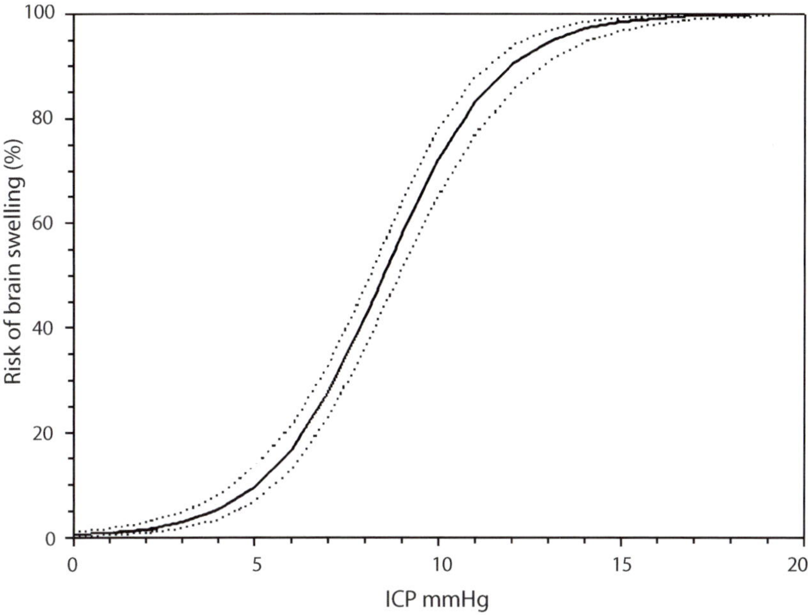

Fig. 6.2 Logistic regression curve with 95% point-wise confidence intervals depicting the relationship between subdural ICP and the percentage risk of brain swelling after opening of dura in 692 patients

The degree of midline shift (OR=1.06, 95% CI=1.02–1.11, P=0.008), a histo-pathological diagnoses of glioblastoma (OR=2.1, 95% CI=1.01–4.3, P=0.047) and metastasis (OR=2.9, 95% CI=1.3–6.9, P=0.01) were independent pre-dictors of brain swelling. The relation between ICP and the risk of moderate and severe brain swelling including 95% confidence intervals is shown in Figure 6.2. At ICP < 5 mmHg brain swelling rarely occurred (5% probability). At ICP > 13 mmHg brain swelling occurred with 95% probability.

Conclusion Subdural ICP is the strongest predictor of intraoperative brain swelling. It is possible to define thresholds of cerebral swelling. At a subdural ICP < 5 mmHg, brain swelling rarely occurred (5% probability); at ICP > 13 mmHg, brain swelling occurred with 95% probability.

Discussion

In the first study we demonstrated that the subdural ICP levels at which cere-bral swelling occurred were independent of pathology (cerebral tumour contra aneurysm), anaesthetic regime (propofol-fentanyl contra isofluranc-nitrous oxide-fentanyl) and level of $PaCO_2$. In the second study we demonstrated that subdural ICP and, to a lesser degree midline shift and histopathological diagnosis (glioblastoma and metastasis), significantly predicted the risk of cerebral swelling after opening of dura in patients with supratentorial cerebral tumours. Furthermore, subdural ICP threshold levels for moderate and severe brain swelling were defined.

In preliminary studies including patients subjected to craniotomy for supra- and infratentorial tumours, a significant correlation was found between subdural ICP and the degree of cerebral swelling (Cold et al. 1996; Jørgensen et al. 1999). In the first study, including 178 patients undergoing craniotomy for supratentorial tumours or subarachnoid haemorrhage, a good correlation was found between subdural ICP and the degree of cerebral swelling after opening of dura mater (Bundgaard et al. 1998). Thus, at subdural ICP < 7 mmHg cerebral swelling rarely occurred, while at ICP > 10 mmHg cerebral swelling occurred with high probability. These thresholds were independent of the pathophysiology (tumour contra subarachnoid haemorrhage), the anaesthetic agents (propofol-fentanyl contra isoflurane-fentanyl) and the $PaCO_2$ level obtained during the subdural ICP measurement. The upper threshold defined in the first study is in accordance with the threshold defined in the second study where an ICP > 10 mmHg was associated with an 83% risk of cerebral swelling (Rasmussen et al. 2004). Furthermore, at ICP > 13 mmHg brain swelling occurred with a 95% probability. However, in contrast to the first study cerebral swelling rarely occurred at ICP < 5 mmHg (5% probability), and ICP < 7 mmHg was associated with a 16% risk of brain swelling. These differences may be explained by the different statistical methods and the number of patients analysed.

The surgical access during craniotomy is impeded when severe brain swelling occurs. In the second study severe brain swelling occurred with a 95% probability at ICP > 26 mmHg. This threshold is higher than reported by Todd et al. (1993) where an ICP of 18 (SD~18) mmHg was associated with severe brain swelling in a sample of 11 patients. The large difference in standard deviation, ICP measurement technique (see below) and a small patient sample size may account for this difference.

Studies of epidural ICP measured through the first burr hole correlates significantly with the degree of cerebral swelling in patients with supratentorial tumours (Todd et al. 1993). The epidural ICP threshold at which cerebral swelling occurs appears to be higher compared with the thresholds obtained with subdural ICP. The ICP technique (epidural contra subdural ICP) may account for this difference. However, other factors may contribute. In the second study a considerable number of patients received ICP-reducing therapy prior to opening of dura. In all of these cases ICP readings were performed repeatedly in an attempt to reduce ICP to ≤ 10 mmHg. In most cases we observed that these therapies reduced ICP to a certain extent. We were, however, only able to estimate the degree of cerebral swelling once in each patient and therefore we cannot provide data whether these interventions reduced the degree of brain swelling. Because we only included the last subdural ICP measurement before opening of the dura, it is likely that the 5% and 95% ICP thresholds for brain swelling would be lower in a patient population which did not receive ICP-reducing therapy. The time interval between epidural ICP measurement through the first burr hole and opening of dura, roughly estimated at about 10–20 min, may interfere because factors influencing ICP, including level of $PaCO_2$ and blood pressure, may differ. Furthermore, cerebral decompression after removal of the bone flap is accompanied by a fall in ICP (Rasmussen et al. 2003), with the size of the craniotomy being likely to influence subdural ICP recordings. After removal of the bone flap subdural ICP is influenced by gravity (Bundgaard and Cold 2000). Thus, ICP in the most declive part of the craniotomy is highest. Furthermore, subdural ICP is influenced by the mass-expanding lesion, being highest if measured in the immediate vicinity of the tumour. Moreover, subdural ICP measurement is a better predictor for the occurrence of brain swelling compared with estimation of dural tension by the neurosurgeon (Cold et al. 1996; Bundgaard et al. 1998). Taking these observations into consideration we therefore hypothesize that subdural ICP is a better estimate of risk of cerebral swelling than estimation of dural tension, intraventricular ICP and epidural ICP, which is measured in the fringe of the craniotomy opening, and consequently at a certain distance from the mass-expanding lesion.

The safety of our ICP measurement technique requires comments. A small subarachnoid haemorrhage after opening of the dura was observed in 0.6% of our patient population. This may be caused by the surgical incision, but we cannot exclude that the haemorrhage was caused by the insertion of the needle. However, in all of these cases ICP was within acceptable limits (mean value of 8 mmHg, data not shown) and the operation progressed without complications. Thus, the incidence of traumatic subarachnoid haemorrhage did not affect the operating conditions. In addition, no visible traumatic lesions of the cortical tissue below the insertion point of the needle was observed.

In previous studies of patients with supratentorial brain tumours, tumour size, ventricular effacement and shift of midline structures are not reliable predictors of elevated ICP measured during craniotomy (Bedford et al. 1982; Todd et al. 1993). In contrast, the degree of cerebral oedema, surrounding the tumour is correlated to ICP (Bedford et al. 1982). Likewise, contralateral ventricular dilatation is an early indicator of intracranial hypertension (Narotam et al. 1993). The significant predictive value of midline shift as well as the non-predictive value of tumour size, found in the present study, must be regarded critically. A mean of 1 week elapsed between the CT scanning and the craniotomy. In this period, the growth of tumour and the formation of cerebral oedema may increase midline shift. On the other hand, corticosteroid treatment may decrease shift of midline structures. We did not estimate the degree of cerebral oedema or the degree of contralateral ventricular dilatation, which in other studies have been documented to correlate to ICP, because estimation would be based on a graduation and not an exact area or volume. Thus, findings from study 2 do not mitigate the need for a more meticulous CT scan-based estimation of tumour size and degree of cerebral oedema immediately before craniotomy; such data would provide more valuable predictive information about the predictive value of CT findings and the related occurrence of degree of brain swelling.

In the second study we demonstrated that patients with glioblastoma and metastasis had a significantly higher odds ratio compared with a diagnosis of meningioma. This observation is explained by the benign nature of the slow-growing meningioma, where cerebral oedema rarely contributes to the mass effect of the tumour.

Unfortunately, we are not able to provide data concerning outcome in these patients. Parameters such as tumour type, tumour location, preoperative morbidity, age and sex may have a strong influence on outcome. Thus, to assess whether prediction of cerebral swelling with measurement of subdural ICP has any influence on surgical outcome would require a large-scale randomized study.

References

Bedford RF, Morris L, Jane JA (1982) Intracranial hypertension during surgery for supratentorial tumour: correlation with preoperative computed tomography scans. Anesth Analg 61:430–433

Bundgaard H, Cold GE (2000) Studies of regional subdural pressure gradients during craniotomy. Br J Neurosurg 14:229–234

Bundgaard H, Landsfeldt U, Cold GE (1998) Subdural monitoring of ICP during craniotomy: thresholds of cerebral swelling/herniation. Acta Neurochir Suppl 71:276–278

Cold GE, Tange M, Jensen TM et al (1996) Subdural pressure measurement during craniotomy. Correlation with tactile estimation of dural tension and brain herniation after opening of dura. Br J Neurosurg 10:69–75

Jorgensen HA, Bundgaard H, Cold GE (1999) Subdural pressure measurement during posterior fossa surgery. Correlation studies of brain swelling/herniation after dural incision with measurement of subdural pressure and tactile estimation of dural tension. Br J Neurosurg 13:449–453

Narotam PK, van Dellen JR, Gouws E (1993) The role of contralateral ventricular dilatation following surgery for intracranial mass lesions. Br J Neurosurg 7:281–286

Rasmussen M, Tankisi T, Cold GE (2004) The effects of indomethacin on intracranial pressure and cerebral haemodynamics in patients undergoing craniotomy. A randomised prospective study. Anaesthesia 59:229–236

Rasmussen M, Bundgaard H, Cold GE (2004) Craniotomy for supratentorial brain tumours: risk factors for brain swelling after opening of dura mater. J Neurosurg 101:621–626

Todd MM, Warner DS, Sokoll MD et al (1993) A prospective, comparative trial of three anesthetics for elective supratentorial craniotomy: propofol/fentanyl, isoflurane/nitrous oxide, and fentanyl/nitrous oxide. Anesthesiology 78:1005–1020

Chapter 7
Subdural Intracranial Pressure, Cerebral Haemodynamics, Dural Tension and Degree of Swelling After Opening of Dura in Patients with Infratentorial Tumours

Mads Rasmussen and Georg Emil Cold

Abstract

The prone position is often recommended for surgery in patients with space-occupying lesions localized in the occipital region or the posterior fossa. Compared to the supratentorial compartment, space-occupying lesions in the smaller infratentorial compartment may have a different influence on subdural ICP and the tendency to brain swelling. In addition, positioning the patient in either the supine, lateral or prone position may influence the level of subdural ICP.

In this chapter we present two studies. In the first study we present data concerning the relationship between the ICP and the degree of brain swelling in patients undergoing infratentorial surgery. In the second study we focus on whether placing the patient in the supine, lateral or prone position has any influence on subdural ICP during surgery for occipital tumours.

The prone position is often recommended for surgery in patients with space-occupying lesions localized in the occipital region or the posterior fossa. However, it has repeatedly been observed that subdural ICP in supine-positioned patients with supratentorial tumours (Rolighed Larsen et al. 2002; Haure et al. 2003; Petersen et al. 2003) is lower compared with ICP in prone-positioned patients subjected to posterior fossa surgery (Jørgensen et al. 1999; Tankisi et al. 2002) or surgery for tumours localized in the occipital region (Tankisi et al. 2002). Theoretically, the prone position causes a higher pressure in the intracerebral venous system, due to the declive position of the head. This suggestion is in accordance with studies indicating a fall in cerebral blood volume during head-up position in awake and anaesthetized subjects (Lovell et al. 2000). Other studies indicate that the prone position results in an increase in abdominal pressure (Hering et al. 2001), and experimental studies have demonstrated that raised intraabdominal pressure increases ICP (Halverson et al. 1998; Rosenthal et al. 1998). Another possibility is that a space-occupying lesion in the smaller infratentorial compartment causes a higher increase in ICP compared with space-occupying lesions in the greater supratentorial compartment. Accordingly, the volume/pressure curve in the infratentorial segment, compared with the supratentorial compartment, is displaced to the left.

In patients with supratentorial tumours a significant relationship was found between the degree of cerebral swelling after opening of dura mater and subdural ICP measured immediately before opening of dura (Rasmussen et al. 2004). In 32 patients subjected to fossa posterior surgery in the prone position the degree of cerebral swelling was related to the level of subdural ICP (Jørgensen et al. 1999). The results indicated that at subdural ICP < 10 mmHg brain swelling rarely occurred, while at ICP > 10 mmHg some degree of cerebral swelling occurred with high probability (Jørgensen et al. 1999). In the present study, which included 109 patients, the relationship between the degree of cerebral swelling after opening of dura and subdural ICP measured immediately before opening of dura was studied in patients subjected to infratentorial cerebral surgery.

In this chapter two studies of patients subjected to craniotomy for infratentorial tumours are presented.

Study 1: The Relationship Between Intracranial Pressure and the Degree of Brain Swelling in Patients Subjected to Infratentorial Surgery

Aim To study the relationship between ICP and the occurrence of brain swelling and to define thresholds for ICP associated with brain swelling in a larger population of adult patients undergoing infratentorial craniotomy.

Method One hundred and nine adult patients subjected to infratentorial surgery were studied. The material included 98 patients with infratentorial tumours, 3 patients with arteriovenous malformations and 8 patients subjected to craniotomy for trigeminus neuralgia. Nine patients were operated in the supine position, 19 patients in the lateral position and 81 patients in the prone position. Propofol-fentanyl was used in 79 patients, propofol- remifentanil in 24 patients and isoflurane-fentanyl in 6 patients. Subdural ICP was measured immediately before opening of dura. Cerebral Perfusion Pressure was calculated as the difference between MABP and ICP. Arterial blood was analysed for $PaCO_2$ and PaO_2. The maximal area and the volume of the intracerebral process were calculated from CT/MRI scans. The degree of dural tension before opening of dura and the degree of cerebral swelling after opening of dura were estimated by the neurosurgeon. Accordingly, four groups were defined: group 1: the brain below the opening of dura mater; group 2: the brain does not swell, but the surface of the brain is at the same level as the opening of

dura mater; group 3: there is moderate swelling of the brain without strangulation at the border of dura mater; group 4: pronounced swelling of the brain
with strangulation of brain tissue.

Statistical analysis Between groups normality test and equal variance test were
applied. If normality tests were passed, one-way analysis of variance was used.
Tukey's test was used for pair-wise multiple comparison procedures. The
Kruskal-Wallis analysis of variance on ranks and multiple comparisons (Dunn's
method) were used for statistical analysis when the normality test or equal variance test were not passed. Means (SD) are indicated for normally distributed
data and median (range) for non-normally distributed data. $P<0.05$ was considered statistically significant. In order to define thresholds for ICP associated
with brain swelling the outcome variable (brain swelling) was dichotomized as
the presence (patients classified as having either moderate or pronounced brain
swelling) or absence (patients classified with brain below or at the level of dura)
of cerebral swelling through the dural opening. Subsequently, a logistic regression curve was calculated using the equation $P = P(x_1) = \exp(b_0 + b_1x_1)/[1 + \exp$
$(b_0 + b_1x_1)]$ where P is the probability of brain swelling, b_0 and b_1 are the intercept
and slope estimates from the logistic regression analysis and x is the ICP.

Results With the exception of the weight of the patients, where patients in
group 4 had a higher weight compared to patients in group 2, no significant differences were disclosed as regards age of the patients, male/female distribution,
the level of $PaCO_2$, PaO_2, rectal temperature, MABP or CPP (Tables 7.1 and 7.4).

The maximal area of the intracranial processes increased from group 1 over
group 2 to group 3, the median levels being 5.2, 5.9 and 11.2 cm^2 in the respective groups and 8.8 cm^2 in group 4. The differences in area in the respective
groups were not significant. The volume of the processes followed the same
tendency, the median (range) being 4.0 (0–13) cm^3 in group 1, 5.1 (0–40) cm^3
in group 2, 13 (0–79) cm^3 in group 3, against 9.3 (2–29) cm^3 in group 4, the
only significant difference being between group 1 and group 3 (Table 7.2).

Table 7.1 Demographic and neuroradiologic data correlated to estimated brain swelling.
The number of patients in each group is shown in the first row. The percentage of total is
indicated in parentheses. Demographic data (age, weight) are given as mean ± SD. Neuroradiological data (tumor area and tumor volume) are given as median (range).

	Group 1 (brain below dura)	Group 2 (brain at the level of dura)	Group 3 (moderate swelling)	Group 4 (pronounced swelling)
Number	10 (9.2%)	35 (32.1%)	42 (38.5%)	22 (20.2%)
Male/female	5/5	18/17	19/23	11/11
Age	51±15	48±17	50±13	49±13
Weight	71±18	70±15	71±15	83±18*
Tumour area (cm^2)	5.2 (0–13)	5.9 (0–26)	11.2 (0–35)	8.8 (3–22)
Tumour volume (cm^3)	4.0 (0–13)	5.1 (0–40)	13 (0–79)#	9.3 (2–29)

*P<0.05 compared to group 2
#P<0.05 compared to group 1

Table 7.2 Maximal tumour area and volume of tumours related to the degree of cerebral swelling after opening of dura. Medians (ranges) are indicated

	Group 1 (brain below dura)	Group 2 (no swelling)	Group 3 (moderate swelling)	Group 4 (pronounced swelling)
Maximal area of tumour (cm^2)	5.2 (0–13)	5.9 (0–26)	11.2 (0–35)	8.8 (3–22)
Volume of tumour (cm^3)	4.0 (0–13)	5.1 (0–40)	13* (0–79)	9.3 (2–29)

*$P<0.05$ between groups 1 and 3

The major groups of pathological diagnosis included metastasis, meningioma and angioma. Astrocytoma was only diagnosed in groups 2, 3 and 4, and patients with trigeminus neuralgia were not represented in group 4. The number of patients in each group was too small to recognize significant differences in distribution (Table 7.3).

The level of ICP increased significantly with increasing degrees of dural swelling. The median (range) being 0.5 (–1 to 7) mmHg in group 1, 6.0 (–1 to 13) mmHg in group 2, 13.5 (7–24) mmHg in group 3 and 21.0 (15–37) mmHg in group 4. The difference in ICP between groups 1 and 2 was not significant, but between the groups 2, 3 and 4 and the groups 1, 3 and 4 significant differences in ICP were disclosed (Table 7.4).

At ICP levels < 7 mmHg cerebral swelling was not observed. Moderate cerebral swelling was observed in all patients when ICP exceeded 13 mmHg. Pronounced cerebral swelling was observed in all patients at ICP > 24 mmHg. In order to identify specifically the thresholds of ICP for the occurrence of brain swelling a logistic regression analysis was performed. The logistic regression analysis identified that an ICP equal to or greater than 13 mmHg was associated with a 95% probability of brain swelling. At an ICP less than 6 mmHg, brain swelling occurred with a 5% probability (Figure 7.1).

Table 7.3 Pathology of infratentorial tumours related to the degree of cerebral swelling after opening of dura

	Group 1 (brain below dura)	Group 2 (no swelling)	Group 3 (moderate swelling)	Group 4 (pronounced swelling)
Metastasis	4	10	22	8
Meningioma	1	3	4	4
Angioma	1	7	3	7
Astrocytoma	0	5	0	1
Trigeminus neuralgia	2	3	3	0
Arteriovenous malformation	0	2	1	0
Other pathology	2	5	7	2

Table 7.4 The levels of rectal temperature, $PaCO_2$, PaO_2, MABP, CPP and ICP related to the degree of brain swelling after opening of dura. Mean±SD are indicated for normally distributed data and median (range) for non-normally distributed data

	Group 1 (brain below dura)	Group 2 (no swelling)	Group 3 (moderate swelling)	Group 4 (pronounced swelling)
Temperature (°C)	36.2±0.9	35.8±0.4	35.8±0.6	36.0±0.5
$PaCO_2$ (kPa)	4.5±0.5	4.4±0.6	4.3±0.4	4.4±0.4
PaO_2 (kPa)	23.0±5.9	28.0±9.5	28.0±8.3	27.0±6.6
MABP (mmHg)	77.0±13.0	84.0±15.0	87.0±15.0	89.0±17.0
Median ICP (mmHg) (range)	0.5 (−1.0 to 7.0)	6.0 (−1.0 to 13.0)	13.5* (7.0–24.0)	21.0* (15.0–27.0)
CPP (mmHg)	76.0±13.0	79.0±16.0	72.0±13.0	68.0±19.0

*$P<0.05$ compared with all lower groups

Conclusion   In this study a significant relationship was found between subdural ICP and the degree of cerebral swelling after opening of dura. In patients with ICP below 7 mmHg no swelling of the brain was observed. Moderate brain swelling was found if ICP exceeded 13 mmHg, and pronounced swelling developed at ICP exceeding 24 mmHg. Specific thresholds for ICP were calculated. A 95% and 5% risk of brain swelling was observed at ICP ≥ 13 mmHg and at ICP < 6 mmHg. Thresholds for ICP associated with brain swelling are close to thresholds defined in patients undergoing supratentorial surgery.

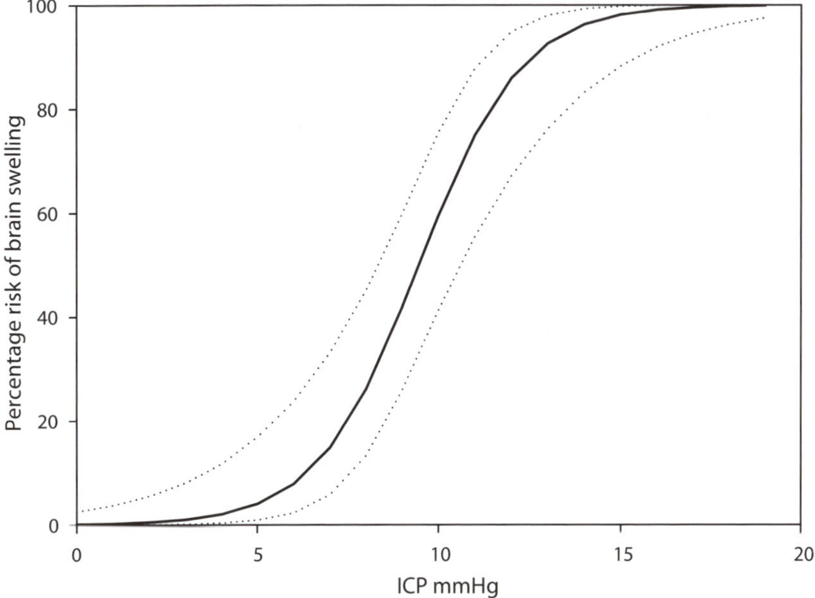

Fig. 7.1   Risk of brain swelling after opening of the dura at different ICP levels

Study 2: Patients Subjected to Craniotomy for Occipital Tumours with Special Reference to Position

Aim To measure subdural ICP in anaesthetized patients with occipital tumours positioned in the supine, lateral or prone position.

Method Thirty-three patients were operated in the prone position, 9 in the supine position and 20 in the lateral position. Anaesthesia was maintained with either propofol-fentanyl or propofol-remifentanil. As regards anaesthetic methods, neuroradiological and pathological data, monitoring of subdural ICP and cerebral haemodynamics, see Chapter 3. Subdural ICP and JBP were measured before opening of dura. CPP was calculated as the difference between MABP and ICP. The neurosurgeon estimated the degree of dural tension before opening of dura and the degree of cerebral swelling immediately after opening of dura.

Statistical analysis Between groups normality test and equal variance test were applied. If the normality tests were passed, one-way analysis of variance was used. Tukey's test was used for pair-wise multiple comparison procedures. The Kruskal-Wallis analysis of variance on ranks and multiple comparisons (Dunn's method) were used for statistical analysis when the normality test or equal variance test were not passed. Means (SD) are indicated. $P<0.05$ was considered statistically significant.

Results No significant difference was found between the three positions as regards demographic data (age, height, weight, sex), neuroradiological data (maximal area of tumour, volume of the tumour or midline shift). Neither did the maintenance dose of propofol differ significantly (Table 7.5).
No significant difference was found as regards $PaCO_2$ or CPP. ICP averaged 18.7, 13.2 and 11.0 mmHg in prone-positioned, supine-positioned and laterally positioned patients, respectively ($P<0.001$ between positions). In the prone position JBP averaged 10.9 mmHg against 6.1 mmHg in the lateral position and 6.0 mmHg in the supine position. ICP and JBP were significantly higher in the prone position compared with the values observed in the lateral position. Likewise, ICP and JBP were significantly higher in prone-positioned patients compared with patients positioned otherwise (Table 7.6). Dural tension and degree of swelling were significantly more pronounced in the prone position compared with patients positioned otherwise (Table 7.7). In both propofol- fentanyl- and propofol-remifentanil-anaesthetized patients the level of ICP followed the same tendency with higher ICP levels in the prone position compared with the supine and lateral positions. The differences in ICP between positions were significant in propofol-remifentanil- anaesthetized patients ($P<0.001$), but not in propofol-fentanyl-anaesthetized patients ($P=0.07$). In prone-positioned patients a significant positive correlation was disclosed between JBP and subdural ICP ($ICP = 5.762 + 1.13 \times JBP$; $r=0.6541$, $P=0.002$, power 0.897). In the combined group of laterally and supine-positioned patients, the correlation between JBP and ICP was insignificant ($P=0.405$).

Table 7.5 Data concerning demography, neuroradiological findings and anaesthesia in prone-, laterally, supine- and lateral + supine-positioned patients with occipital tumours. Mean±SD are indicated

	Prone position	Lateral position	Supine position	Lateral+supine position
Number	33	20	9	29
Men/women	15/18	16/4	4/5	20/9
Age (years)	52.8±16.2	46.0±20.6	55.7±12.2	52.7±15.6
Weight (kg)	74.3±17.0	72.2±11.3	75.7±11.5	74.6±11.4
Height (cm)	172.0±7.0	172.0±8.0	176.0±9.0	175.0±8.0
Radiology				
Maximal area of tumour (cm^2)	13.5±7.6	11.3±6.3	11.3±6.3	11.5±6.9
Volume of tumour (cm^3)	23.6±17.8	19.8±16.5	19.8±16.5	19.8±15.3
Midline shift (mm)	4.9±5.9	3.8±4.9	2.9±4.6	3.5±4.7
Anaesthesia				
Propofol (mg/h)	618.0±199.0	552.0±246.0	656.0±174.0	584.0±192.0

Table 7.6 $PaCO_2$, ICP, CPP and JBP in prone-, laterally, supine- and lateral + supine-positioned patients with occipital tumours. Mean±SD are indicated

	Prone position	Lateral position	Supine position	Lateral+supine position
$PaCO_2$ (kPa)	4.4±0.5	4.7±0.4	4.4±0.6	4.6±0.5
ICP (mmHg)	18.7±6.8*	11.0±5.4	13.2±7.5	11.7±6.1
CPP (mmHg)	64.1±14.0	69.3±13.0	73.6±11.3	70.6±19.0
JBP (mmHg)	10.9±4.8*	6.1±5.1	6.0±1.4	6.1±4.8

*$P<0.05$ from prone position

Table 7.7 Degree of dural tension and degree of cerebral swelling after opening of dura in prone-, laterally, supine- and lateral + supine-positioned patients with occipital tumours. Number of patients is indicated (*$P<0.05$ from normal tension)

	Prone position	Lateral position	Supine position	Lateral+supine position
Tension of dura				
Normal	6	3	10	13
Increased	12	4	9	13
Pronounced	15*	2	1	3
Cerebral swelling				
None	4	3	9	12
Moderate	6	4	10	14
Pronounced	22*	2	1	3

Conclusion In the present study ICP and JBP were significantly higher in the prone position compared with the supine and lateral position. These findings suggest that the high ICP found in prone-positioned patients is partially caused by an increase in cerebral venous blood volume.

Discussion

The level of ICP is of importance in the surgical management of space-occupying cerebral lesions. At high ICP surgical access to deep cerebral structures is impeded, and pressure by self-retaining specula may decrease cerebral perfusion regionally (Albin et al. 1977; Hongo et al. 1987; Rosenørn 1987). Likewise, swelling/herniation of cerebral tissue through the opening of dura may be deleterious by preventing venous outflow from brain tissue. Thereby, a vicious circle may develop with increasing cerebral oedema and ischaemia, and surgical access is impeded or even prevented.

In preliminary studies in patients with supratentorial tumours (Cold et al. 1996; Bundgaard et al. 1997) and infratentorial tumours (Jørgensen et al. 1999) of the relationship between subdural ICP, the degree of dural tension and the degree of cerebral swelling after opening of dura, it has been documented that the subdural ICP correlates better to the degree of cerebral swelling/herniation as compared with the tactile estimation of dural tension by the neurosurgeon. One reason may be the experience of the neurosurgeon; another reason may be that the thickness of dura makes interpretation of dural tension, as an indicator of intracranial hypertension, difficult. If ICP is below 5–7 mmHg cerebral swelling rarely occurs, while subdural ICP above 13 mmHg is accompanied by moderate cerebral swelling, and at ICP above 26 mmHg pronounced cerebral swelling occurs after opening of dura (Cold et al. 1996; Jørgensen et al. 1999; Rasmussen et al. 2004). The threshold of swelling is independent of the level of $PaCO_2$, choice of anaesthesia and diagnosis (tumour versus aneurysm surgery) (Bundgaard et al. 1997).

In recent studies subdural ICP was high in prone-positioned patients with infratentorial space-occupying lesions (Jørgensen et al. 1999; Tankisi et al. 2002), compared with subdural ICP observed in patients with supratentorial space-occupying processes (Petersen et al. 2003; Rolighed Larsen et al. 2002).

The first study included 109 patients subjected to infratentorial surgery. One hundred and one patients had mass lesions due to tumour ($n=98$) or arteriovenous malformation ($n=2$), while 8 patients were without space-occupying lesions, being operated for trigeminus neuralgia. In patients with ICP below 7 mmHg no swelling of the brain was observed. Moderate brain swelling was found if ICP exceeded 13 mmHg and pronounced swelling developed at ICP exceeding 24 mmHg. It is remarkable that these thresholds are similar or very close to those found in patients subjected to surgery for supratentorial space-occupying lesions where the respective thresholds for swelling were as follows: At ICP < 5 mmHg brain swelling occurred with 5% probability, at ICP exceeding 13 mmHg brain swelling occurred with 95% probability and at an ICP exceeding 26 mmHg severe cerebral swelling occurred with 95% probability (Rasmussen et al. 2004). The percentage of patients in the respective swelling groups were 9.2%, 32.1%, 35.5%, and 20.2%. In comparison the percentages in patients with supratentorial brain tumours were 8.5%, 55.8%, 29.6% and 6.1% (Rasmussen et al. 2004). The proportions of observations in the two studies vary significantly ($P<0.001$), indicating that the occurrence of cerebral swelling in infratentorial surgery is higher compared with supratentorial tumour surgery, but that the corresponding levels of ICP in each group are identical in patients subjected to infratentorial and supratentorial surgery. In patients subjected to craniotomy in the prone position, ICP averaged 18.3 mmHg for patients with occipital tumours and 21.0 mmHg for those with infratentorial tumours (Tankisi et al. 2002). These levels of ICP were identical with the ICP levels observed in another study of infratentorial tumours (Jørgensen et al. 1999). In comparison, the levels of ICP are considerably lower in patients subjected to supratentorial surgery in the supine position, where subdural ICP averaged 7.5, 7.0 and 10.9 mmHg (Haure et al. 2003; Petersen et al. 2003; Rasmussen et al. 2004). Likewise, an increase in ICP occurs in head injury patients when turned from the supine to the prone position (Lee 1989).

The high levels of ICP found during intracranial surgery in prone-positioned patients are associated with a high jugular venous pressure averaging 14.3 and 12.1 mmHg in patients with occipital tumours and infratentorial tumours, respectively (Tankisi et al. 2002). In comparison JBP averaged 8 mmHg in patients operated on in the supine position (Rolighed Larsen et al. 2002). During change in position to 10° rTp a decrease in ICP and jugular venous pressure is observed within 1 min (Tankisi et al. 2002). These findings suggest that the high jugular venous pressure partly causes the high ICP found in prone-positioned patients. Accordingly, a fall in cerebral blood volume during head-up position in awake and anaesthetized subjects has been demonstrated (Lovell et al. 2000). The prone position also results in an increase in ICP and a fall in CPP in patients with subarachnoid haemorrhage and acute respiratory distress syndrome (ARDS) (Reinprecht et al. 2003). Furthermore, the abdominal pressure increases (Hering et al. 2001), and in experimental studies an increase in intraabdominal pressure increases ICP (Halverson et al. 1998; Rosenthal et al. 1998). Accordingly, in patients with severe head injury ICP is higher in prone-positioned patients compared with supine-positioned patients (Lee 1989), and a rise in ICP occurs when patients with subarachnoid haemorrhage and ARDS are turned from the supine to the prone position (Reinprecht et al. 2003). One reason could be that the gravity of the brain increases ICP in the underlying brain tissue in prone-positioned patients. This has been documented in supine-positioned patients subjected to craniotomy for supratentorial tumours (Bundgaard and Cold 2000). However, it cannot be the reason in prone-positioned patients with occipital tumours, because the occipital lobe is positioned superior to other supratentorial brain structures. Another reason could be that tumour size in the smaller infratentorial compartment gives rise to a more pronounced ICP increase. A third reason might be that intracranial blood volume increases in the prone position, because of the declive position of the head. This reason is supported by the observation that the abdominal pressure increases in prone-positioned patients (Hering et al. 2001; Reinprecht et al. 2003), and by experimental studies showing that an increase in intraabdominal pressure is accompanied by an increase in ICP (Halverson et al. 1998; Rosenthal et al. 1998).

In the second study presented in this chapter, the position of the space-occupying lesion in the infra- contra supratentorial compartment is eliminated, because only patients with occipital processes were included. At the neurosurgeons discretion three different positions, including supine, lateral and prone, were analysed, and the values of subdural ICP and JBP were compared. Significantly higher subdural ICP and JBP were observed in prone-positioned patients, compared with patients positioned laterally, or patients positioned in a combined group including both laterally positioned patients and supine-positioned patients. In prone-positioned patients the correlation between JBP and ICP was positive and significant. Furthermore, the degree of dural tension and the degree of cerebral swelling was more pronounced in prone-positioned patients, compared with patients in the supine position and the lateral position. The use of two anaesthetic procedures, including propofol-fentanyl and propofol-remifentanil, might influence the significant differences in ICP. However, ICP in the respective anaesthetic groups followed the same tendency, with a higher ICP in prone-positioned patients compared with ICP in supine- and laterally positioned patients, and with a significant difference in ICP in propofol-remifentanil-anaesthetized patients, but not in propofol-fentanyl-anaesthetized patients.

A positive correlation between JBP and ICP has previously been documented in patients subjected to supratentorial craniotomy in either propofol-fentanyl or propofol-remifentanil anaesthesia (Chapter 8, study 3). Furthermore, studies of the effect of rTp in prone-positioned patients (Tankisi et al. 2002) and supine-positioned patients (Haure et al. 2003; Rolighed Larsen et al. 2002) have shown a decrease in both jugular venous pressure and ICP when the operating table is tipped to a head up position.

To avoid cerebral swelling after opening of dura, subdural ICP measurement is a guide. Recently, thresholds of ICP at which moderate or pronounced cerebral swelling occurs have been defined. These thresholds are identical in supratentorial (Rasmussen et al. 2004; Chapter 6) and infratentorial surgery (Chapter 7). Thus at ICP below 5–7 mmHg cerebral swelling rarely occurs, while at ICP exceeding 13 mmHg some degree of cerebral swelling occurs with high probability, and at ICP > 26 mmHg pronounced swelling occurs. Therefore, if ICP exceeds 13 mmHg therapeutic measures to reduce ICP should be initiated. Comparative studies of therapeutic methods in the treatment of perioperative intracranial hypertension are discussed in Chapter 17.

References

Albin MS, Bunegin L, Bennett MH et al (1977) Clinical and experimental brain retractor pressure monitoring. Acta Neurol Scand 56(suppl 64):522–573

Bundgaard H, Cold GE (2000) Studies of regional subdural pressure gradients during craniotomy. Br J Neurosurg 14:229–234

Bundgaard H, Landsfeldt U, Cold GE (1998) Subdural monitoring of ICP during craniotomy: thresholds of cerebral swelling/herniation. Acta Neurochir Suppl 71:276–279

Cold GE, Tange M, Jensen TM et al (1996) Subdural pressure measurement during craniotomy. Correlation with tactile estimation of dural tension and brain herniation after opening of dura. Br J Neurosurg 10:69–75

Halverson A, Buchanan R, Jacobs L et al (1998) Evaluation of mechanism of increased intracranial pressure with insufflation. Surg Endosc 12:266–269

Haure P, Cold GE, Hansen TM (2003) The ICP-lowering effect of 10° reverse Trendelenburg position during craniotomy is stable during a 1-minute period. J Neurosurg Anesthesiol 15:297–301

Hering R, Wrigge H, Vorwerk R et al (2001) The effects of prone positioning on intraabdominal pressure and cardiovascular and renal function in patients with acute lung injury. Anesth Analg 92:1226–1231

Hongo K, Kabayashi S, Yokoh A (1987) Monitoring retraction pressure in the brain. J Neurosurg 66:270–275

Iversen BN, Rasmussen M, Cold GE (2008) The relationship between intracranial pressure and the degree of brain swelling in patients subjected to infratentorial surgery. Acta Neurochir 150:337–344

Jørgensen HA, Bundgaard H, Cold GE (1999) Subdural pressure measurement during posterior fossa surgery. Correlation studies of brain swelling/herniation after dural incision with measurement of subdural pressure and tactile estimation of dural tension. Br J Neurosurg 13:449–453

Lee ST (1989) Intracranial pressure changes during positioning of patients with severe head injury. Heart Lung 18:411–414

Lovell AT, Marschall AC, Elwell CE et al (2000) Changes in cerebral blood volume with changes in position in awake and anesthetized subjects. Anesth Analg 90:372–376

Petersen KD, Landsfeldt U, Cold GE et al (2003) Intracranial pressure and cerebral hemodynamic in patients with cerebral tumours. Anesthesiology 98:329–336

Rasmussen M, Bundgaard H, Cold GE (2004) Craniotomy for supratentorial brain tumours: risk factors of brain swelling after opening of the dura. J Neurosurg 101:621–626

Reinprecht A, Greher M, Wolfsberger S et al (2003) Prone position in subarachnoid hemorrhage patients with acute respiratory distress syndrome: effects on cerebral tissue oxygenation and intracranial pressure. Crit Care Med 31:1831–1838

Rolighed Larsen JK, Haure P, Cold GE (2002) Reverse Trendelenburg position reduces intracranial pressure during craniotomy. J Neurosurg Anesthesiol 14:16–21

Rosenørn J (1987) Self-retaining brain retractor pressure during intracranial procedures. Acta Neurochir 85:17–22

Rosenthal RJ, Friedman RL, Chidambaram A et al (1998) Effects of hyperventilation and hypoventilation on $PaCO_2$ and intracranial pressure during acute elevation of intraabdominal pressure with CO_2 pneumo-peritoneum: large animal observations. J Am Coll Surg 187:32–38

Tankisi A, Rolighed Larsen J, Rasmussen M et al (2002) The effects of 10° reverse Trendelenburg position of ICP and CPP in prone positioned patients subjected to craniotomy for occipital and cerebellar tumours. Acta Neurochir 144:665–670

Chapter 8
Subdural Intracranial Pressure During General Anaesthesia for Craniotomy in Patients with Supratentorial Cerebral Tumours

Lise Schlünzen and Georg Emil Cold

Abstract

Supratentorial cerebral tumours represent the bulk of intracranial pathological processes presented in most clinics. Some patients have small tumours in important deep areas and others have large tumours creating midline shift but situated close to the surface of the brain. Regardless of pathology the team treating the patient must work to create the best possible environment in the surgical field, thus giving the patient optimal chances for curative surgery. The choice of anaesthetic agent is known to influence both cerebral blood volume and other cerebral haemodynamic parameters.

In this chapter three studies of patients with supratentorial tumours are presented. Two of the studies investigate the anaesthetic techniques and the influence on cerebral haemodynamics, and the third includes the histopathological diagnosis of the tumour and relates this to the measured parameters

Anaesthesia for craniotomy has to be carried out with emphasis on haemodynamic stability, a sufficient CPP and avoidance of agents or procedures that increase the ICP. Experimental and clinical studies of cerebral haemodynamics, including CBF, $CMRO_2$ and ICP, have been carried out during isoflurane (Adams et al. 1981; Madsen et al. 1987a, b; Algotsson et al. 1988; Gordon et al. 1988; Olsen et al. 1994; Talke et al. 1996; Artru et al. 1997), sevoflurane (Scheller et al. 1988; Artru et al. 1997; Bundgaard et al. 1998; Talke et al. 1999) and propofol anaesthesia (Moos and Price 1990; Pinaud et al. 1990; Ramani et al. 1992; Alkire et al. 1995; Oshima et al. 2002). Clinical studies indicate that when isoflurane (Madsen et al. 1987a, b; Algotsson et al. 1988; Olsen et al. 1994) or sevoflurane (Artru et al. 1997; Bundgaard et al. 1998; Mielck et al. 1999) are administered CBF and $CMRO_2$ are reduced as compared to values obtained in awake normocapnic subjects. An increase in ICP has been found during anaesthesia with isoflurane (Adams et al. 1981; Talke et al. 1996) and sevoflurane (Talke et al. 1999), and an increase in CBF has been disclosed during isoflurane (Olsen et al. 1994) and sevoflurane anaesthesia (Bundgaard et al. 1998). However, in other studies of isoflurane (Madsen et al. 1987a, b; Artru et al. 1997) and sevoflurane (Scheller et al. 1988; Artru et al. 1997; Schlünzen et al. 2004), global CBF and ICP are unchanged. In contrast, a dose-related decrease in CBF, $CMRO_2$ and ICP has been found during propofol anaesthesia (Moss and Price 1990; Pinaud et al. 1990; Ramani et al. 1992; Alkire et al. 1995).

Only a few clinical comparative studies of ICP are available. In a prospective trial of three anaesthetic techniques for elective supratentorial craniotomy (isoflurane-nitrous oxide, fentanyl-nitrous oxide and propofol-fentanyl), epidural ICP measured through the first burr hole did not differ significantly, but more patients in the isoflurane-nitrous oxide group had ICP $\geq 24\,mmHg$ than in the other two groups (Todd et al. 1993). In contrast, a significantly lower ICP and higher CPP were found in tumour patients anaesthetized with propofol-fentanyl compared with isoflurane-fentanyl or sevoflurane-fentanyl, and in the same study the degree of dural tension and brain swelling after opening of dura were less pronounced in patients allocated to propofol-fentanyl (Petersen et al. 2003). Other studies of lumbar CSF pressure for neurosurgical anaesthesia disclosed contrasting results, no difference during propofol versus thiopental-isoflurane (Ravussin et al. 1991), but significantly lower ICP during propofol anaesthesia compared to isoflurane and sevoflurane anaesthesia (Moss and Price 1990; Talke et al. 1996).

In this presentation the randomized study by Petersen et al. (2003) is recapitulated. Moreover, based on our database, further studies are presented where special attention has been paid to the relation between pathology and ICP (the second part of the study), and the level of ICP related to jugular venous pressure (the third part of the study).

Study 1: Subdural Intracranial Pressure and Cerebral Haemodynamics in Patients with Supratentorial Cerebral Tumours Randomized to Either Propofol-Fentanyl, Isoflurane-Fentanyl or Sevoflurane-Fentanyl Anaesthesia

Aims The primary aims of the present study were to investigate whether significant differences in subdural ICP and cerebral haemodynamics existed between the three anaesthetic regimes (propofol-fentanyl, isoflurane-fentanyl and sevoflurane-fentanyl) and to study the incidence of cerebral swelling after opening of dura.

Method One hundred and seventeen patients were enrolled in the study. Forty-one patients were allocated to the propofol-fentanyl group, and the isoflurane-fentanyl and sevoflurane-fentanyl groups were allocated 38 patients each. Concerning neuroradiological findings, anaesthetic maintenance doses and monitoring, see Chapter 3.

Statistical analysis Data within groups were tested for normal distribution. Within groups the paired t-test or Wilcoxon signed rank test was used. Between groups the normality test and equal variance test were applied. Intergroup analyses included one-way analysis of variance. The Tukey test was used for pair-wise multiple comparison procedures. The Kruskal-Wallis analysis of variance on ranks, and multiple comparisons versus control groups (Dunn's method) were used for statistical analysis when the normality test or equal variance test were not passed. The chi-square test was used for statistical analysis of proportions of observation within neuroradiological, histopathological findings and the degrees of dura tension and brain swelling. Medians (ranges) are indicated. $P<0.05$ was considered statistically significant.

Results Data concerning neuroradiological findings, pathology and anaesthesia are summarized in Table 8.1. No significant differences were found as regards demographic, histopathology and neuroradiological findings. Data obtained after removal of the bone flap are indicated in Table 8.2. Subdural ICP and jugular saturation were significantly lower while MABP and CPP were significantly higher during propofol-fentanyl compared to isoflurane-fentanyl and sevoflurane-fentanyl. The distributions of the tactile estimate of dural tension are indicated in Table 8.3. Dural tension was significantly lower during propofol-fentanyl compared with the isoflurane-fentanyl.

Table 8.1 Data including demographics, neuroradiological data, pathology and anaesthesia. Numbers or mean (SD) are indicated

	Propofol-fentanyl	Isoflurane-fentanyl	Sevoflurane-fentanyl
Number of patients	41	38	38
Men/women	20/21	16/22	20/18
Age (years)	55 (14)	55 (10)	53 (11)
Midline shift (mm)	5.5 (5.4)	4.2 (4.0)	4.4 (4.1)
Maximal area of tumour (cm^2)	13.7 (3.4)	13.9 (14.7)	14.8 (13.7)
Glioblastoma	16	10	16
Meningioma	8	12	12
Glioma	10	8	3
Metastasis	4	5	6
Other tumours	3	3	1
Maintenance of propofol (mg/kg/h)	9.2 (1.8)	0	0
Fentanyl (µg/kg/h)	2.2 (0.7)	1.9 (0.4)*	2.0 (0.4)
MAC of volatile agent	0	0.9 (0.1)	1.0 (0.0)

*$P<0.05$ compared with propofol-fentanyl

Table 8.2 Data obtained in patients subjected to craniotomy for cerebral tumours after removal of the bone flap. Mean (SD) are indicated

	Propofol-fentanyl	Isoflurane-fentanyl	Sevoflurane-fentanyl
Rectal temperature (°C)	35.8 (0.4)	36.0 (0.6)	35.9 (0.7)
$PaCO_2$ (mmHg)	34.5 (3.0)	34.5 (3.0)	36.0 (3.0)
PaO_2 (mmHg)	203 (68)	197 (66)	179 (67)
MABP (mmHg)	86 (14)	73 (10)	76 (10)
Subdural ICP (mmHg)	7.5 (4.9)	13.0 (7.5)*	13.2 (7.1)*
CPP (mmHg)	78 (15)	60 (12)*	63 (8)*
Jugular saturation (%)	57 (10)	65 (11)*	65 (12)*

*$P<0.05$ compared with propofol-fentanyl

Table 8.3 Degree of dural tension in patients subjected to craniotomy for cerebral tumours after removal of the bone flap. Numbers (%) are indicated

Dural tension	Propofol-fentanyl	Isoflurane-fentanyl*	Sevoflurane-fentanyl
Dura very slack	4 (9.8)	1 (2.6)	1 (2.6)
Normal tension	22 (53.7)	11 (28.9)	14 (36.8)
Increased tension	13 (31.7)	20 (52.6)	21 (55.3)
Pronounced increased	2 (4.9)	6 (15.8)	2 (5.3)

*$P<0.05$ compared with propofol-fentanyl

Conclusion The study indicates that subdural ICP and jugular saturation are significantly lower and CPP higher in propofol-fentanyl-anaesthetized patients compared with patients anaesthetized with isoflurane-fentanyl or sevoflurane-fentanyl. Moreover, the degree of dural tension was less pronounced in patients subjected to propofol-fentanyl anaesthesia compared with isoflurane-fentanyl anaesthesia.

Study 2: Subdural Intracranial Pressure and Cerebral Haemodynamics in Patients Operated on in the Supine Position for Supratentorial Glioblastoma, Meningioma and Metastasis

Aim To investigate whether the histopathology of supratentorial brain tumours (glioblastoma, meningioma and metastasis) influenced the level of subdural ICP and cerebral haemodynamics during maintenance anaesthesia with propofol-fentanyl, isoflurane-fentanyl and sevoflurane-fentanyl.

Method Data from supine-positioned patients with supratentorial cerebral tumours, including glioblastoma ($n=272$), metastasis ($n=250$) or meningioma ($n=163$), were included in the present study. Four anaesthetic procedures were compared: Propofol-fentanyl ($n=393$), propofol-remifentanil ($n=128$), isoflurane-fentanyl (n=107) and sevoflurane-fentanyl (n=57). Concerning histopathology, neuroradiological findings, anaesthesia maintenance doses and monitoring during anaesthesia, see Chapter 3.

Statistical analysis   Data within groups were tested for normal distribution. Within groups the paired t-test or Wilcoxon signed rank test was used. Between groups the normality test and equal variance test were applied. Intergroup analyses included one-way analysis of variance. The Tukey test was used for pair-wise multiple comparison procedures. The Kruskal-Wallis analysis of variance on ranks, and multiple comparisons versus control groups (Dunn's method) were used for statistical analysis when the normality test or equal variance test were not passed. The chi-square test was used for statistical analysis of proportions of observation within neuroradiological, histopathological findings and the degrees of dura tension and brain swelling. Medians (ranges) are indicated. $P<0.05$ was considered statistically significant.

Results   In Table 8.4 the distribution of localization of the tumours in the four different diagnostic groups are indicated. Frontal and temporal localization dominated, followed by parietal localization. In patients with meningioma basal localization was represented. In each anaesthetic group the percentage of glioblastoma was highest. Thus, in the propofol-fentanyl group 43.8% were operated on for glioblastoma, in the propofol-remifentanil group 36.3%, in the isoflurane-fentanyl group 37.6% and in the sevoflurane-fentanyl group 50%. In total 685 patients were included in the study.

In Table 8.5 the maintenance doses of anaesthetics are indicated. In all diagnostic groups the doses of propofol were significantly lower in the propofol-remifentanil group compared with the propofol-fentanyl group. The degrees of dural tension are indicated in Table 8.6. The percentages of patients with pronounced dural tension were generally lower with propofol-fentanyl (4.5–9.2%) or propofol-remifentanil (7.3–14.3%) anaesthesia compared with isoflurane-fentanyl (12.5–28%) or sevoflurane-fentanyl (9.5–21.5%) anaesthetia. Conversely, the percentages of patients with normal dural tension were higher in patients anaesthetized with propofol-fentanyl (52.4–60%) and propofol-remifentanil (61.0–71.4%) compared with isoflurane-fentanyl (34.3–46.9%) or sevoflurane-fentanyl (28.6–50%).

In Table 8.7 the level of midline shift, maximal area of tumour, volume of tumour, $PaCO_2$, PaO_2, rectal temperature, MABP, ICP and CPP are related to diagnostic groups and anaesthetic technique. Within each diagnostic group no significant differences in neuroradiological parameters were found between anaesthetic groups. No significant differences as regards $PaCO_2$, PaO_2 or rectal temperature were found between the four anaesthetic techniques. In patients with glioblastoma significant differences between ICP were found. The mean values of ICP during isoflurane-fentanyl (12.7 mmHg) or sevoflurane-fentanyl anaesthesia (13.1 mmHg) were significantly higher than during propofol-fentanyl (9.7 mmHg), which was significantly higher compared with propofol-remifentanil (6.7 mmHg). In patients with meningioma anaesthetized

Table 8.4 Histopathology and localization of tumour in patients subjected to craniotomy. Four different anaesthetic techniques were used.

Anaesthesia	Diagnosis	Frontal	Parietal	Temporal	Central	Hemispheric	Basal	Total	Percent
Propofol	Glioblastoma	56	32	65	12	5	0	170	43.3
-fentanyl	Metastasis	32	30	32	3	0	0	97	24.6
	Meningioma	55	32	21	3	0	15	126	32.1
Propofol	Glioblastoma	16	11	16	2	1	0	46	35.9
-remifentanil	Metastasis	15	7	10	1	0	0	33	25.8
	Meningioma	21	10	5	0	0	13	49	38.3
Isoflurane	Glioblastoma	11	12	11	0	0	0	34	31.8
-fentanyl	Metastasis	8	9	3	1	0	2	23	21.5
	Meningioma	20	12	13	1	0	4	50	46.7
Sevoflurane	Glioblastoma	8	7	7	0	0	0	22	38.6
-fentanyl	Metastasis	2	4	4	0	0	0	10	17.5
	Meningioma	9	10	3	0	0	3	25	43.9
Total		253	176	190	23	6	37	685	

Table 8.5 Maintenance dose of anaesthesia related to diagnosis (glioblastoma, metastasis or meningioma) in patients with supratentorial tumours. Four different anaesthetic techniques were used

Anaesthesia	Diagnosis	Maintenance dose of propofol (mg/h)	Maintenance dose of fentanyl (µg/h)	Maintenance dose of remifentanil (mg/h)	Isoflurane (MAC)	Sevoflurane (MAC)
Propofol -fentanyl	Glioblastoma	669±186	133±34	0	0	0
	Metastasis	603±170	127±35	0	0	0
	Meningioma	610±186	129±36	0	0	0
Propofol -remifentanil	Glioblastoma	397±88*	0	2.25±0.65	0	0
	Metastasis	396±106*	0	1.94±0.72	0	0
	Meningioma	385±107*	0	1.86±0.66	0	0
Isoflurane -fentanyl	Glioblastoma	0	125±36		0.71±0.29	
	Metastasis	0	113±40		0.86±0.31	
	Meningioma	0	120±42		0.89±0.23	
Sevoflurane -fentanyl	Glioblastoma	0	128±33	0	0	0.76±0.16
	Metastasis	0	156±68	0	0	0.70±0.12
	Meningioma	0	135±37	0	0	0.87±0.18

*P<0.05 compared with propofol-fentanyl

Table 8.6 Histopathology related to estimation of dural tension. The patients were subjected to four different anaesthetic procedures. Number (%) of patients are indicated

Anaesthesia	Diagnosis	Total number	Normal tension	Increased tension	Pronounced increased tension
Propofol -fentanyl	Glioblastoma	170	88 (51.8)	70 (41.2)	12 (7.0)
	Metastasis	97	55 (56.7)	37 (38.1)	5 (5.1)
	Meningioma	126	75 (59.5)	42 (33.3)	9 (7.1)
	Total	393	218 (55.5)	149 (37.9)	26 (6.6)
Propofol -remifentanil	Glioblastoma	46	29 (63.0)	14 (30.4)	3 (6.5)
	Metastasis	33	23 (69.7)	7 (21.1)	3 (9.1)
	Meningioma	49	38 (77.6)	7 (14.3)	4 (8.2)
	Total	128	90 (70.3)	28 (21.9)	10 (7.8)*
Isoflurane -fentanyl	Glioblastoma	34	11 (32.4)	13 (38.2)	10 (29.4)
	Metastasis	23	8 (34.8)	10 (43.5)	5 (21.7)
	Meningioma	50	20 (40.0)	22 (44.0)	8 (16.0)
	Total	107	39 (36.4)	45 (42.1)	23 (21.5)*,**
Sevoflurane -fentanyl	Glioblastoma	22	6 (27.3)	13 (59.1)	3 (13.6)
	Metastasis	10	4 (40.0)	5 (50.0)	1 (10.0)
	Meningioma	25	13 (52.0)	5 (20.0)	7 (28.0)
	Total	57	23 (40.4)	23 (40.4)	11 (19.3)*,**

*Significantly different distribution compared with propofol-fentanyl
**Significantly different distribution compared with propofol-remifentanil

with either isoflurane-fentanyl or sevoflurane-fentanyl ICP averaged 11.3 and 12.2 mmHg, respectively. These values were significantly higher compared with the ICP registered in propofol-remifentanil-anaesthetized patients (7.6 mmHg). In the same diagnostic group sevoflurane-fentanyl-anaesthetized patients had a significantly higher ICP (12.2 mmHg) compared with patients subjected propofol-fentanyl anaesthesia (8.0 mmHg). In all diagnostic groups, except patients with metastasis anaesthetized with isoflurane-fentanyl, the levels of CPP were significantly higher in propofol-fentanyl-anaesthetized patients. Within each anaesthetic group no significant differences in subdural ICP or cerebral haemodynamics were disclosed. Table 8.8 indicates the pooled data, irrespective of diagnosis. The four anaesthetic groups are indicated. No significant intergroup differences were disclosed as regards neuroradiological data (maximal tumour area, tumour volume and midline shift) or levels of $PaCO_2$. The level of ICP was significantly lower during propofol-remifentanil (6 mm Hg) and propofol-fentanyl anaesthesia (8 mmHg) compared with isoflurane-fentanyl (11.0 mmHg) and sevoflurane-fentanyl anaesthesia (11.0 mm Hg). Furthermore, the level of ICP in propofol-remifentanil-anaesthetized patients was lower than during propofol-fentanyl anaesthesia. The level of CPP was significantly higher during propofol-fentanyl anaesthesia (74 mmHg) compared with propofol-remifentanil (65 mmHg), isoflurane-fentanyl (65 mm Hg) and sevoflurane-fentanyl anaesthesia (62 mmHg).

Table 8.7 The levels of midline shift, volume of tumour, $PaCO_2$, PaO_2, rectal temperature, MABP, ICP and CPP in supratentorial cerebral tumours (glioblastoma, metastasis and meningioma). Four anaesthetic techniques were used. Mean±SD are indicated

	Diagnosis	Midline shift (mm)	Volume of tumour (cm^3)	$PaCO_2$ (kPa)	PaO_2 (kPa)	Rectal temperature (°C)	MABP (mmHg)	ICP (mmHg)	CPP (mmHg)
Propofol	Glioblastoma	8.4±5.8	33±22	4.5±0.5	27±9.6	35.9±0.6	85±13	9.8±6.2	75±14
-fentanyl	Metastasis	4.5±5.1	14±16	4.6±0.5	25±8.0	35.9±0.5	82±15	9.0±5.4	73±15
	Meningioma	5.7±7.0	31±49	4.4±0.4	26±8.6	36.1±0.5	85±14	8.0±6.7	77±15
Propofol	Glioblastoma	7.3±6.5	30±19	4.5±0.4	24±6.3	35.9±0.3	74±13*	6.8±4.5*	67±14*
-remifentanil	Metastasis	4.8±6.5	20±21	4.6±0.4	23±7.7	35.9±0.5	75±12	7.8±5.2	67±14*
	Meningioma	5.2±7.2	37±58	4.4±0.3	26±7.4	35.8±0.5	70±10*	7.0±7.9	63±13*
Isoflurane	Glioblastoma	4.6±4.1	29±21	4.6±0.4	26±9.0	36.2±0.5	75±7.4*	12.6±7.6**	63±8.9*
-fentanyl	Metastasis	3.6±4.1	11±10	4.6±0.6	23±7.8	36.2±0.4	74±9.4	11.7±6.0**	62±11*
	Meningioma	2.4±4.1	31±64	4.5±0.4	27±8.3	35.9±0.6	77±11*	11.0±6.1*,**	66±13*
Sevoflurane	Glioblastoma	4.5±4.4	27±20	4.6±0.7	23±6.5	36.0±0.6	77±10*	13.3±7.8**	64±11*
-fentanyl	Metastasis	3.6±4.0	16±17	4.6±0.6	27±10	35.8±0.6	69±12*	9.8±5.9	59±11*
	Meningioma	4.0±4.8	23±16	4.5±0.3	29±13	36.0±0.6	74±11*	12.6±6.0*,**	61±12*

*Significant difference from propofol-fentanyl
**Significant difference from propofol-remifentanil

Table 8.8 Patients with supratentorial tumours (glioblastoma, meningioma and metastasis). Neuroradiological data (maximum areas of tumour, volume of tumour and midline shift), $PaCO_2$, MABP, ICP and CPP are indicated. Mean±SD are indicated

Anaesthesia	Number of patients	Women/Men	Tumour volume (cm^3)	Midline shift (mm)	$PaCO_2$ (kPa)	MABP (mmHg)	ICP (mmHg)	CPP (mmHg)
Propofol -fentanyl	393	207/186	28.0±33.0	6.6±6.3	4.5±0.5	84.0±14.0	9.0±6.3	75.0±15.0
Propofol -remifentanil	128	79/49	30.0±31.0	6.3±6.8	4.5±0.4	73.0±12.0*	7.2±6.1*	66.0±14.0*
Isoflurane -fentanyl	107	58/49	26.0±21.0	4.9±4.1	4.6±0.5	76.0±10.0*	11.6±6.6*,**	64.0±11.0*
Sevoflurane -fentanyl	57	34/23	23.0±18.0	4.1±4.5	4.6±0.4	74.0±11.0*	12.4±6.7*,**	62.0±11.0*

*Significant difference ($P<0.05$) compared with propofol-fentanyl
**Significant difference compared with propofol-remifentanil

Conclusion   During supratentorial tumour surgery ICP and dural tension are lowest during propofol-remifentanil anaesthesia, followed by propofol-fentanyl and anaesthesia with either isoflurane-fentanyl or sevoflurane-fentanyl. CPP, however, is significantly higher during propofol-fentanyl compared with the other three groups. Within each anaesthetic group no significant differences in subdural ICP or cerebral haemodynamics were disclosed.

Study 3: Studies of Subdural Intracranial Pressure and Jugular Bulb Pressure in Patients with Supratentorial Tumours Anaesthetized with Propofol-Fentanyl or Propofol-Remifentanil

Aim   To investigate the relationship between JBP and subdural ICP/cerebral haemodynamics in patients anaesthetized with either propofol-fentanyl or propofol-remifentanil.

Method   Patients with supratentorial tumours (glioblastoma, meningioma or metastasis) received either maintenance anaesthesia with propofol-fentanyl ($n=188$) or propofol-remifentanil ($n=85$). Subdural ICP, MABP and JBP were monitored immediately before opening of the dura. Arterial blood and jugular venous blood were analysed for $PaCO_2$, PaO_2, venous saturation (SATv) and $AVDO_2$. CPP was calculated as MABP – ICP. Rectal temperature was monitored. From the preoperative CT scan the maximal area of the tumour and the volume of the tumour were calculated. For details concerning histopathology, neuroradiological findings, maintenance of anaesthesia and monitoring, see Chapter 3.

Statistical analysis   Data within groups were tested for normal distribution. Within groups the paired *t*-test or Wilcoxon signed rank test were used. Between groups the normality test and equal variance test were applied. Intergroup analyses included one-way analysis of variance. The Tukey test was used for pair-wise multiple comparison procedures. The Kruskal-Wallis analysis of variance on ranks, and multiple comparisons versus control groups (Dunn's method) were used for statistical analysis when the normality test or equal variance test were not passed. The chi-square test was used for statistical analysis of proportions of observation within neuroradiological, histopathological findings and the degrees of dura tension and brain swelling. Median and ranges are indicated. $P<0.05$ was considered statistically significant.

Results   No significant difference was found as regards demographic data (age, weight, height, sex), serum-Na^+, serum-K^+, $PaCO_2$, PaO_2 or rectal temperature. The propofol maintenance dose was significantly lower in propofol-remifentanil-anaesthetized patients. The distribution of tumour diagnosis, localization of tumour, the midline shift and the area and volume of the tumours did not differ significantly between propofol-fentanyl and propofol-remifentanil-anaesthetized patients.

During propofol-fentanyl anaesthesia the median (ranges) of MABP 84 (52–128) mmHg, ICP 8.0 (2–38) mmHg, CPP 75 (36–118) mmHg and JBP 5.0 (4–17) mmHg were significantly higher than the values obtained during propofol-remifentanil: MABP 70 (52–118) mmHg, ICP 6.0 (−3 to 36) mmHg, CPP 65 (27–115) mmHg and JBP 2.0 (−4 to 13) mm Hg, respectively. Jugular venous oxygen saturation (SATv) was significantly higher in the propofol-fentanyl group 55.5% (36–91%) compared with the propofol-remifentanil group 51.4% (34–80%). In contrast the values of $AVDO_2$ were significantly lower during propofol-fentanyl 3.2 (0.9–5.7) mmol/L compared with the propofol-remifentanil group 3.5 (1.4–4.8) mmol/L (Table 8.9).

The estimation of tension of dura and the degrees of brain swelling after opening of dura are indicated in Table 8.10. In the propofol-fentanyl group the percentages of patients with normal tension of dura (52.1%) and patients without swelling after opening of dura (53.2%) were significantly different from the propofol-remifentanil group, where 70.6% had normal tension of dura and 70.6% were without swelling. In both groups the correlations between maximal area of tumour and ICP, the correlations between midline shift and ICP, and the correlations between JBP and ICP were significant (Table 8.11). In contrast, the correlations between CPP and jugular venous saturation, and between CPP and $AVDO_2$ were insignificant in both groups (Table 8.11).

Table 8.9 Median and ranges of MABP, subdural ICP, CPP, JBP, jugular venous saturation (SATv) and $AVDO_2$ in patients with supratentorial tumours anaesthetized with either propofol-fentanyl or propofol-remifentanil

Anaesthesia		MABP (mmHg)	ICP (mmHg)	CPP (mmHg)	JBP (mmHg)	SATv (%)	$AVDO_2$ (mmol/L)
Propofol	Median	84	8.0	75	5.0	55.5	3.2
-fentanyl	Range	52–128	2–38	36–118	4–17	36–91	0.9–5.7
Propofol	Median	70*	6.0*	65*	2.0*	51.4*	3.5*
-remifentanil	Range	52–118	−3 to 36	27–115	−4 to 13	34–80	1.4–4.8

*$P<0.05$

Table 8.10 Tension of dura and degree of brain swelling after opening of dura in patients with supratentorial tumour anaesthetized with either propofol-fentanyl or propofol-remifentanil. Number (%) of patients is indicated

	Propofol-fentanyl	Propofol-remifentanil
Tension of dura		
Normal tension	98 (52.1)	60 (70.6)
Increased tension	76 (40.4)	17 (20.0)
Pronounced increased tension	14 (7.5)	8 (9.4)
Degree of brain swelling		
No swelling	100 (53.2)	60 (70.6)
Moderate swelling	61 (32.4)	18 (21.2)
Pronounced swelling	27 (14.4)	7 (8.2)

Table 8.11 Linear regression, correlation coefficient r and P values for the relationship between ICP contra neuroradiological findings (maximal area, volume and midline shift of tumour) and JBP

		Propofol-fentanyl	Propofol-remifentanil
Number of patients		188	85
ICP contra maximal area of tumour (cm^2)	Linear regression	ICP=5.52 + 0.24 × area	ICP=5.24 + 0.18 × area
	Coefficient (r)	0.3283	0.2471
	Significance	$P<0.001$	$P=0.0230$
ICP contra volume of tumour (cm^3)	Linear regression	ICP=7.01 + 0.07 × volume	Not significant
	Coefficient (r)	0.2670	Not significant
	Significance	$P<0.001$	Not significant
ICP contra midline shift (mm)	Linear regression	ICP=7.05 + 0.29 × midline shift	ICP= 4.74 + 0.48 × midline shift
	Coefficient (r)	0.2580	0.4295
	Significance	$P<0.001$	$P<0.001$
ICP contra JBP (mmHg)	Linear regression	ICP=6.49+0.46 × JBP	ICP=5.42+0.73 × JBP
	Coefficient (r)	0.2822	0.3411
	Significance	$P<0.001$	$P<0.001$

Conclusion In this prospective but non-randomized study significant differences between propofol-fentanyl- and propofol-remifentanil-anaesthetized patients were disclosed, comprising significantly lower ICP, CPP, JBP and jugular venous saturation values in patients anaesthetized with propofol combined with remifentanil. The results suggest that the low jugular venous pressure and the low CPP may influence ICP, and that the low $AVDO_2$ is a result of a low CPP during propofol-remifentanil anaesthesia.

Discussion

A dose-related decrease in CBF, $CMRO_2$ and ICP has been found during propofol anaesthesia (Moss and Price 1990; Pinaud et al. 1990; Ramani et al. 1992; Alkire et al. 1995). Cerebral autoregulation is better preserved during propofol anaesthesia than with isoflurane (Strebel et al. 1995) or sevoflurane (McCulloch et al. 2000). The CBV is higher during inhalation anaesthesia compared with propofol anaesthesia (Todd and Weeks 1996; Cenic et al. 2002), and jugular venous saturation is lower during propofol compared with isoflurane (Jansen et al. 1999; Petersen et al. 2003) or sevoflurane anaesthesia (Nandate et al. 2000; Petersen et al. 2003; Kawano et al. 2004; Yoshitani et al. 2005). The first randomized study presented here strongly suggests that in the clinical situation propofol-fentanyl anaesthesia for cerebral tumour surgery is superior to anaesthesia with both isoflurane or sevoflurane both combined with fentanyl, because ICP is significantly lower and CPP significantly higher, and the degree of dural tension and degree of cerebral swelling after opening of dura are less pronounced (Petersen et al. 2003).

After a bolus dose of remifentanil ICP is unchanged but MABP and CPP fall (Warner et al. 1996). Compared with fentanyl both blood pressure and heart rate are lower during remifentanil anaesthesia (Twersky et al. 2001). Remifentanil in anaesthetic doses reduces regional CBF (Klimscha et al. 2003), transcranial flow velocity (Paris et al. 1998) and preserves CO_2 reactivity (Baker et al. 1997; Ostapkovich et al. 1998; Klimscha et al. 2003), which is not significantly different from anaesthesia with fentanyl as analgesic (Ostapkovich et al. 1998).

Three comparable studies of the effects of fentanyl and remifentanil in patients with supratentorial tumours are available. In a randomized study, including 18 patients, nitrous oxide-oxygen 2/1 was used as anaesthesia. The effects of continuous infusion of either fentanyl or remifentanil on CBF, measured by the intravenous ^{133}Xe method, and brain relaxation were compared. With no significant difference in $PaCO_2$, CBF was 37 ml and 36 ml/ 100 g/min in the remifentanil and fentanyl groups, respectively, and brain relaxation was comparable between groups (Ostapkovich et al. 1998). In another study where nitrous oxide was used as anaesthesia, 16 patients were allocated to fentanyl and 17 patients to remifentanil. Epidural ICP averaged 14 and 13 mmHg, CPP 76 and 78 mmHg and $PaCO_2$ 29 and 28 mmHg, and cerebral swelling was recorded in 65% and 58% of patients, respectively (Guy et al. 1997). In comparison, significant differences in ICP, CPP and both dura tension and the degree of brain swelling were found in the present study. Differences in anaesthetic technique (nitrous oxide contra propofol), dosages of fentanyl and remifentanil, number of patients and level of mean blood pressure might explain the discrepancy between the two studies. In the second prospective, but non-randomized study, including in total 619 patients, comparisons of ICP, CPP and dural tension were performed in patients with supratentorial tumours subjected to either propofol-fentanyl, propofol-remifentanil, isoflurane-fentanyl or sevoflurane-fentanyl. ICP were significantly higher and CPP significantly lower with isoflurane-fentanyl- or sevoflurane-fentanyl-anaesthetized patients compared with patients anaesthetized with propofol-fentanyl or propofol-remifentanil. Furthermore, ICP and CPP were significantly lower in patients subjected to propofol-remifentanil anaesthesia (mean values 7.6 and 65 mmHg, respectively), compared with patients anaesthetized with propofol-fentanyl (mean values 9.0 and 75 mmHg, respectively). The average maintenance doses of propofol, fentanyl and remifentanil were comparable with the doses used in the present study. Likewise, the levels of $PaCO_2$, ICP and CPP during propofol-fentanyl and propofol-remifentanil anaesthesia were identical with those obtained in the present study. The significantly higher values of ICP and CPP found in the propofol-fentanyl-anaesthetized patients, compared with the propofol-remifentanil group were not caused by differences in $PaCO_2$, tumour size or midline shift. Recent studies indicate that the

CO_2 reactivity is preserved during remifentanil-nitrous oxide anaesthesia (Baker et al. 1997), and the CO_2 reactivity is similar during remifentanil-nitrous oxide and fentanyl-nitrous oxide anaesthesia (Ostapkovich et al. 1998). The difference in ICP was surprising because the maintenance dose of propofol was significantly lower in the propofol-remifentanil group. According to experimental and clinical studies, propofol induces a dose-related decrease in $CMRO_2$ and CBF (Moss and Price 1990; Pinaud et al. 1990; Ramani et al. 1992; Alkire et al. 1995). Consequently, lower CBV and a lower ICP level should be expected in the propofol-fentanyl group.

The significant difference in subdural ICP might be explained by the difference in CPP, which, dependent on the status of cerebral autoregulation, might influence ICP. If cerebral autoregulation is abolished a low CPP is accompanied by a decrease in ICP. Cerebral autoregulation is not influenced by propofol (Strebel et al. 1995) or fentanyl (Hoffman et al. 1992). It is well known that cerebral autoregulation is abolished close to the site of cerebral tumours (Kuroda et al. 1982), but loss of cerebral autoregulation remote from the tumour site is also common (Endo et al. 1977) while global loss of autoregulation rarely occurs (Pálvölgyi 1969). As cerebral autoregulation was not tested in the present study, it is impossible to deny that the difference in ICP was caused by differences in CPP. In favour of this explanation is the observation that the median value of CPP was very close to the lower point of cerebral autoregulation, which otherwise is considered to be 60 mmHg, but higher values have been demonstrated in healthy volunteers (Schmidt et al. 1991; Olsen et al. 1994). At CPP below the lower value of cerebral autoregulation, CBF and CBV are positively correlated to CPP, and collapse of cerebral vessels with reduction of CBV and ICP might occur.

Differences in ICP might also be caused by a difference in JBP between the two anaesthetic groups. It has been demonstrated that tilting of the operating table to rTp in supine-positioned patients (Rolighed Larsen et al. 2002; Haure et al. 2003; Tankisi et al. 2006) and in prone-positioned patients (Tankisi et al. 2002) is accompanied by a decrease in ICP and JBP. The mechanism is supposed to be a decrease in intracranial blood volume caused by drainage of blood from the intracerebral compartment. In the third study presented here a significant difference in JBP was found, with a median of 5 mmHg in the propofol-fentanyl group against 2 mmHg in the propofol-remifentanil group. Furthermore, significant correlations between JBP and ICP were found in both anaesthetic groups. It therefore seems reasonable to suggest that the lower ICP observed in propofol-remifentanil-anaesthetized patients to some degree was caused by a lower JBP in this group.

In the third study, jugular venous oxygen saturation was lower and $AVDO_2$ higher in the propofol-remifentanil group and values of venous saturation as low as 36% and 34% were observed in the propofol-fentanyl and propofol-remifentanil groups, respectively. Although the correlations between CPP and jugular venous saturation, and CPP and $AVDO_2$ were insignificant, it cannot be excluded that the lower values of venous saturation and high values of $AVDO_2$ in the propofol-remifentanil group were caused by the lower level of CPP in the remifentanil group. In some patients the value of jugular venous saturation was considerably below 40%, which otherwise is supposed to be associated with development of cerebral ischaemia (Gopinath et al. 1996). A re-definition of the lower limit of jugular venous saturation during propofol seems justified. At least in studies of diffusion-weighted MRI jugular venous saturation below 40% is not associated with evidence of cerebral ischaemia damage in patients anaesthetized with propofol (Rasmussen et al. 2004).

Two of the presented studies have limitations because they were not randomized. Data, however, were collected prospectively and continuously between the years 1997 and 2005. In this period subdural ICP monitoring was performed in 1,151 patients with supratentorial tumour, 685 of which had glioblastoma, metastasis or meningioma. The anaesthetic groups were not of equal size, propofol-fentanyl being the largest group. Propofol-remifentanil was used over the period 2000–2005, while propofol-fentanyl was used over the entire period. The maintenance dose of propofol and CPP differed significantly, which made interpretation of the results difficult. The staff of neurosurgeons and anaesthesiologists involved in craniotomy, however, was almost the same over the period. The same applies to preoperative care, principles of steroid treatment and the operating and monitoring conditions.

The clinical implications are as follows: The first two studies indicate that as regards ICP, CPP, dural tension and degree of swelling after opening of dura, propofol-fentanyl and propofol-remifentanil anaesthesia are the be preferred to isoflurane-fentanyl or sevoflurane-fentanyl. The third study indicates a preference for propofol-remifentanil compared with propofol-fentanyl because ICP was lower and the degree of dural tension and degree of swelling were less pronounced during propofol-remifentanil compared with propofol-fentanyl anaesthesia. However, CPP was also lower and close to or below the lower point of autoregulation defined elsewhere. Furthermore, jugular venous saturation was lower and $AVDO_2$ higher in propofol-remifentanil-anaesthetized patients. The third study also suggests that the low ICP in propofol-remifentanil-anaesthetized patients might be caused by a lower jugular venous bulb pressure, but the low CPP theoretically also might be a causal factor. Thus, further comparative studies of the effect of propofol-fentanyl and propofol-remifentanil on ICP seem justified, especially, studies where the doses of propofol are comparable and studies where MABP is adjusted to the same level during anaesthesia.

References

Adams RW, Cucchiara RF, Gronert GA et al (1981) Isoflurane and cerebrospinal fluid pressure in neurosurgical patients. Anesthesiology 54:97–99

Algotsson L, Messeter K, Nordström CH (1988) Cerebral blood flow and oxygen consumption during isoflurane and halothane anaesthesia in man. Acta Anaestheiol Scand 32:15–20

Alkire MT, Haier RJ, Barker SJ et al (1995) Cerebral metabolism during propofol anesthesia in humans studied with positron emission tomography. Anesthesiology 82:393–403

Artru AA, Lam AM, Johnson JO et al (1997) Intracranial pressure, middle cerebral artery flow velocity, and plasma inorganic fluoride concentrations in neurosurgical patients receiving sevoflurane or isoflurane. Anesth Analg 85:587–592

Baker KZ, Ostapkovich N, Sisti MB et al (1997) Intact cerebral blood flow reactivity during remifentanil/nitrous oxide anesthesia. J Neurosurg Anesthesiol 9:134–140

Bundgaard H, von Oettingen G, Larsen KM et al (1998) Effects of sevoflurane on intracranial pressure, cerebral blood flow, and cerebral metabolism. A dose-response study in patients subjected to craniotomy for cerebral tumours. Acta Anaesthesiol Scand 42:621–627

Cenic A, Craen RA, Lee TY et al (2002) Cerebral blood volume and blood flow responses to hyperventilation in brain tumours during isoflurane or propofol anesthesia. Anesth Analg 94:661–666

Endo H, Larsen B, Lassen NA (1977) Regional cerebral blood flow alterations remote from the site in intracranial tumours. J Neurosurg 46: 271–281

Gopinath SP, Cormio M, Ziegler J et al (1996) Intraoperative jugular desaturation during surgery for traumatic intracranial hematomas. Anesth Analg 83:1014–1021

Gordon E, Lagerkranser M, Rudehill A et al (1988) The effect of isoflurane on cerebrospinal fluid pressure in patients undergoing neurosurgery. Acta Anaesthesiol Scand 32:108–112

Guy J, Hindman BJ, Baker KZ et al (1997) Comparison of remifentanil and fentanyl in patients undergoing craniotomy for supratentorial space-occupying lesions. Anesthesiology 86:514–524

Haure P, Cold GE, Hansen TM et al (2003) The ICP-lowering effect of 10° reverse Trendelenburg position during craniotomy is stable during a 10-minute period. J Neurosurg Anesthesiol 15:297–301

Hoffman WE, Werner C, Kochs E et al (1992) Cerebral and spinal cord blood flow in awake and fentanyl-N_2O anaesthetized rats: evidence for preservation of blood flow autoregulation during anesthesia. J Neurosurg Anesthesiol 4:31–35

Jansen GF, van Praagh BH, Kedaria MB (1999) Jugular bulb oxygen saturation during propofol and isoflurane/nitrous oxide anesthesia in patients undergoing brain tumour surgery. Anesth Analg 89:358–363

Kawano Y, Kawaguchi M, Inoue S et al (2004) Jugular bulb oxygen saturation under propofol or sevoflurane/nitrous oxide anesthesia during deliberate mild hypothermia in neurosurgical patients. J Neurosrug Anesthesiol 16:6–10

Klimscha W, Ullrich R, Nasal C et al (2003) High dose remifentanil does not impair cerebrovascular carbon dioxide reactivity in healthy male volunteers. Anesthesiology 99:834–840

Kuroda K, Olsen TS, Lassen NA (1982) Regional cerebral blood flow in various types of brain tumour. Acta Neurol Scand 66:160–171

Madsen JB, Cold GE. Hansen ES et al (1987a) Cerebral blood flow and metabolism during isoflurane-induce hypotension in patients subjected to surgery for cerebral aneurysms. Br J Anaesth 59:1204–1207

Madsen JB, Cold GE, Hansen ES (1987b) The effect of isoflurane on cerebral blood flow and metabolism in humans during craniotomy for small supratentorial cerebral tumours. Anesthesiology 66:332–336

McCulloch TJ, Visco E, Lam AM (2000) Graded hypercapnia and cerebral autoregulation during sevoflurane or propofol anesthesia. Anesthesiology 93:1205–1209

Mielck F, Stephan H, Weyland A (1999) Effects of one minimum alveolar anesthesic concentration sevoflurane on cerebral metabolism, blood flow, and CO_2 reactivity in cardiac patients. Anesth Analg 89:364–369

Moss E, Price DJ (1990) Effect of propofol on brain retraction pressure and cerebral perfusion pressure. Br J Anaesth 65:823–825

Nandate K, Vuylsteke A, Ratsep I et al (2000) Effects of isoflurane and propofol anaesthesia on jugular venous oxygen saturation in patients undergoing coronary artery bypass surgery. Br J Anaesth 84:631–633

Olsen KS, Henriksen L, Owen-Falkenberg A et al (1994) Effect of 1 and 2 MAC isoflurane with or without ketanserin on cerebral blood flow autoregulation in man. Br J Anaesth 72:66–71

Oshima T, Karasawa F, Satoh T (2002) Effects of propofol on cerebral blood flow and the metabolic rate of oxygen in humans. Acta Anaesthesiol Scand 46:831–835

Ostapkovich ND, Baker KZ, Fogarty-Mack P et al (1998) Cerebral blood flow and CO_2 reactivity is similar during remifentanil/N_2O and fentanyl/N_2O anesthesia. Anesthesiology 89:358–363

Pálvölgyi R (1969) Regional cerebral blood flow in patients with intracranial tumours. J Neurosurg 31:149–163

Paris A, Scholz J, von Knobelsdorff G et al (1998) The effect of remifentanil on cerebral blood flow velocity. Anesth Analg 87:569–573

Petersen KD, Landsfeldt U, Cold GE et al (2003) Intracranial pressure and cerebral hemodynamic in patients with cerebral tumours. Anesthesiology 98:329–336

Pinaud M, Lelausque JN, Chetanneau A et al (1990) Effects of propofol on cerebral hemodynamics and metabolism in patients with brain trauma. Anesthesiology 73:404–409

Ramani R, Todd MM, Warner DS (1992) A dose-response study of the influence of propofol on cerebral blood flow, metabolism and the electroencephalogram in the rabbit. J Neurosurg Anesthesiol 4:110–119

Rasmussen M, Østergaard L, Juul N et al (2004) Does indomethacin and propofol cause cerebral ischemia? Anesthesiology 101:872–878

Ravussin P, Tempelhoff R, Modica PA et al (1991) Propofol vs. thiopenthal-isoflurane for neurosurgical anesthesia: comparison of hemodynamics, CSF pressure and recovery. J Neurosurg Anesthesiol 3:85–95

Rolighed Larsen JK, Haure P, Cold GE (2002) Reverse Trendelenburg position reduces intracranial pressure during craniotomy. J Neurosurg Anesthesiol 14:16–21

Scheller MS, Tateishi A, Drummond JC et al (1988) The effects of sevoflurane on cerebral blood flow, cerebral metabolic rate for oxygen, intracranial pressure, and electroencephalogram are similar to those of isoflurane in the rabbit. Anesthesiology 68:548–551

Schlünzen L, Vafaee MS, Cold GE et al (2004) Effects of subanaesthetic and anaesthetic doses of sevoflurane on regional cerebral blood flow in healthy volunteers. A positron emission tomographic study. Acta Anaesthesiol Scand 48:1268–1276

Schmidt JF, Olsen KS, Waldemar G et al (1991) Effect of ketanserin on cerebral blood flow autoregulation in healthy volunteers. Acta Neurochir 111:138–142

Strebel S, Lam AM, Matta B et al (1995) Dynamic and static cerebral autoregulation during isoflurane, desflurane, and propofol anesthesia. Anesthesiology 83:66–76

Talke P, Caldwell J, Dodsont B et al (1996) Desflurane and isoflurane increase lumbar cerebrospinal fluid pressure in normocapnic patients undergoing transsphenoidal hypophysectomy. Anesthesiology 85:999–1004

Talke P, Caldwell JE, Richardson CA (1999) Sevoflurane increases lumbar cerebrospinal fluid pressure in normocapnic patients undergoing transsphenoidal hypophysectomy. Anesthesiology 91:127–130

Tankisi A, Rolighed Larsen J, Rasmussen M et al (2002) The effects of 10 degrees reverse Trendelenburg position on ICP and CPP in prone positioned patients subjected to craniotomy for occipital or cerebellar tumours. Acta Neurochir (Wien) 144:665–670

Tankisi A, Rasmussen M, Juul N (2006) The effects of 10° reverse Trendelenburg position (rTp) on subdural intracranial pressure and cerebral perfusion pressure in patients subjected to craniotomy for cerebral aneurysm. J Neurosurg Anesthsiol 18:11–17

Todd MM, Weeks J (1996) Comparative effects of propofol, pentobarbital, and isoflurane on cerebral blood flow and blood volume. J Neurosurg Anesthesiol 8:296–303

Todd MM, Warner DS, Sokoll MD et al (1993) A prospective, comparative trial of three anesthetics for elective supratentorial craniotomy. Anesthesiology 78:1005–1020

Twersky RS, Jamerson B, Warner DS et al (2001) Hemodynamics and emergence profile of remifentanil versus fentanyl prospectively compared in a large population of surgical patients. J Clin Anesth 13:407–416

Warner DS, Hindman BJ, Todd MM et al (1996) Intracranial pressure and hemodynamic effects of remifentanil versus anfentanil in patients undergoing supratentorial craniotomy. Anesth Analg 83:348–353

Yoshitani K, Kawaguchi M, Iwata M et al (2005) Comparison of changes in jugular venous bulb oxygen saturation and cerebral oxygen saturation during variations of haemoglobin concentration under propofol and sevoflurane anaesthesia. Br J Anaesth 94:341–346

Chapter 9
Effect of Sevoflurane on Subdural Intracranial Pressure and Cerebral Haemodynamics During Craniotomy

Georg Emil Cold and Helle Bundgaard

Abstract

Volatile anaesthetics act as cerebral vasodilators with the potential to increase cerebral blood flow, cerebral blood volume and ICP. In experimental studies sevoflurane is a less potent vasodilator than isoflurane and halothane, and sevoflurane has been advocated for neurosurgical anaesthesia. However, concerning the effect of ICP, the results in experimental studies are conflicting.

In this chapter we discusses sevoflurane and the dose-related changes in cerebrovascular resistance, cerebral blood flow, subdural ICP and relative CO_2 reactivity in patients undergoing craniotomy for cerebral tumour.

Volatile anaesthetics act as cerebral vasodilators with the potential to increase CBF, CBV, ICP (Drummond et al. 1986). In experimental studies, sevoflurane is a less potent vasodilator than isoflurane and halothane, and sevoflurane has been advocated for neurosurgical anaesthesia (Scheller et al. 1988, 1990; Takahashi et al. 1993; Baker 1997). However, concerning the effect of ICP, the results in experimental studies are conflicting. In rabbits (Scheller et al. 1988) and cats (Kotani et al. 1992; Sugioka 1992) sevoflurane elicits an increase in ICP. In dogs with normal intracranial compliance, however, the changes in ICP are not significant (Takahashi et al. 1993). The results of clinical studies are also conflicting. A dose-related increase in the CBF equivalent $1/AVDO_2$ has been reported (Kuroda et al. 1996). In patients undergoing transsphenoidal hypophysectomy without evidence of mass effect, sevoflurane at 0.5 and 1 MAC increases lumbar CSF pressure (Talke et al. 1999). In contrast, no dose-related changes in velocity of the middle cerebral artery were found (Kuroda et al. 1997), and ICP is unchanged from baseline during administration of 0.5–1.5% sevoflurane (Artru et al. 1997).

In patients without cerebral diseases autoregulation is intact during 1.2 MAC sevoflurane (Cho et al. 1996). In a study of hypotensive anaesthesia induced by prostaglandin E_1 autoregulation was intact as well (Kitaguchi et al. 1992). In another study, in patients subjected to extra-intracranial by-pass anastomosis, cerebral autoregulation was intact (Kitaguchi et al. 1993). Studies of dynamic cerebral autoregulation with transcranial Doppler sonographics indicate that during 1.5 MAC sevoflurane dynamic autoregulation was better preserved during sevoflurane than during isoflurane anaesthesia (Summors et al. 1999).

In patients without cerebral diseases (Cho et al. 1996), cardiac patients (Mielck et al. 1999), patients with cerebral tumours (Inada et al. 1996) and patients subjected to extra-intracranial by-pass anastomosis (Kitaguchi et al. 1993) the CO_2 reactivity is intact during sevoflurane anaesthesia. In patients subjected to craniotomy for supratentorial cerebral tumours, the CO_2 reactivity was higher for sevoflurane and isoflurane, compared with propofol-anaesthetized patients (Petersen et al. 2003).

In the present study, the dose-related changes in CVR, CBF, $CMRO_2$, subdural ICP and relative CO_2 reactivity were analysed in patients undergoing craniotomy for cerebral tumour.

Effect of Sevoflurane on Intracranial Pressure, Cerebral Blood Flow and Cerebral Metabolism

Data from this study are based on Bungaard et al. (1998).

Aim The dose-response of CVR, CBF, $CMRO_2$, CO_2 reactivity and subdural ICP of sevoflurane was studied in patients undergoing craniotomy for cerebral tumour.

Method Twenty adult patients undergoing craniotomy for supratentorial cerebral tumour participated in the study. Only patients with midline shift < 10 mm on preoperative CT were included. The patients were randomized into two groups according to the anaesthetic procedure. In group 1 ($n=10$) 0.7 MAC sevoflurane supplemented with Fentanyl 2 µg/kg/h was used for maintenance of anaesthesia. In group 2 ($n=10$) sevoflurane 1.3 MAC with the same fentanyl dose was used. CBF was measured with ^{133}Xe as tracer with two angular detectors placed on each side of the head. CBF was calculated as the initial slope index. The average values of CBF from the two detectors were used. A jugular catheter was inserted according to Chapter 3. Samples of arterial and jugular bulb blood were analysed for oxygen content and $AVDO_2$ was calculated as the difference in oxygen content between arterial blood and jugular bulb blood. $CMRO_2$ was calculated as the product of $AVDO_2$ and CBF. CVR was calculated according to the formula CPP = CBF × CVR. The relative CO_2 reactivity was calculated as the % change $AVDO_2$/change $PaCO_2$ (%/mmHg).

Table 9.1 Parameters in two groups of patients measured during maintenance anaesthesia with 0.7 MAC sevoflurane (group 1) and 0.7 followed by 1.3 MAC sevoflurane (group 2)

	$PaCO_2$ (kPa)	MABP (mmHg)	ICP (mmHg)	CPP (mmHg)	$AVDO_2$ (mmol/L)	CBF (ml/100 g/min)	CVR (mmHg/ml min 100 g)	$CMRO_2$ (ml O_2/100 g/min)
Group 1								
0.7 MAC	4.8±0.3	69±6	11±7	58±11	2.4±0.7	31±10	2.2±1.0	1.7±0.6
0.7 MAC	4.9±0.3	68±4	11±8	57±10	2.2±0.7	30±10	2.2±0.7	1.5±0.6
Group 2								
0.7 MAC	5.0±0.3	80±11	11±7	69±15	2.1±0.9	29±10	2.7±1.2	1.3±0.3
1.3 MAC	5.0±0.4	77±9	12±8	66±15	1.9±0.9	34±12*	2.3±1.2*	1.3±0.4

*$P<0.05$ within group

Table 9.2 Changes in $PaCO_2$, $AVDO_2$ and subdural ICP before and after 5 min hyperventilation in patients undergoing anaesthesia with 0.7 and 1.3 MAC sevoflurane. The relative CO_2 reactivity is also shown. Mean±SD are indicated

	$\Delta PaCO_2$ (mmHg)	$\Delta AVDO_2$ (mmol/L)	ΔICP (mmHg)	Relative CO_2 reactivity (%/mmHg)
Sevoflurane 0.7 MAC	5.6±1.8	0.6±0.5	3.0±2.1	3.3±3.1
Sevoflurane 1.3 MAC	6.1±0.9	0.3±0.3	3.0±2.7	2.2±1.8

The duration of hyperventilation was 5 min. Subdural ICP, CBF and $CMRO_2$ were measured twice as follows: In group 1 both measurements were performed with 0.7 MAC sevoflurane. In group 2, the first measurement was performed with 0.7 MAC sevoflurane and the second with 1.3 MAC sevoflurane.

Statistic analysis Mean±SD are calculated. The unpaired t-test was used to analyse intergroup difference, and the paired t-test for intragroup changes. If the test for normal distribution failed, Mann-Whitney's test and the Wilcoxon test were used for unpaired and paired data.

Results No intergroup differences were found as regards demographic data, perioperative values of $PaCO_2$, PaO_2, rectal temperature, neuroradiological examination (tumour size and midline shift) or data concerning histopathology. In group 1 no time-dependent changes in subdural ICP, CPP, CBF, CVR, $AVDO_2$ and $CMRO_2$ were found. In group 2, an increase in sevoflurane concentration from 0.7 to 1.3 MAC resulted in a significant increase in CBF from 29±10 to 34±12 ml/100 g/min, and a significant decrease in CVR from 2.7±0.9 to 2.3±1.2 mmHg/ml min 100 g (Table 9.1, see page 149). During hyperventilation $PaCO_2$ decreased significantly in both groups. This was accompanied by a significant decrease in $AVDO_2$ and ICP. The relative CO_2 reactivities were 3.3±3.1 and 2.2±1.8%/mmHg during 0.7 and 1.3 MAC sevoflurane, respectively (Table 9.2).

Conclusion The present study confirms that sevoflurane is a cerebral vasodilator, as sevoflurane increases CBF and decreases CVR in a dose-dependent manner. However, in the present study the cerebral vasodilatation was not accompanied by an increase in subdural ICP. The CO_2 reactivity is preserved during 0.7 as well as 1.3 MAC sevoflurane maintenance anaesthesia.

Discussion

The major findings in this study were as follows: During normocapnic maintenance anaesthesia with 0.7 MAC sevoflurane supplemented with fentanyl no time-dependent alterations in CBF, subdural ICP, CVR and $CMRO_2$ were observed. However, a significant increase in CBF and a significant decrease in CVR were shown when sevoflurane concentration was increased from 0.7 to 1.3 MAC.

These values of CBF and $CMRO_2$ are comparable to CBF and $CMRO_2$ measured by the Kety and Schmidt technique with argon as tracer in normocapnic patients with ischaemic cerebrovascular disease anaesthetized with 1.5% sevoflurane (Kitaguchi et al. 1993). Furthermore, CBF and $CMRO_2$ were approximately 40% lower than CBF measured by the Kety and Schmidt technique in awake healthy volunteers (Madsen et al. 1993). These findings indicate that sevoflurane, supplemented with fentanyl, even in low MAC concentration induces a substantial suppression of cerebral oxygen uptake. A dose-dependent decrease in $CMRO_2$, following increase in MAC concentration from 0.7 to 1.3 MAC, was expected because anaesthetics in general suppress $CMRO_2$ dose dependently (Michenfelder 1974; Newberg et al. 1983). Accordingly, CBF and $CMRO_2$ are coupled with a reduction of flow and metabolism averaging 38% and 47%, respectively, during 1 MAC sevoflurane in cardiac patients (Mielck et al. 1999). However, with these low values of $CMRO_2$ a dose-dependent decrease was not found, probably because a 50% decrease is accompanied by isoelectric activity, and oxygen consumption is only used for maintenance of cellular membrane potential.

In accordance with Kuroda et al. (1997) time-dependent alterations in CBF, $CMRO_2$ and subdural ICP were not observed in the present study. A dose-related increase in CBF and a decrease in CVR, however, were disclosed, while subdural ICP and CPP were unchanged. The increases in CBF and the fall in CVR indicate that sevoflurane is a cerebral vasodilator. Under these circumstances, the reason for the unchanged subdural ICP might be a favourable cerebral compliance, where changes in CBV, caused by the increased sevoflurane concentration, did not elicit a measurable ICP increase. A reasonable explanation may also be that all patients were fully conscious, that only patients with midline shift < 10 mm were included, that the individual levels of subdural ICP were relatively low, meaning that the actual ICP pressures were localized on the flat part of the volume/pressure curve, and that the majority of patients were in treatment with steroid.

In clinical studies in patients without cerebral diseases (Cho et al. 1996) and in patients subjected to extra-intracranial by-pass anastomosis, cerebral autoregulation was intact during sevoflurane anaesthesia (Kitaguchi et al. 1993). It is well known, however, that cerebral autoregulation is abolished regionally and globally in patients with brain tumour. The status of cerebral autoregulation might not seem to influence the results in the present study because CPP was unchanged in both groups.

The relative CO_2 reactivity was calculated as % change $AVDO_2$/change in $PaCO_2$ in accordance with Obrist et al. (1984). CBF is inversely proportional to $AVDO_2$ on the assumption that $CMRO_2$ is constant during hyperventilation (Michenfelder and Theye 1969), and hyperventilation has been reported to have no effect on $CMRO_2$ (Åkeson et al. 1993). The relative CO_2 reactivity averaged 3.3 and 2.2%/mmHg at 0.7 and 1.3 MAC sevoflurane, respectively. These values are less than the values obtained with the initial slope ^{133}Xe method in awake subjects during normocapnic conditions (average 4%/mmHg) (Olesen et al. 1971) and in patients undergoing craniotomy for cerebral tumour in 1 MAC sevoflurane supplemented with fentanyl, where the relative CO_2 reactivity averaged 4.6%/mmHg (Petersen et al. 2003). Higher CO_2 reactivities during sevoflurane anaesthesia have also been documented patients with ischaemic cerebral disease (Kitaguchi et al. 1993) and in another study in patients with cerebral tumour (Inada et al. 1996). Methodological differences, differences in level of $PaCO_2$, blood pressure and the use of nitrous oxide may explain the discrepancy. Using the definition proposed by Obrist et al. (1984), the relative CO_2 reactivity is preserved at values > 1%/mmHg. Accordingly, in the present study the CO_2 reactivity was preserved at 0.7 as well as 1.3 MAC sevoflurane.

References

Åkeson J, Messeter K, Rosen I (1993) Cerebral haemodynamic and electrocortical CO_2 reactivity in pigs anaesthetized with fentanyl, nitrous oxide and pancuronium. Acta Anaesthesiol Scand 37:85–91

Artru AA, Lam AM, Johnson JO et al (1997) Intracranial pressure, middle cerebral artery flow velocity, and plasma inorganic fluoride concentrations in neurosurgical patients receiving sevoflurane or isoflurane. Anesth Analg 85:587–592

Baker KZ (1997) Desflurane and sevoflurane are valuable additions to the practice of neuroanaesthesiology. J Neurosurg Anesthesiol 9:66–68

Bundgaard H, von Oettingen G, Larsen KM et al (1998) Effects of sevoflurane on intracranial pressure, cerebral blood flow and cerebral metabolism. Acta Anaesthesiol Scand 42:621–627

Cho S, Fujigaki T, Uchiyama Y et al (1996) Effects of sevoflurane with and without nitrous oxide on human cerebral circulation. Anesthesiology 85:755–760

Drummond JC, Todd MM, Scheller MS et al (1986) A comparison of the direct vasodilating potencies of halothane and isoflurane in the New Zealand white rabbit. Anesthesiology 65:462–467

Inada T, Shingu K, Uchida M et al (1996) Changes in the cerebral arteriovenous oxygen content difference by surgical incision are similar during sevoflurane and isoflurane anaesthesia. Can. J Anaesth 43:1019–1024

Kitaguchi K, Kuro M, Nakajia T et al (1992) The change in cerebral blood flow during hypotensive anesthesia induced by prostaglandin E1. Masui 41:766–771

Kitaguchi K, Ohsumi H, Kuro M et al (1993) Effects of sevoflurane on cerebral circulation and metabolism in patients with ischemic cerebrovascular disease. Anesthesiology 79:704–709

Kotani J, Sugioka S, Momota Y et al (1992) Effect of sevoflurane on intracranial pressure, sagittal sinus pressure, and the intracranial volume-pressure relation in cats. J Neurosurg Anesthesiol 4:194–198

Kuroda Y, Murakami M, Tsuruta J et al (1996) Preservation of the ratio of cerebral blood flow/metabolic rate of oxygen during prolonged anesthesia with isoflurane, sevoflurane, and halothane in humans. Anesthesiology 84:555–561

Kuroda Y, Murakami M, Tsuruta J et al (1997) Blood flow velocity of middle cerebral artery during prolonged anesthesia with halothane, isoflurane, and sevoflurane in humans. Anesthesiology 87:527–532

Madsen PL, Holm S, Herning M (1993) Average blood flow and oxygen uptake in the human brain during resting wakefulness: a critical appraisal of the Kety-Schmidt technique. J Cereb Blood Flow Metab 13:646–655

Michenfelder JD (1974) The interdependency of cerebral function and metabolic effects following massive doses of thiopental in the dog. Anesthesiology 41:231–237

Michenfelder JD, Theye RA (1969) The effects of prolonged hypocapnia and dilutional anemia on canine cerebral metabolism and blood flow. Anesthesiology 31:449–457

Mielck F, Stephan H, Weyland A et al (1999) Effect of one minimum alveolar anesthesic concentration sevoflurane on cerebral metabolism, blood flow, and CO_2 reactivity in cardiac patients. Anesth Analg 89:364–369

Newberg L, Milde J, Michenfelder J (1983) The cerebral metabolic effects of isoflurane at and above concentrations that suppress cortical electrical activity. Anesthesiology 59:23–28

Obrist WD, Langfitt TW, Jaggi JL et al (1984) Cerebral blood flow and metabolism in comatose patients with head injury. Relationship to intracranial hypertension. J Neurosurg 61:241–253

Olesen J, Paulson OB, Lassen NA (1971) Regional cerebral blood flow in man determined by the initial slope of the clearance of the intra-arterially injected [133]Xe. Stroke 2:519–540

Petersen KD, Landsfeldt U, Cold GE et al (2003) Intracranial pressure and cerebral hemodynamic in patients with cerebral tumours. A randomised prospective study of patients subjected to craniotomy in propofol-fentanyl, sioflurane-fentanyl, or sevoflurane-fentanyl anesthesia. Anesthesiology 98:329–336

Scheller MS, Tateichi A, Drummond JC et al (1988) The effects of sevoflurane on cerebral blood flow, cerebral metabolic rate for oxygen, intracranial pressure, and the electroencephalogram are similar to those of isoflurane in the rabbit. Anesthesiology 68:548–551

Scheller MS, Nakakimura K, Fleischer JE et al (1990) Cerebral effects of sevoflurane in the dog: comparison with isoflurane and enflurane. Br J Anaesth 65:388–392

Sugioka S (1992) Effects of sevoflurane on intracranial pressure and formation and absorption of cerebrospinal fluid in cats. Masui 41:1434–1442

Summors AC, Gupta AK, Matta BF (1999) Dynamic cerebral autoregulation during sevoflurane anesthesia: a comparison with isoflurane. Anesth Analg 88:341–345

Takahashi H, Murata K, Ikeda K (1993) Sevoflurane does not increase intracranial pressure in hyperventilated dogs. Br J Anaesth 71:551–555

Talke P, Caldwell JE, Richardson CA (1999) Sevoflurane increases lumbar cerebrospinal fluid pressure in normocapnic patients undergoing transsphenoidal hypophysectomy. Anesthesiology 91:127–130

Chapter 10
Effect of Hyperventilation on Subdural Intracranial Pressure

Lise Schlünzen and Georg Emil Cold

Abstract

Hyperventilation has been used in the treatment of patients with intracranial pathologies for decades. In the neurointensive care unit the use of hyperventilation is on retreat due to the risk of cerebral ischaemia. During surgery the situation is somewhat different because of the shorter duration of hyperventilation and the close monitoring of physiological parameters.

In this chapter the results of three studies regarding the effect of hyperventilation on subdural ICP and cerebral haemodynamics during four anaesthetic regimes are presented. The inhalation agents most often used in western countries, isoflurane and sevoflurane, as well as the total intravenous anaesthetic regimes of propofol-fentanyl and propofol-remifentanil, and the influence on ICP during hyperventilation are discussed.

In Chapter 8 studies of ICP and cerebral haemodynamics in patients subjected to craniotomy for cerebral tumours are summarized. Four anaesthetic regimes, including propofol-fentanyl, isoflurane-fentanyl, sevoflurane-fentanyl and propofol-remifentanil, were studied. As regards ICP at the time of opening of dura ICP was significantly higher during isoflurane-fentanyl and sevoflurane-fentanyl compared with propofol-fentanyl, but lower during propofol-remifentanil than during propofol-fentanyl.

Continuous remifentanil infusion combined with propofol provides stable central haemodynamics, but clinical data concerning ICP and other measures of cerebral haemodynamics are few. In clinical practice in our clinic the maintenance dose of propofol is higher during propofol-fentanyl- compared with propofol-remifentanil-anaesthetized patients subjected to craniotomy. As a consequence it is expected that the suppression of cerebral metabolism and thereby CBF is more pronounced during propofol-fentanyl anaesthesia. Consequently, ICP theoretically should be lower. Moreover, the lower blood pressure during propofol-remifentanil anaesthesia should decrease CPP. If cerebral autoregulation is predominantly intact this decrease should increase

ICP. In contrast, ICP should decrease if cerebral autoregulation is lost. As the effect of hyperventilation on ICP is influenced by cerebral autoregulation as well as the depression of cerebral oxygen uptake, and anaesthetics influence both factors, studies of hyperventilation during different anaesthetic regimes seem justified. Moreover, studies of the combination of hyperventilation, which acts via cerebral vasoconstriction, and mannitol treatment, acting via osmotic forces, are of interest, and especially in cases where hyperventilation alone does not reduces ICP below the threshold for occurrence of brain swelling after opening of dura.

In this chapter the results of three studies of the effect of hyperventilation on subdural ICP and cerebral haemodynamics during four anaesthetic regimes are presented. Results of the first study have been presented by Petersen et al. in Anesthesiology (2003) 98:329–336.

Study 1: Comparative Study of the Effect of Hyperventilation During Propofol-Fentanyl, Isoflurane-Fentanyl and Sevoflurane-Fentanyl Anaesthesia on Cerebral Haemodynamics

Aim To study the effect of hyperventilation on cerebral haemodynamics in patients subjected to craniotomy for supratentorial cerebral tumours during anaesthesia with propofol-fentanyl, isoflurane-fentanyl or sevoflurane-fentanyl.

Method In an open label study 117 patients with supratentorial cerebral tumours were randomized to propofol-fentanyl (group 1), isoflurane-fentanyl (group 2) or sevoflurane-fentanyl anaesthesia (group 3). Principles for anaesthesia (induction and maintenance) are indicated in Chapters 3 and 8. Principles for neuroradiological and pathological findings and monitoring are indicated in Chapter 3. Normo- to moderate hypocapnia was applied, the target level of $PaCO_2$ being 30–40 mmHg. MABP was stabilized with i.v. ephedrine (2.5–5 mg), if necessary. Subdural ICP, MABP, CPP, $AVDO_2$ and internal jugular vein oxygen saturation (SjO_2) were monitored before and after a 10-min period of hyperventilation, and the CO_2 reactivity was calculated. Furthermore, the tension of dura before and during hyperventilation, and the degree of cerebral swelling during hyperventilation and after opening of dura were estimated by the neurosurgeon. Data concerning neurological findings, pathology and demographics are summarized in Chapter 8, study 1.

Statistical analysis Based on a previous non-randomized study of ICP during three different anaesthetic techniques, given a minimum detectable difference of 3.6 mmHg, expected SD of 5.0 mmHg, power of 0.80 and a significance level of $P<0.05$, the total number of patients was calculated to be 114 patients. Data within groups were tested for normal distribution. The normality test and equal variance test were applied, one-way ANOVA was used for analysis if these tests were passed, and Tukey's test was used for pair-wise multiple comparison procedures. The Kruskal-Wallis one-way analysis of variance on ranks and multiple comparisons versus control groups (Dunn's method) were used for statistical analysis when the normality test or equal variance test were not passed. These data included subdural ICP, MABP and $AVDO_2$. Bonferroni's test was applied for statistical analysis. The chi-square test was used for statistical analysis of demographic data, localization, size and histopathological diagnosis of the tumours, preoperative steroid administration and position of the head between the groups. Difference in tension of dura and the degree of cerebral swelling were tested by the chi-square test. For correlation studies Pearson's product moment correlation and linear regression were performed. Mean±SD were calculated. $P<0.05$ was considered statistically significant.

Results No significant differences between the three anaesthetic groups were disclosed as regards neurological findings, pathology and demographics. During hyperventilation ICP decreased significantly in all groups. ICP was sinificantly lower while MABP and CPP were significantly higher during propofol-fentanyl compared to isoflurane-fentanyl and sevoflurane-fentanyl

Table 10.1 Data obtained before and during hyperventilation, changes in parameters before and during hyperventilation, and CO_2 reactivity. Mean±SD are indicated. No significant differences were disclosed between the isoflurane and sevoflurane groups

	Propofol	Isoflurane	Sevoflurane
Before hyperventilation			
MABP (mmHg)	86.0±14.0	73.0±10.0	76.0±10.0
ICP (mmHg)	7.5±4.9	13.0±7.5*	13.2±7.1*
CPP (mmHg)	78.0±15.0	60.0±12.0*	63.0±8.0*
JBP (mmHg)	7.0±3.5	8.5±4.3	8.9±3.9
$PaCO_2$ (mmHg)	34.5±3.0	34.5±3.0	36.0±3.0
PaO_2 (mmHg)	203.0±68.0	197.0±66.0	179.0±67.0
SATv (%)	57.0±10.0	65.0±11.0*	65.0±12.0*
$AVDO_2$ (mmol/L)	3.1±0.8	2.5±0.8*	2.5±0.8*
Temperature (°C)	35.8±0.4	36.0±0.6	35.9±0.7
During hyperventilation			
MABP (mmHg)	87.0±13.0	71.0±12.0	74.0±11.0
ICP (mmHg)	5.8±4.6	9.8±6.3*	9.4±6.6*
CPP (mmHg)	82.0±14.0	61.0±11.0*	64.0±10.0*
JBP (mmHg)	6.3±3.4	8.1±4.0	8.4±4.2
$PaCO_2$ (mmHg)	28.5±3.0	29.3±2.3	30.8±3.0*
SATv (%)	52.0±11.0	57.0±12.0*	56.0±12.0*
$AVDO_2$ (mmol/L)	3.6±0.9	3.0±0.9*	3.2±0.8
ΔICP (mmHg)	1.7±2.2	3.2±3.7*	3.4±3.7*
$ΔPaCO_2$ (mmHg)	6.1±2.0	5.0±2.0*	4.9±2.2*
ΔCPP (mmHg)	3.3±6.1	1.5±7.4	0.2±8.7
CO_2 reactivity (% change $AVDO_2/ΔPaCO_2$ (mmHg))	2.0±1.4	3.6±2.6*	4.6±3.2*

*$P<0.05$ compared with the propofol group

anaesthesia. Hyperventilation was accompanied by a significant increase in $AVDO_2$ in all groups. During propofol-fentanyl anaesthesia $AVDO_2$ was significantly higher compared with isoflurane-fentanyl anaesthesia, but not significantly different from sevoflurane-fentanyl anaesthesia. $PaCO_2$ was significantly higher in the sevoflurane group compared with the propofol group.

The CO_2 reactivity was significantly lower during propofol-fentanyl compared with isoflurane-fentanyl and sevoflurane-fentanyl anaesthesia. Although the difference in $PaCO_2$ was significantly greater during propofol-fentanyl anaesthesia, the reduction in ICP during hyperventilation was significantly smaller compared with isoflurane-fentanyl and sevoflurane-fentanyl anaesthesia, respectively (Table 10.1).

The distributions of the tactile estimate of dural tension before and during hyperventilation, and the estimates of brain swelling after opening of dura are indicated in Table 10.2. Before and during hyperventilation dural tension was significantly lower during propofol-fentanyl compared with isoflurane-fen-

Table 10.2 Degree of dural tension before hyperventilation and during hyperventilation, and the degree of brain swelling after opening of dura. Number and percentage are indicated. No significant differences between the isoflurane and sevoflurane groups were disclosed

	Propofol	Isoflurane	Sevoflurane
Tension of dura before hyperventilation			
Dura slack	4 (9.8%)	1 (2.6%)	1 (2.6%)
Normal tension	22 (53.7%)	11 (28.9%)	14 (36.8%)
Moderately increased tension	13 (31.7%)	20 (52.6%)	21 (55.3%)
Pronounced increase in tension	2 (4.9%)	6 (15.8%)	2 (5.3%)
Significance compared with propofol		$P<0.05$	Not significant
Tension of dura during hyperventilation			
Dura slack	7 (17.1%)	2 (5.3%)	2 (5.3%)
Normal tension	24 (58.5%)	16 (42.1%)	23 (60.5%)
Moderately increased tension	8 (19.5%)	14 (36.8%)	13 (34.2%)
Pronounced increase in tension	2 (4.9%)	6 (15.8%)	0 (0.0%)
Significance compared with propofol		$P<0.05$	Not significant
Brain swelling			
No swelling	30 (73.2%)	16 (42.1%)	21 (53.3%)
Moderate swelling	11 (26.8%)	16 (42.1%)	14 (36.8%)
Pronounced swelling	0 (0.0%)	6 (15.8%)	3 (7.9%)
Significance compared with propofol		$P<0.05$	Not significant

tanyl anaesthesia. After opening of the dura the degree of cerebral swelling was found to be more prominent during isoflurane-fentanyl and sevoflurane-fentanyl anaesthesia compared with propofol-fentanyl anaesthesia.

Correlation studies No significant correlations were found between $PaCO_2$ and ICP, between $\Delta PaCO_2$ and ΔICP or between MABP and ICP in the respective groups. Neither did we find any significant correlation between neuroradiological data (tumour size, midline shift) and subdural ICP obtained before hyperventilation, or between the anaesthetic maintenance dose of fentanyl and subdural ICP.

Conclusion The study indicates that before as well as during hyperventilation, subdural ICP and $AVDO_2$ are lower and CPP higher in propofol-anaesthetized patients compared with patients anaesthetized with isoflurane or sevoflurane. These findings were associated with less tendency for cerebral swelling after opening of dura in the propofol group. The CO_2 reactivity in patients anaesthetized with isoflurane and sevoflurane was significantly higher than in the propofol group. The differences in subdural ICP between the groups are presumed to be caused by differences in the degree of vasoconstriction elicited by the anaesthetic agents, but autoregulatory mechanisms caused by differences in CPP cannot be excluded.

Study 2: Comparative Study of the Effect of Hyperventilation During Propofol-Fentanyl and Propofol-Remifentanil Anaesthesia on Cerebral Haemodynamics

Aim To study the effect of hyperventilation on cerebral haemodynamics in patients subjected to craniotomy for supratentorial cerebral tumours in anaesthesia with either propofol-fentanyl or propofol-remifentanil.

Method Subdural ICP, MABP, CPP, $PaCO_2$, SATv, JBP, and $AVDO_2$ were compared in 52 patients scheduled to propofol-fentanyl (P/F) anaesthesia and 53 patients to propofol-remifentanil (P/R) anaesthesia. The measurements were performed before and immediately after a 5-min period of hyperventilation. Principles for anaesthesia (induction and maintenance), and principles for neuroradiological and pathological findings and monitoring are indicated in Chapter 3.

Statistical analysis Based on a previous non-randomized study of ICP during three different anaesthetic techniques, given a minimum detectable difference of 3.6 mmHg, expected SD of 5.0 mmHg, power of 0.80 and a significance level of $P<0.05$, the total number of patients was calculated to be 114 patients. Data within groups were tested for normal distribution. The normality test and equal variance test were applied, one-way ANOVA was used for analysis if these tests were passed, and Tukey's test was used for pair-wise multiple comparison procedures. The Kruskal-Wallis one-way analysis of variance on ranks and multiple comparisons versus control groups (Dunn's method) were used for statistical analysis when the normality test or equal variance test were not passed. These data included subdural ICP, MABP and $AVDO_2$. Bonferroni's test was applied for statistical analysis. The chi-square test was used for statistical analysis of demographic data, localization, size and histopathological diagnosis of the tumours, preoperative steroid administration and position of the head between the groups. Difference in tension of dura and the degree of cerebral swelling were tested by the chi-square test. For correlation studies Pearson's product moment correlation and linear regression were performed. Mean±SD were calculated. $P<0.05$ was considered statistically significant.

Results   Demographic data, neurological findings, including maximal area of the tumour and midline shift, were comparable between the two groups. Neither did electrolytes, haemoglobin, blood pressure on admission, histopathological data nor distribution of tumour localization differ significantly between groups. The maintenance dose of propofol was 8.9 mg/kg/h in the

Table 10.3   Data obtained before and during hyperventilation, changes in parameters before and during hyperventilation, and CO_2 reactivity. Mean±SD are indicated

	Propofol -fentanyl	Propofol -remifentanil	*P* values
Before hyperventilation			
Temperature (°C)	35.8±0.5	35.8±0.4	0.924
$PaCO_2$ (kPa)	4.6±0.4	4.5±0.3	0.289
PaO_2 (kPa)	27.2±8.3	25.2±7.0	0.196
MABP (mmHg)	86.0±13.0	76.0±14.0	<0.001
ICP (mmHg)	6.8±4.8	6.2±3.9	0.690
CPP (mmHg)	80.0±14.0	69.0±14.0	<0.001
JBP (mmHg)	6.8±4.0	2.7±3.4	<0.001
Jugular oxygen saturation (%)	56.8±9.6	53.2±10.5	0.044
$AVDO_2$ (mmol/L)	3.2±0.7	3.4±0.7	0.262
During hyperventilation			
$PaCO_2$ (kPa)	3.8±0.5	3.9±0.3	0.641
MABP (mmHg)	87.0±13.0	74.0±13.0	<0.001
ICP (mmHg)	5.1±4.6	4.3±3.8	0.475
CPP (mmHg)	82.0±14.0	70.0±13.0	<0.001
JBP (mmHg)	6.2±4.0	2.6±3.3	<0.001
Jugular oxygen saturation (%)	51.2±10.6	47.7±10.8	0.070
$AVDO_2$ (mmol/L)	3.6±0.8	3.7±0.7	0.402
$\Delta PaCO_2$ (kPa)	0.74±0.26	0.70±0.20	0.615
ΔICP (mmHg)	1.6±1.6	2.0±1.4	0.088
ΔCPP (mmHg)	1.8±5.3	2.0±1.4	0.670
CO_2 reactivity (% change $AVDO_2/\Delta PaCO_2$ (mmHg))	2.0±1.4	1.9±1.4	0.670

propofol-fentanyl group, against 5.8 mg/kg/h in the propofol-remifentanil group ($P<0.001$). No significant differences between groups were found as regards $PaCO_2$, PaO_2, $AVDO_2$ or rectal temperature.

During hyperventilation ICP averaged 5.1 and 4.3 mmHg in the propofol-fentanyl and propofol-remifentanil groups, respectively ($P=0.475$). MABP and CPP were 87 and 82 mmHg in the propofol-fentanyl group against 74 and 70 mmHg in the propofol-remifentanil group. In intergroups, differences in MABP and CPP were significant ($P<0.001$). SATv or $AVDO_2$ did not differ significantly between groups. As regards changes in $PaCO_2$ ($\Delta PaCO_2$ mmHg), MABP ($\Delta MABP$ mmHg), ICP (ΔICP mmHg), CPP (ΔCPP mmHg) and the CO_2 reactivity no significant intergroup differences were disclosed (Table 10.3). No significant differences as regards the degree of dural tension or the degree of cerebral swelling after opening of dura were disclosed either before or during hyperventilation.

Conclusion   No difference in ICP during hyperventilation between patients anaesthetized with propofol-fentanyl or propofol-remifentanil was found. MABP and CPP were significantly lower in the patients anaesthetized with propofol-remifentanil.

Study 3: Is It Possible to Reduce Subdural Intracranial Pressure Below 10 mmHg by Hyperventilation Eventually Supplemented with Mannitol Treatment?

Aim   To evaluate if hyperventilation eventually supplemented with mannitol treatment is able to reduce subdural ICP below 10 mmHg in patients subjected to craniotomy for supratentorial cerebral tumours.

Method   Twenty-nine patients with supratentorial cerebral tumours (glioblastoma ($n=12$), meningioma ($n=6$), astrocytoma ($n=7$), other tumours ($n=4$)) were included in the study. For maintenance of anaesthesia propofol-fentanyl was used. After exposure of dura subdural ICP, MABP and arterial gas analyses were performed. These measurements were repeated after 5 min hyperventilation. If subdural ICP was ≥ 10 mmHg, mannitol 1 g/kg was administered over 5 min, and the measurements were repeated 15 min after the start of mannitol treatment. After opening of dura the degree of brain swelling was evaluated by the surgeon.

Statistical analysis   Median and range are presented. Mann-Whitney's test was used for intergroup analyses. $P<0.05$ signifies statistical significance.

Results   Before hyperventilation, the median level of subdural ICP was 9 mmHg (range −2 to 20 mmHg). In 16 of 29 patients (55%) subdural ICP < 10 mmHg was observed, and the tension of dura was estimated as normal. In the remaining 13 patients with subdural ICP ≥ 10 mmHg, dural tension was normal in 5 patients and increased in 8 patients. After 5 min hyperventilation

Table 10.4 $PaCO_2$, MABP, subdural ICP and CPP in 29 patients with cerebral tumours before and during hyperventilation

Variable	Before hyperventilation	During hyperventilation	Significance
$PaCO_2$ (kPa)	4.9 (4.1–5.6)	4.1 (3.2–4.8	$P<0.05$
MABP (mmHg)	81.0 (58.0–118.0)	83.0 (59.0–155.0)	Not significant
ICP (mmHg)	9.0 (−2.0 to 20.0)	7.0 (−3.0 to 14.0)	$P<0.05$
CPP (mmHg)	72.0 (49.0–98.0)	76.0 (54.0–103.0)	$P<0.05$

Table 10.5 $PaCO_2$, MABP, subdural ICP and CPP before mannitol and 15 min after mannitol (1 g/kg) combined with hyperventilation in 7 patients with ICP $\geq$ 10 mmHg

Variable	Before mannitol	After mannitol	Significance
$PaCO_2$ (kPa)	3.9 (3.5–4.8)	3.6 (3.3–4.4)	$P<0.05$
MABP (mmHg)	86.0 (71.0–99.0)	85.0 (70.0–106.0)	Not significant
ICP (mmHg)	13.0 (10.0–14.0)	9.0 (4.0–12.0)	$P<0.05$
CPP (mmHg)	73.0 (57.0–103.0)	76.0 (58.0–112.0)	$P<0.05$

a significant decrease in the median level of subdural ICP from 9 mmHg (−2 to 20 mmHg) to 7 mmHg (−3 to 14 mmHg) was observed (Table 10.4). In total, hyperventilation elicited a decrease in subdural ICP in 24 of 29 patients. Dural tension was still increased in 6 patients. In 7 patients with a median subdural ICP of 13 mmHg (10–14 mmHg) mannitol (1 g/kg) was administered, while hyperventilation continued. After 15 min a significant decrease in subdural ICP to median 9 mmHg (4–12 mmHg) was observed (Table 10.5). Two patients still had subdural ICP $\geq$ 10 mmHg (12 mmHg), and in these patients pronounced brain swelling was observed after opening of dura. In the other patients brain swelling did not occur. In total, moderate brain swelling was observed in 4 patients and pronounced swelling in 2 patients.

Conclusion Addition of mannitol to hyperventilation decreases ICP during craniotomy.

Discussion

In this review the effect of hyperventilation on subdural ICP and cerebral haemodynamics has been analysed during four different anaesthetic procedures, including propofol-fentanyl, propofol-remifentanil, isoflurane-fentanyl and sevoflurane-fentanyl. The principal findings were that hyperventilation decreased subdural ICP significantly independent of anaesthetic method, but the effect differed. Thus, the ICP-reducing effect of hyperventilation was most pronounced during isoflurane-fentanyl and sevoflurane-fentanyl anaesthesia, while the ICP-reducing effect was less pronounced during propofol-fentanyl and propofol-remifentanil anaesthesia. Accordingly, the relative CO_2 reactivity calculated as the % change $AVDO_2/\Delta P_aCO_2/mmHg$ was higher during isoflurane and sevoflurane anaesthesia compared with the CO_2 reactivities obtained during propofol-fentanyl and propofol-remifentanil anaesthesia. These findings correspond to experimental and clinical studies. During isoflurane-nitrous oxide anaesthesia for supratentorial cerebral tumours the CO_2 reactivity is preserved, averaging 4.4%/mmHg $PaCO_2$ (Madsen et al. 1987). In another study including patients subjected to craniotomy for supratentorial cerebral tumours, the relative CO_2 reactivity averaged 3.3% and 2.2% change $AVDO_2/$ $\Delta PaCO_2/mmHg$ at concentrations of 0.7 and 1.3 MAC sevoflurane (Bundgaard et al. 1998). In patients without cerebral diseases (Cho et al. 1996), patients with cerebral tumours (Inada et al. 1996), patients with cardiac disease (Mielck et al. 1999) and patients subjected to extra-intracranial by-pass anastomosis (Kitaguchi et al. 1993) the CO_2 reactivity is intact during sevoflurane anaesthesia. In another study it was documented that the CO_2 reactivity in young adults, ranging from 20 to 40 years, is greater than in adults in the range 50–70 years of age (Nishiyama et al. 1999). In dogs subjected to low and moderate doses of propofol, the cerebral autoregulation and CO_2 reactivity were preserved. In contrast, high-dose propofol decreased CPP below the lower point of cerebral autoregulation (Artru et al. 1992). In rabbit's subjected to propofol anaesthesia the cerebrovascular reactivity of blood flow and CBV are markedly decreased during hypocapnia, but maintained during hypercapnia (Cenic et al. 2000). After propofol bolus injection the CO_2 reactivity was preserved (Stephan et al. 1987). This finding was also confirmed in studies with the Doppler technique (Jansen and Kagenaar 1993; Strebel et al. 1994; Ederberg 1998). In a study including healthy adults the slope of the CBF versus $PaCO_2$ was 1.56 ml/100 g/ min/mmHg $PaCO_2$ (Fox et al. 1992). During continuous propofol infusion in patients without brain disorders the CO_2 reactivity was also found to be intact (Harrison et al. 1999). In other studies the CO_2 reactivity based on flow velocity was attenuated (Mirzai et al. 2004). Hyperventilation to end-tidal CO_2 values less than 30 mmHg is without effect because flow velocity is unchanged below this level (Karsli et al. 2004).

The low CO_2 reactivity found during propofol-remifentanil and propofol-fentanyl anaesthesia may be for the following reasons. One explanation, at least during propofol-remifentanil anaesthesia, is that the CPP was significantly lower compared with the other three anaesthetic procedures, and close to the lower point of cerebral autoregulation of 60 mmHg. In dogs the CO_2 reactivity is sustained during drug-induced hypotension (Artru and Colley 1984), and during propofol-fentanyl anaesthesia nicardipine-, nitroglycerin- and prostaglandin E_1-induced hypotension attenuate the CO_2 reactivity (Endoh et al. 1999). Studies in rats subjected to intracranial hypertension also indicate that reduced CPP seems to be followed by a decreased CO_2 reactivity (Hauerberg et al. 2001). The low CO_2 reactivity found during hypotension might be considered as a sign of threatening cerebral ischaemia and as such is accompanied by an increase in $AVDO_2$ and a low SATv. In awake healthy humans SjO_2 averages 62% (range 55–75%). In acute head injury $SjO_2 < 50\%$

suggests hypoperfusion, and readings $< 40\%$ are supposed to be associated with cerebral ischaemia (Gopinath et al. 1996). In comparison with isoflurane and sevoflurane low values of SATv were disclosed during propofol anaesthesia in patients undergoing coronary by-pass (Nandate et al. 2000), and during craniotomy a 50% incidence of $SjO_2 < 50\%$ was found in patients subjected to propofol-fentanyl anaesthesia, but not in patients anaesthetized with isoflurane-nitrous oxide (Moss et al. 1995; Jansen et al. 1999). In the studies presented in this chapter venous saturations were significantly lower during propofol-fentanyl and propofol-remifentanil compared with isoflurane-fentanyl and sevoflurane-fentanyl anaesthesia. After hyperventilation the incidences of low venous saturation (high $AVDO_2$) increased in all groups. The differences in SjO_2 between the respective groups were not explained alone by the difference in the level of blood pressure or CPP, the latter being higher in the propofol-fentanyl group. It must be stressed that a threshold value of SjO_2 indicating impeding cerebral ischaemia has not been defined during clinical anaesthesia. Propofol is generally accepted as an agent with neuroprotective properties and propofol-induced neurological deterioration has never been described. In a recent clinical PET study, no indication of propofol-induced diffusion-weighted ischaemic changes were observed in patients with cerebral tumours (Rasmussen et al. 2004).

In the third study hyperventilation and the combined use of hyperventilation and mannitol treatment were studied in patients with supratentorial cerebral tumours. Although both treatment modalities reduced subdural ICP significantly during the 20-min study, it was not possible to reduce subdural ICP to $< 10\,mmHg$ in all patients, and pronounced swelling after opening of dura was observed in two patients. If cerebral swelling is to be omitted, other measures to reduce subdural ICP, such as the use of rTp (Haure et al. 2003; Tankisi and Cold 2007), indomethacin (Bundgaard et al. 1996), surgical decompression, drainage of CSF or evacuation of fluid from cystic processes (see Chapter 17), might be considered appropriate.

References

Artru AA, Coley PS (1984) Cerebral blood flow responses to hypocapnia during hypotension. Stroke 15:878–883

Artru AA, Shapira Y, Bowdle A (1992) Electroencephalogram, cerebral metabolism, and vascular responses to propofol anesthesia in dogs. J Neurosurg Anesthesiol 4:99–109

Bundgaard H, Jensen K, Cold GE et al (1996) Effects of perioperative indomethacin on intracranial pressure, cerebral blood flow, and cerebral metabolism in patients subjected to craniotomy for cerebral tumours. J Neurosurg Anesthesiol 8:273–279

Bundgaard H, vonOettingen G, Larsen KM et al (1998) Effect of sevoflurane on intracranial pressure, cerebral blood flow and cerebral metabolism. Acta Anaesthesiol Scand 42:621–627

Cenic A, Craen RA, Howard-Lech VL et al (2000) Cerebral blood volume and blood flow at varying arterial carbon dioxide tension levels in rabbits during propofol anaesthesia. Anesth Analg 90:1376–1383

Cho S, Fujigaki T, Uchiyama Y et al (1996) Effects of sevoflurane with and without nitrous oxide on human cerebral circulation. Anesthesiology 85:755–760

Ederberg S, Westerlind A, Houltz E et al (1998) The effects of propofol on cerebral blood flow velocity and cerebral oxygen extraction during cardiopulmonary bypass. Anesth Analg 86:1201–1206

Endoh H, Honda T, Komura N, et al (1999) Effects of nicardipine-, nitroglycerin- and prostaglandin E_1-induced hypotension on human cerebrovascular carbon dioxide reactivity during propofol-fentanyl anesthesia. J Clin Anesth 11:545–549

Fox J, Gelb AW, Enns J et al (1992). The responsiveness of cerebral blood flow to changes in arterial carbon dioxide is maintained during propofol-nitrous oxide anesthesia in humans. Anesthesiology 77:453–456

Gopinath SP, Cormio M, Ziegler J et al (1996) Intraoperative jugular desaturation during surgery for traumatic intracranial hematomas. Anesth Analg 83:1014–1021

Harrison JM, Girling KJ, Mahajan RP(1999) Effects of target-controlled infusion of propofol on the transient hyperaemic response and carbon dioxide reactivity in the middle cerebral artery. Br J Anaesth 83:839–844

Hauerberg J, Ma X, Bay-Hansen R et al (2001) Effects of alterations in arterial CO_2 tension on cerebral blood flow during acute intracranial hypertension in rats. J Neurosurg Anesthesiol 13:213–221

Haure P, Cold GE, Hansen TM et al (2003) The ICP-lowering effect of 10° reverse Trendelenburg position during craniotomy is stable during a 10-minute period. J Neurosurg Anesthesiol 4:297–301

Inada T, Shingu K, Uchida M et al (1996) Changes in the cerebral arteriovenous oxygen content difference by surgical incision are similar during sevoflurane and isoflurane anaesthesia. Can J Anaesth 43:1019–1024

Jansen GF, Kagenaar D (1993) Effects of propofol in the relation between CO_2 and cerebral blood flow velocity. Anesth Analg 76:S163

Jansen GF, van Praagh BH, Kedaria MB et al (1999) Jugular bulb oxygen saturation during propofol and isoflurane/nitrous oxide anesthesia in patients undergoing brain tumor surgery Anesth Analg 89:358–363

Karsli C, Luginbuehl I, Bissonnette B (2004) The cerebrovascular response to hypocapnia in children receiving propofol. Anesth Analg 99:1049–1052

Kitaguchi K, Ohsumi H, Kuro M et al (1993) Effects of sevoflurane on cerebral circulation and metabolism in patients with ischemic cerebrovascular disease. Anesthesiology 79:704–709

Madsen JB, Cold GE, Hansen ES et al (1987) The effect of isoflurane on cerebral blood flow and metabolism in humans during craniotomy for small supratentorial cerebral tumours. Anesthesiology 66:332–336

Mielck F, Stephan H, Weyland A et al (1999) Effects of one minimum alveolar anesthesic concentration sevoflurane on cerebral metabolism, blood flow, and CO_2 reactivity in cardiac patients. Anesth Analg 89:364–369

Mirzai H, Tekin I, Tarhan S et al (2004) Effect of propofol and clonidine on cerebral blood flow velocity and carbon dioxide reactivity in the middle cerebral artery. J Neurosurg Anesthesiol 16:1–5

Moss E, Dearden NM, Berridge JC (1995) Effects of changes in mean arterial pressure on SjO_2 during cerebral aneurysm surgery. Br J Anaesth 75:527–530

Nandate K, Vuylsteke A, Ratsep I et al (2000) Effects of isoflurane, sevoflurane and propofol anaesthesia on jugular venous oxygen saturation in patients undergoing coronary artery by-pass surgery. Br J Anaesth 84:631–633

Nishiyama T, Matsukawa T, Yokoyama T et al (1999) Cerebrovascular carbon dioxide reactivity during general anaesthesia: a comparison between sevoflurane and isoflurane. Anesth Analg 89:1437–1441

Rasmussen M, Østergaard L, Juul N et al (2004) Do indomethacin and propofol cause cerebral ischemic damage? Anesthesiology 101:872–878

Stephan H, Sonntag H, Schenk HD (1987) Einfluss von Disoprivan (Propofol) auf die Durchblutung und Sauerstoffverbrauch des Gehirns and die CO_2 Reaktivität der Hirngefässe beim Menschen. Anaesthetist 36:60–65

Strebel S, Kaufmann M, Guardiola P-M (1994) Cerebral vasomotor responsiveness to carbon dioxide is preserved during propofol and midazolam anaesthesia in humans. Anaesth Analg 78:884–888

Tankisi A, Cold GE (2007) Optimal reverse Trendelenburg position in patients undergoing craniotomy for cerebral tumours. J Neurosurg 106:239–244

Effect of Indomethacin on Subdural Intracranial Pressure and Cerebral Haemodynamics

Mads Rasmussen and Georg Emil Cold

Abstract

Treatment options for increased ICP during craniotomy include hyperventilation, bolus injection of barbiturate or other hypnotic agents, mannitol administration and head elevation. However, these interventions are not consistently successful. Indomethacin acts as a potent cerebral vasoconstrictor and decreases cerebral blood flow and ICP without affecting cerebral oxygen consumption. Previous studies in patients with severe head injury suggested that indomethacin may be effective in lowering high ICP resistant to the traditional methods of managing elevated ICP. Administration of indomethacin may be an alternative option for managing increased ICP in patients undergoing craniotomy.

In this chapter two studies concerning indomethacin are presented. The first study includes the effect of perioperative indomethacin on subdural ICP, cerebral blood flow and cerebral metabolic rate of oxygen in patients subjected to craniotomy for cerebral tumour. The second study is a randomized study where we investigated the effect of indomethacin on ICP and cerebral haemodynamics in patients undergoing supratentorial craniotomy.

Treatment options for increased ICP during craniotomy include hyperventilation, bolus injection of barbiturate or other hypnotic agents, mannitol administration and head elevation (Miller and Leech 1975; Bedford et al. 1980; Cenic et al. 2000; Tankisi et al. 2002). Intracranial hypertension can also be treated by surgical drainage of CSF or evacuation of cystic intracranial processes if present. However, these interventions are not consistently successful. Controlled hyperventilation is often of limited value; patients with intracerebral space-occupying lesions may have impaired or abolished cerebrovascular reactivity to changes in $PaCO_2$. The effect of hyperventilation are subject to adaptation (Raichle and Plum 1972) and adverse effects have been reported (Cold 1989; Muizelaar et al. 1991). The effect of mannitol has also been questioned (Kaufmann and Cardoso 1992). Barbiturates may induce cardiovascular depression with a decrease in CPP, and CSF drainage is often impossible because of difficult access to the ventricular system. In experimental and human studies indomethacin, a fatty acid cyclooxygenase inhibitor, acts as a potent cerebral vasoconstrictor and decreases CBF without affecting cerebral oxygen consumption (Pichard and MacKenzie 1973; Wennmalm et al. 1981; Jensen et al. 1993). In patients with severe head injury and otherwise intractable intracranial hypertension, indomethacin reduces ICP substantially and within a few minutes. This effect is accompanied by a decrease in CBF, while $CMRO_2$ is unchanged (Jensen et al. 1991). In another study of patients with severe acute head injury, the ICP-reducing effect of indomethacin was comparable with the effect of hyperventilation (Dahl et al. 1996). In some patients, however, the ICP-reducing effect of indomethacin was more pronounced than hyperventilation and vice versa (Dahl et al. 1996).

Two studies are presented in this chapter: the first has been presented by Bundgaard et al. in J Neurosurg Anesthesiol (1996) 8:273–279 and the second has been presented by Rasmussen et al. in Anaesthesia (2004) 59:1–9.

Study 1: Effect of Perioperative Indomethacin on Intracranial Pressure, Cerebral Blood Flow and Cerebral Metabolism in Patients Subjected to Craniotomy for Cerebral Tumours

Aim   To examine the effect of perioperatively administered indomethacin on subdural ICP, CBF and $CMRO_2$ in patients subjected to craniotomy for supratentorial cerebral tumours.

Methods   Twenty adult patients, age 18–70 years, with supratentorial cerebral tumours participated in the study. Anaesthesia was maintained with isoflurane-nitrous oxide-fentanyl. The patients were randomized to receive intravenous indomethacin 50 mg or placebo (0.9% saline) administered after exposure of the dura mater. Subdural ICP was measured after removal of the bone flap and exposure of the dura mater as previously described. Subdural ICP, MABP and CPP were recorded simultaneously and continuously. CBF was measured by the ^{133}Xe method and calculated as the initial slope index using 10-min clearance curves. For measurement of $AVDO_2$ and jugular bulb oxygen saturation (SjO_2) a jugular bulb catheter was inserted. Measurements of ICP, CPP, CBF and $AVDO_2$ were performed before and after administration of indomethacin/placebo. All measurements were performed before opening of dura mater.

Statistical analysis   Medians and range were calculated. The Mann-Whitney test was used to analyse data between the two groups, and the Wilcoxon test was used to analyse data within groups. Statistical significance was considered to be $P<0.05$.

Results   No significant differences between the two groups were found, as regards demographics (age, weight, gender), tumour volume, time until opening of dura, number of patients receiving preoperative steroid, anaesthetic doses, rectal temperature and $PaCO_2$ level.

Physiological data are shown in Table 11.1 (see page 170). In the placebo group no significant differences were observed in ICP, CBF, CPP, SjO_2 or $AVDO_2$. Indomethacin bolus was accompanied by: an increase in MABP from median 69 mmHg (range 65–83) to 82 mmHg (range 78–93), $P<0.05$; a decrease in subdural ICP from 6.5 mmHg (range 2–27) to 1.5 mmHg (range −1 to 18), $P<0.05$; a decrease in CBF from 39 ml/100 g/min (range 20–31) to 20 ml/100 g/min (range 14–31), $P<0.05$; a decrease in SjO_2 from 69% (range 45–89) to 49% (range 38–83), $P<0.05$; and an increase in $AVDO_2$ from 1.7 mmol/L (range 0.7–2.9) to 3.2 mmol/L (range 1.2–4.2), $P<0.05$.

Conclusion Indomethacin effectively reduces ICP by a cerebral vasoconstrictive effect giving rise to a fall in CBF and SjO_2 and an increase in $AVDO_2$. The effect of i.v. indomethacin on ICP occurs within 1 min, and is accompanied by an increase in MABP and CPP.

Study 2: Effect of Indomethacin on Intracranial Pressure and Cerebral Haemodynamics in Patients Undergoing Craniotomy: A Randomized Prospective Study

Aim To investigate the perioperative effect of indomethacin, administered immediately before induction of anaesthesia, on subdural ICP in patients subjected to craniotomy for supratentorial tumours.

Method We compared the effect of indomethacin (bolus of 0.2 mg/kg followed by infusion of 0.2 mg/kg/h) and placebo on ICP and cerebral haemodynamics in 30 patients undergoing craniotomy for supratentorial brain tumours in propofol-fentanyl anaesthesia. Indomethacin was administered beore induction of anaesthesia and the infusion was terminated after opening of dura. Subdural ICP was measured through the first burr hole and before opening of dura. CBF velocity, CPP, SjO_2), $AVDO_2$ and CO_2 reactivity were measured and dural tension and the degree of brain swelling were estimated.

Statistical analysis Non-parametric data are reported as median (interquartile range). The Mann-Whitney test was used to analyse data between the two groups and the Wilcoxon signed rank test was used to analyse data within groups. Parametric data are reported as mean±SD and Student's *t*-test was used to analyse data between groups. The chi-square test was used for statistical analysis of demographic data, tumour localization, histopathological diagosis, preoperative steroid administration, difference in dural tension and the degree of swelling (no swelling contra swelling).

Table 11.1 Physiological parameters measured before and after administration of indomethacin 50 mg i.v (group 1) or placebo (group 2)

		$PaCO_2$ (kPa)	MABP (mmHg)	ICP (mmHg)	CPP (mmHg)	SjO_2 (%)	CBF (ml/100g/min)	$AVDO_2$ (mmol/L)	$CMRO_2$ (mlO_2/100 g/min)
Group 1									
Before indomethacin	Median	4.8	69	6.5	63	69	39	1.7	1.6
	Range	3.6–5.6	65–83	2–27	43–71	45–89	20–41	0.7–2.9	0.4–2.6
After indomethacin	Median	4.8	82*	1.5*	80*	49*	20*	3.2*	1.8
	Range	3.4–5.6	78–93	−1 to 18	60–82	38–83	14–31	1.2–4.2	0.4–2.4
Group 2									
Before saline	Median	4.8	75	9.5	67	69	34	2.6	1.6
	Range	4.5–5.6	66–87	4–25	54–74	43–90	11–44	0.9–3.9	0.7–2.5
After saline	Median	4.8	78	8.5	70	70	33	2.2	1.8
	Range	4.5–5.7	68–89	1–22	55–83	46–89	13–39	0.8–3.6	0.6–2.4

*$P<0.05$

Table 11.2 Transcranial Doppler measurements: MABP, $PaCO_2$, SjO_2 and $AVDO_2$ before and after the start of indomethacin infusion and after induction of anaesthesia. Values are median and interquartile range

	Indomethacin ($n=15$)	Placebo ($n=14$)
Before start of indomethacin		
Mean middle cerebral artery blood flow velocity (cm/s)	66.0 (56.0–90.0)	70.0 (50.0–73.0)
MABP (mmHg)	101.0 (90.0–112.0)	102.0 (87.0–113.0)
$PaCO_2$ (kPa)	5.2 (4.8–5.5)	5.3 (5.0–5.6)
After start of indomethacin		
Mean middle cerebral artery blood flow velocity (cm/s)	48.0 (37.0–59.0)**	68.0 (53.0–74.0)
MABP (mmHg)	110.0 (101.0–118.0)*	104.0 (86.0–112.0)
$PaCO_2$ (kPa)	5.2 (4.4–5.5)	5.3 (5.1–5.6)
After induction of anaesthesia		
SjO_2 (%)	48.5 (42.9–56.3)*	57.2 (50.2–62.9)
$AVDO_2$ (mmol/L)	4.0 (3.2–4.5)	3.6 (3.3–4.4)
Mean middle cerebral artery blood flow velocity (cm/s)	41.0 (29.0–46.0)*	35.0 (31.0–38.0)*
MABP (mmHg)	80.0 (70.0–84.0)*	76.0 (70.0–91.0)*
$PaCO_2$ (kPa)	4.8 (4.5–5.0)	4.7 (4.4–5.0)*

*$P<0.05$ within groups
**$P<0.05$ between groups

Results Patient characteristics and preoperative and anaesthesia data were similar in the two groups. Before induction of anaesthesia indomethacin administration was associated with a significant decrease in CBF velocity and a significant increase in MABP (Table 11.2). After induction of anaesthesia, CBF velocity and the MABP decreased significantly in both groups (Table 11.2). No significant differences in ICP or CPP were seen during the measurements performed through the first burr hole (Table 11.3). After removal of the bone flap, a significant decrease in ICP was observed in both groups without differences between the groups (Table 11.3). Hyperventilation caused a derease in ICP and SjO_2 and an increase in $AVDO_2$ in both groups without intergroup differences (Table 11.3). There was no intergroup difference in CPP, dural tension and degree of brain swelling. CO_2 reactivity measured after induction of anaesthesia was significantly lower in the indomethacin group ($P<0.05$). After removal of the bone flap no significant difference in CO_2 reactivity was observed (Table 11.4).

Conclusion This study indicates that the ICP-decreasing effect of an indomethacin infusion during propofol-fentanyl anaesthesia is attenuated or absent and is likely to be caused by propofol-induced cerebral vasoconstriction and the subsequent decrease in CBF.

Table 11.3 Subdural ICP, MABP, CPP and other physiological variables measured at the drilling of the first burr hole, after removal of the bone flap, and before and after a 5-min period of hyperventilation. Values are median and interquartile range

Variables	First burr hole		After removal of bone flap		After hyperventilation	
	Indomethacin	Placebo	Indomethacin	Placebo	Indomethacin	Placebo
ICP (mmHg)	9.0 (7.0–13.0)	9.0 (5.0–17.0)	8.0 (5.0–10.0)*	7.0 (4.0–9.0)*	7.0 (5.0–10.0)*	6.0 (2.0–9.0)*
MABP (mmHg)	86.0 (76.0–90.0)	84.0 (77.0–94.0)	87.0 (76.0–94.0)	86.0 (76.0–100.0)	87.0 (76.0–93.0)	90.0 (77.0–102.0)
CPP (mmHg)	77.0 (66.0–85.0)	74.0 (58.0–85.0)	81.0 (58.0–87.0)	80.0 (67.0–93.0)	80.0 (70.0–89.0)	79.0 (72.0–93.0)
Temperature (°C)	35.6 (35.1–36.0)	35.7 (35.2–35.9)	35.8 (35.2–36.1)	35.6 (35.2–36.0)	35.7 (35.2–36.1)	35.6 (35.2–36.0)
$PaCO_2$ (kPa)	4.5 (4.1–4.9)	4.6 (4.3–5.1)	4.4 (4.1–5.1)	4.7 (4.6–5.1)	3.7 (3.4–3.9)*	3.9 (3.7–4.2)*
PaO_2 (kPa)	24.7 (22.2–33.5)	22.1 (19.4–31.4)	23.5 (22.2–27.6)	23.9 (19.7–29.9)	27.5 (24.8–40.7)*	24.3 (20.2–30.7)*
SjO_2 (%)	49.0 (43.0–62.0)	54.0 (49.0–62.0)	46.0 (42.0–57.0)	55.0 (47.0–61.0)	41.0 (38.0–58.0)*	46.0 (41.0–55.0)*
$AVDO_2$ (mmol/L)	3.8 (2.8–5.0)	3.4 (2.6–4.1)	3.6 (2.9–5.0)	3.4 (3.0–4.2)	4.5 (3.5–5.3)*	4.3 (2.9–4.6)*

*$P<0.05$ within groups

Table 11.4 Change in $PaCO_2$, $AVDO_2$ and CO_2 reactivity after induction of anaesthesia and after removal of the bone flap. Values are median and interquartile range

	Indomethacin ($n=15$)	Placebo ($n=15$)
After induction of anaesthesia		
Change in $PaCO_2$ (kPa)	1.0 (0.8–1.2)	1.0 (0.5–1.0)
Change in $AVDO_2$ (mmol/L)	0.4 (0.1–0.6)	0.7 (0.3–1.0)
CO_2 reactivity (%/kPa)	9.8 (2.3–14.3)	17.3 (10.5–27.1)**
After removal of bone flap		
Change in $PaCO_2$ (kPa)	0.8 (0.6–1.3)	0.8 (0.7–1.0)
Change in $AVDO_2$ (mmol/L)	0.3 (0.0–0.7)	0.5 (0.1–0.8)
CO_2 reactivity (%/kPa)	12.0 (3.8–16.5)	15.8 (0.0–20.3)

**$P<0.05$ between groups

Discussion

During craniotomy for cerebral tumours a high ICP may result in cerebral swellng after opening of dura mater (Rasmussen et al. 2004a). This condition can seriously jeopardize surgical access and may increase the risk of cerebral ischaemia with a poor outcome. In the study by Bundgaard et al. (1996) administration of indomethacin was associated with a significant fall in ICP from 6.5 mmHg (median) to 1.5 mmHg (median) and an increase in CPP from 63 to 80 mmHg (median) within 1 min. The reduction in ICP was associated with a significant decrease in CBF from 39 to 20 ml/100 g/min (Bundgaard et al. 1996). The authors did not report whether indomethacin affected the degree of brain swelling through the craniotomy. These findings are in good agreement with previous studies where indomethacin caused a significant reduction in ICP in patients with head injury (Jensen et al. 1991; Biestro et al. 1995; Dahl et al. 1996), in patients with plateau waves associated with head injury (Imberti et al. 2005) and in patients with fulminant hepatic failure (Tofteng and Larsen 2004).

The findings by Bundgaard et al. (1996) in previous studies are in contrast to the study by Rasmussen et al. (2004a) where indomethacin administration immediately before induction of anaesthesia did not influence the level of ICP in propofol-fentanyl-anaesthetized patients with cerebral tumours. Moreover, in the study by Rasmussen et al. the occurrence of brain swelling after opening of dura mater demonstrated a tendency to be higher in the indomethacin group compared with the control group. The two studies also differ by choice of anaesthesia, indomethacin dose and the time interval between administration of indomethacin and the ICP measurements.

A number of studies have demonstrated that the percentage reduction of CBF after administration of propofol is larger than the reduction of $CMRO_2$. These findings suggest that propofol may have a direct cerebral vasoconstricting effect, beyond the associated decrease in $CMRO_2$ leading to a decrease of the $CBF/CMRO_2$ ratio (Vandesteene et al. 1988; Van Hemelrijck et al. 1990; Ederberg et al. 1998; Jansen et al. 1999). The consequence is a shift to the left on the ICP compliance curve, where changes in CBV by cerebral vasoconstricting agents have less impact on ICP. The study by Rasmussen et al. supports these findings indicated by the substantial decrease in CBF velocity in both groups after induction of propofol-fentanyl anaesthesia without intergroup difference. Thus, additional treatment with indomethacin may have little or no impact on ICP, as observed in this study.

This hypothesis was not supported by a recent experimental study where sheep were randomized to receive indomethacin during either propofol or isoflurane anaesthesia (Rasmussen et al. 2006). Changes in CBF, ICP, MABP, $AVDO_2$ and $PaCO_2$ were measured at specific time points before and after a bolus dose of indomethacin (0.2 mg/kg). Indomethacin caused a reduction in ICP within 15 s during both anaesthetic regimes with the decrease in ICP being significantly more pronounced during isoflurane. Several factors may explain this difference. First, in the human study by Rasmussen et al. (2004a) the indomethacin infusion was administered before anaesthesia induction and terminated after opening of dura mater. The mean time interval between indomethacin administration and the first ICP measurement was 117 min. Baseline recordings of ICP were not performed and the possibility exists that indomethacin initially lowered ICP but failed to sustain the effect during the long infusion time. The authors suggested that indomethacin-induced cerebral vasoconstriction shows adaptation, however, this has not previously been demonstrated (Rasmussen et al. 2004a). Secondly, Rasmussen et al. (2004a) demonstrated a 50% decrease in CBF after induction with propofol compared to a 35% reduction in CBF observed in the experimental study. Thus, propofol-induced cerebral vasoconstriction was possibly near maximal in the study by Rasmussen et al. (2004a), with limited room for further vasoconstriction by indomethacin. Consequently, the differences in the reduction of CBF and degree of vasoconstriction observed in the two studies may explain how indoethacin in the experimental study managed to constrict the resistance vessels further and reduce ICP. Thirdly, differences regarding species, dose-reponse relationships and methods of measuring ICP (subdural versus epidural) may have influenced the results.

The rapid ICP-reducing effect of indomethacin observed in the studies by Bundgaard et al. (1996) and Rasmussen et al. (2006) is similar to that obtained with barbiturates. Thiopentone, however, is accompanied by a fall in CPP (Shapiro et al. 1973). In contrast the effects of hyperventilation and mannitol are only maximal after 10–15 min and 30–60 min, respectively (James 1980; Ravussin et al. 1988). Thus, compared to other treatments of high ICP, indomethacin is unique in effecting an immediate decrease in ICP associated with an increase in CPP.

The dose of indomethacin administered in the study by Rasmussen et al. (2004a) is based on a study in healthy volunteers where indomethacin (bolus 0.2 mg/kg followed by 0.2 mg/kg/h) caused a significant decrease in CBF, ranging between 29% and 37% (Jensen et al. 1996). In the study by Rasmussen et al. (2004a) indomethacin induced a 29% median decrease in CBF velocity compared to the control group. This finding is in agreement with a clinical study in head-injured patients where indomethacin (bolus of 30 mg followed by 30 mg/h) reduced ICP and caused a reduction in CBF averaging 15–26% (Jensen et al. 1991). However, the reduction in CBF velocity observed in this study was lower compared to the study by Bundgaard et al. (1996) in isoflurane-anaesthetized tumour patients where indomethacin (bolus of 50 mg) induced a 48% median decrease in CBF accompanied by a decrease in ICP. Thus, the effect on CBF velocity induced by the administered dose of indomethacin is comparable to the effects of equal or higher doses administred in other clinical studies where significant decreases in CBF and ICP were observed.

The use of indomethacin is controversial because several studies have demnstrated marked reductions in CBF which may cause cerebral ischaemia (Jensen et al. 1991; Bundgaard et al. 1996; Dahl et al. 1996). To examine whether indomethacin induces severe cerebral ischaemia, diffusion-weighted magnetic resonance imaging (DWI) was performed in nine patients subjected to craniotomy for cerebral tumours (Rasmussen et al. 2004b). DWI is an established MRI technique that is widely used in the diagnosis of acute stroke due to its extreme sensitivity to acute ischaemic damage (Warach et al. 1992). The technique detects the diffusion of water molecules. Due to the altered hindrance of their Brownian motions caused by cytotoxic oedema following ATP depletion, DWI hyperintensities appear within minutes of ischaemic tissue damage. DWI sequences were performed: (1) the day before surgery; (2) before administration of indomethacin; (3) 20 min after administration of indomethacin (bolus of 0.2 mg/kg followed by infusion of 0.2 mg/kg/h) in the propofol-fentanyl-anaesthetized patient; and (4) 2 days after surgery. SjO_2 decreased from an average of 51% to 43% comparable to the findings in the study by Bundgard et al. (1996). However, no ischaemic lesions were detected on the DWI images. This observation is in accordance with Biestro et al. (1995) who reported no evidence of cerebral ischaemia or infarctions on follow-up CT scans after indomethacin administration in patients with severe head injury.

References

Bedford RF, Persing JA, Pobereskin L et al (1980) Lidocaine or thiopental rod rapid control of intracranial hypertension? Anesth Analg 59:435–437

Biestro AA, Alberti RA, Soca AE et al (1995) Use of indomethacin in brain-injured patients with cerebral perfusion pressure impairment: preliminary report. J Neurosurg 83:627–630

Bundgaard H, Jensen K, Cold GE et al (1996) Effects of perioperative indomethacin on intracranial pressure, cerebral blood flow, and cerebral metabolism in patients subjected to craniotomy for cerebral tumours. J Neurosurg Anesthesiol 8:273–279

Cenic A, Craen RA, Lee TY et al (2000) Cerebral blood volume and blood flow responses to hyperventilation in brain tumours during isoflurane or propofol anesthesia. Anesth Analg 90:1376–1383

Cold GE (1989) Does acute hyperventilation provoke cerebral oligaemia in comatose patients after acute head injury? Acta Neurochir 96:100–106

Dahl B, Jensen K, Cold GE et al (1996) CO_2- and indomethacin vasoreactivity in patients with head injury. Acta Neurochir 138:265–273

Ederberg S, Westerlind A, Houltz E et al (1998) The effects of propofol on cerebral blood flow velocity and cerebral oxygen extraction during cardiopulmonary bypass. Anesth Analg 86:1201–1206

Imberti R, Fuardo M, Bellinzona G et al (2005) The use of indomethacin in the treatment of plateau waves: effects on cerebral perfusion and oxygenation. J Neurosurg 102:455–459

James HE (1980) Methodology for the control of intracranial pressure with hypertonic mannitol. Acta Neurochir 51:161–172

Jansen GF, van Praagh BH, Kedaria MB et al (1999) Jugular bulb oxygen saturation during propofol and isoflurane/nitrous oxide anesthesia in patients undergoing brain tumour surgery. Anesth Analg 89:358–363

Jensen K, Öhrström J, Cold GE et al (1991) The effects of indomethacin in intracranial pressure, cerebral blood flow and cerebral metabolism in patients with severe head injury and intracranial hypertension. Acta Neurochir 108:116–121

Jensen K, Freundlich M, Bünemann L et al (1993) The effect of indomethacin upon cerebral blood flow in healthy volunteers. Acta Neurochir 124:114–119

Jensen K, Kjaergaard S, Malte E et al (1996) Effect of graduated intravenous and standard rectal doses of indomethacin on cerebral blood flow in healthy volunteers. J Neurosurg Anesthesiol 8:111–116

Kaufmann AM, Cardoso ER (1992) Aggravation of vasogenic cerebral edema by multiple-dose mannitol. J Neurosurg 77:584–589

Miller JD, Leech P (1975) Effects of mannitol and steroid therapy on intracranial volume-pressure relationship in patients. J Neurosurg 42:274–275

Muizelaar JP, Marmarou A, Ward JD et al (1991) Adverse effects of prolonged hyperventilation in patients with severe head injury: a randomized clinical trial. J Neurosurg 75:731–739

Pichard JD, MacKenzie ET (1973) Inhibition of prostaglandin synthesis and the response of baboon cerebral circulation to carbon dioxide. Nat New Biol 245:187–188

Raichle ME, Plum F (1972) Hyperventilation and cerebral blood flow. Stroke 3:566–575

Rasmussen M, Tankisi A, Cold GE (2004a) The effects of indomethacin on intracranial pressure and cerebral haemodynamics in patients undergoing craniotomy: a randomised prospective study. Anaesthesia 59:229–236

Rasmussen M, Østergaard L, Juul N et al (2004b) Does indomethacin and propofol cause cerebral ischemic damage? Diffusion-weighted magnetic resonance imaging in patients subjected to craniotomy for brain tumours. Anesthesiology 101:872–878

Rasmussen M, Upton RN, Grant C et al (2006) The effects of indomethacin on intracranial pressure and cerebral hemodynamics during isoflurane or propofol anesthesia in sheep with intracranial hypertension. Anesth Analg 102:1823–1829

Ravussin P, Abou-Madi M, Archer D et al (1988) Changes in CSF pressure after mannitol in patients with and without elevated CSF pressure. J Neurosurg 69:869–876

Shapiro HM, Galindo A, Wyte SR et al (1973) Rapid intraoperative reduction of intracranial pressure with thiopentone. Br J Anaesth 45:1057–1062

Tankisi A, Rolighed Larsen J, Rasmussen M et al (2002) The effects of 10 degrees reverse Trendelenburg position on ICP and CPP in prone positioned patients subjected to craniotomy for occipital or cerebellar tumours. Acta Neurochir 144:665–670

Tofteng F, Larsen FS (2004) The effect of indomethacin on intracranial pressure, cerebral perfusion and extracellular lactate and glutamate concentrations in patients with fulminant hepatic failure. J Cereb Blood Flow Metab 24:798–804

Vandesteene A, Trempont V, Engelman E et al (1988) Effect of propofol on cerebral blood flow and metabolism in man. Anaesthesia 43(suppl):42–43

Van Hemelrijck J, Fitch W, Mattheussen M et al (1990) Effect of propofol on cerebral circulation and autoregulation in the baboon. Anesth Analg 71:49–54

Warach S, Chien D, Li W et al (1992) Fast magnetic resonance diffusion-weighted imaging of acute human stroke. Neurology 42:1717–1723

Wennmalm Å, Eriksson S, Wahren J (1981) Effect of indomethacin on basal and carbon dioxide stimulated cerebral blood flow in man. Clin Physiol 1:227–234

Chapter 12
Effect of Dihydroergotamine on Subdural Intracranial Pressure and Cerebral Haemodynamics

Helle Bundgaard and Georg Emil Cold

Abstract

Dihydroergotamine (DHE) acts as a non-competitive agonist at vascular 5-hydroxytryptamine receptors. Experimental studies indicate that DHE is a constrictor of the venous capacitance vessels and, in in vitro studies, DHE induces concentration-dependent contraction in human cerebral arteries and veins. Theoretically, DHE is more effective in the treatment of increased ICP than hyperventilation and is less dangerous because it predominantly acts on the cerebral venous pool, which contains a larger blood volume than the arterial pool.

In this chapter DHE and the results of a study dealing with the effect of DHE on arterial blood pressure, subdural ICP, cerebral perfusion pressure, cerebral blood flow and the cerebral metabolism in patients subjected to craniotomy for supratentorial brain tumours is discussed.

Treatments of increased ICP, tension of dura or brain swelling during craniotomy include therapy that increases CVR, such as hyperventilation and indomethacin, hypnotic agents, such as barbiturates or propofol and osmotic therapy (mannitol and hypertonic saline); also CSF drainage and evacuation of cystic processes, head elevation or rTp can be used (Miller and Leech 1975; Bedford et al. 1980; Bundgaard et al. 1996; Cenic et al. 2000; Tankisi et al. 2002). Each of these measures has advantages and disadvantages. Controlled hyperventilation is often of limited value since patients with intracerebral space-occupying lesions may have impaired or abolished cerebrovascular reactivity to changes in $PaCO_2$. The effect of hyperventilation follows the changes in $PaCO_2$, but maximal effect will only occur after 10–15 min and adaption to the effect takes place during continuous hypocapnia (Raichle and Plum 1972); adverse effects such as serious decrease in CBF have been reported (Cold 1989; Muizelaar et al. 1991). A precipitous decrease in CBF has also been found after i.v. indomethacin, but unlike hyperventilation this drug incrcascs CPP. The effect of repeated mannitol infusion has also been questioned, and a rebound effect at a high repeated dose is well known (Kaufmann and Cardoso 1992). Barbiturates and propofol may induce cardiovascular depression with a decrease in CPP, and CSF drainage is often impossible because of difficult access to the ventricular system.

Dihydroergotamine (DHE) acts as a non-competitive agonist at vascular 5-hydroxytryptamine receptors (Glusa and Markwardt 1984; Müller-Scheweinitzer and Rosenthaler 1987; Müller et al. 1988). Experimental studies indicate that DHE is a constrictor of the venous capacitance vessels (Mellander and Nordenfelt 1970; Müller-Scheweinitzer and Rosenthaler 1987) and, in in vitro studies, DHE induces concentration-dependent contraction in human cerebral arteries and veins (Nilsson et al. 1997). The Lund group have shown that in patients with severe head injury a bolus dose of DHE reduces ICP and increases CPP (Grände 1989; Asgeirsson et al. 1994, 1995). The ICP-reducing effect of DHE starts within 1 min after i.v. injection, reaching its maximal effect after 8–20 min, and the effect remains stable for up to 90 min (Asgeirsson et al. 1995). Theoretically, the effect of DHE is more effective in the treatment of increased ICP than hyperventilation and is less dangerous because it predominantly acts on the cerebral venous pool, which contains a larger blood volume than the arterial pool (Mellander and Johansson 1968; Mellander and Nordenfelt 1970), and because the arterial constrictor effect is less pronounced.

Data in this chapter have been presented by Bundgaard et al. in J Neurosurg Anesthesiol (2001) 3:195–201.

Effect of Dihydroergotamine on Intracranial Pressure, Cerebral Blood Flow and Cerebral Metabolism in Patients Undergoing Craniotomy for Brain Tumours

Aim   To test the effect of a single bolus of DHE on ICP during craniotomy.

Method   Twenty adult patients, median age 49 years (range 23–63 years) underwent craniotomy for supratentorial cerebral tumours in the supine position. Only patients with midline shift < 10 mm at preoperative CT scan participated in the study. For maintenance of anaesthesia isoflurane (end-tidal % 0.2–1.5%) and nitrous oxide (50–60%) supplemented with fentanyl was used. In a double-blind design, the patients were randomized to receive either 0.25 mg DHE as a bolus dose (group 1) or placebo physiological saline (group 2). The measurements were performed after exposure of the dura. CBF was measured by the ^{133}Xe technique and calculated as the initial slope index from 10-min clearance curves. Two angular detectors were placed on each side of the head, and the average CBF of the two detectors was used. Subdural ICP, jugular blood and arterial blood samples were analysed for gas analysis and $AVDO_2$. $CMRO_2$ was calculated as the product of $AVDO_2$ and CBF. The CVR was calculated according to the formula: $CPP = CBF \times CVR$. Subdural ICP and cerebral haemodynamics were measured twice in each patient. The first measurement was performed before administration of DHE or placebo and the second 30 min later. (For details concerning method, see Chapter 3.)

Statistical analysis Median and range were calculated. The Mann-Whitney rank sum test was used to analyse the difference between groups, and the Wilcoxon signed rank test and Friedman repeated measures analysis of variance on ranks were used to analyse data within groups. $P<0.05$ signifies significant difference.

Results No significant differences were found between the two groups as regards demographic (age, weight, gender), neuroradiological findings (maximal area of tumour, midline shift, localization of tumour) or histopathological data. The concentration of anaesthesia was kept constant during the study period. The physiological variables during the measurements are indicated in Table 12.1. Before administration of DHE or placebo, no significant differences were found between the two groups. In group 1 DHE bolus injection was followed by a significant increase in subdural ICP from 9.5 mmHg (range 3–21 mmHg) to 11.5 mmHg (range 5–24 mmHg) and a significant increase in CPP from 65 mmHg (range 49–77 mmHg) to 72 mmHg (range 57–100 mmHg). Simultaneously, a significant increase in MABP was found.

Table 12.1 Parameters obtained in group 1, where measurements were obtained before 0.25 mg DHE and 30 min after DHE administration. In group 2 the variables were measured before and after i.v. administration of normal saline (placebo). Median and range are indicated

	Group 1		Group 2	
	Before DHE	After DHE	Before placebo	After placebo
Temperature (°C)	36.2 (35.6–36.5)	36.2 (35.7–36.5)	36.0 (36.3–37.0)	36.0 (35.3–37.0)
PaCO$_2$ (kPa)	4.8 (4.4–5.1)	4.9 (4.5–5.1)	4.9 (4.4–5.0)	4.9 (4.4–5.1)
MABP (mmHg)	74.0 (67.0–84.0)	87.0* (67.0–112.0)	75.0 (69.0–105.0)	73.0 (62.0–113.0)
ICP (mmHg)	9.5 (3.0–21.0)	11.5* (5.0–24.0)	8.0 (2.0–20.0	8.0 (0.0–11.0)**
CPP (mmHg)	65.0 (49.0–77.0)	72.0* (57.0–100.0)	71.0 (60.0–95.0)	68.0 (56.0–103.0)
CBF (ml/100 g/min)	27.0 (23.0–56.0)	30.0 (24.0–63.0)	30.0 (25.0–54.0)	32.0 (27.0–55.0)
CVR mmHg/ml/min/100 g	2.2 (1.1–3.0)	2.5 (0.9–3.3)	2.4 (1.3–3.3)	2.2 (1.0–3.3)
AVDO$_2$ (mmol/L)	2.4 (1.0–3.5)	2.6 (1.0–3.3)	2.3 (0.6–3.5)	2.3 (0.5–3.5)
CMRO$_2$ (ml O$_2$/100 g/min)	1.8 (1.1–2.3)	2.1 (1.2–2.4)	1.9 (0.8–2.3)	2.0 (1.1–2.3)
Venous saturation (%)	68.0 (53.0–89.0)	67.0 (57.0–88.0)	70.0 (44.0–96.0)	71.0 (45.0–97.0)

*$P<0.05$ within group
**$P<0.05$ between groups

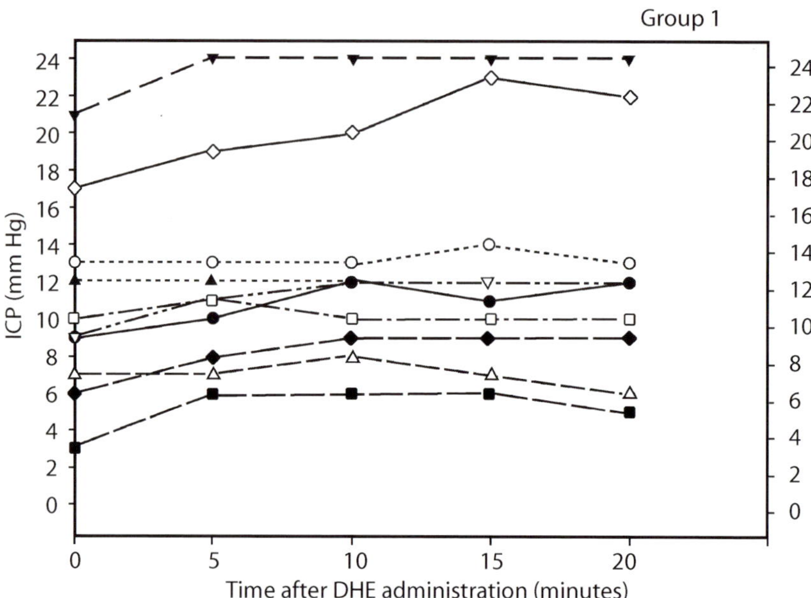

Fig. 12.1 Subdural ICP in relation to time in group 1 patients after 0.25 mg DHE i.v. as bolus

In group 2 (placebo group) no significant differences in the variables were detected.

In group 1 a substantial increase in both subdural ICP and MABP was observed 30 min after administration of DHE, while no changes in subdural ICP or MABP were observed in the placebo group (Figure 12.1).

Conclusion No ICP-decreasing effect of a bolus dose of DHE was found when administered to patients with brain tumours during isoflurane-nitrous oxide anaesthesia. Corresponding increases in MABP and ICP suggest that abolished cerebral autoregulation might explain why DHE was associated with an ICP increase.

Discussion

In the present study it was not possible to confirm the ICP-decreasing effect of a bolus dose DHE, as observed previously in patients with severe head injury (Grände 1989; Asgeirsson et al. 1994, 1995). In contrast, a significant increase in subdural ICP was observed, accompanied by an increase in MABP and CPP.

In a porcine model of intracranial hypertension (Nilsson et al. 1995) and in studies of patients with severe traumatic brain lesion (Grände 1989; Asgeirsson et al. 1994, 1995) DHE effectively reduces ICP and increases MABP, CPP and CVR. These studies suggest that the ICP-reducing effect of DHE results from a reduction in CBV caused predominantly by an increase in constriction of the intracranial venous blood pool. The difference in results in our study was not caused by a change in surgical activity and eventually cerebral stimulation, because surgical activity was postponed during the measuring, and $CMRO_2$ did not change significantly. In addition $PaCO_2$, PaO_2 and rectal temperature did not change significantly after DHE administration. The difference in results may be caused by the difference in sedation (anaesthesia). DHE acts as a non-competitive agonist at vascular 5-hydroxytryptamine receptors (Glusa and Markwardt 1984; Müller-Scheweinitzer and Rosenthaler 1987; Müller et al. 1988) and sensitises venous smooth muscle cells to the vasoconstrictor effect of biogenic amines (Müller-Scheweinitzer 1984). Theoretically, inhalation anaesthetics block this effect. If so, it is unlikely that this effect was caused by nitrous oxide used in the current study, because indirect evidence of a cerebral venous constrictor effect by DHE was found in pigs anaesthetized with nitrous oxide (Nilsson et al. 1995). Furthermore, in the present study an increase in blood pressure was observed that either could be caused by an increase in cardiac output or an increase in peripheral resistance. At least, the dose of DHE was sufficient to increase blood pressure and subdural ICP in the current study, without affecting CVR, CBF or cerebral oxygen consumption. The increase in blood pressure, however, might augment cerebral vasoconstriction via cerebral autoregulation. If cerebral autoregulation predominantly is preserved, an increase in blood pressure elicits cerebral vasoconstriction and thereby a decrease in ICP. In contrast an increase in blood pressure might be accompanied by an increase in ICP when cerebral autoregulation is abolished. Although cerebral autoregulation was not tested in our patients, this possibility exists because abolished cerebral autoregulation has been documented in several studies of patients with cerebral tumour and because both nitrous oxide and isoflurane, by acting as cerebral vasodilators, abolish cerebral autoregulation (Todd and Drummond 1984; van Aken et al. 1986). Both experimental studies (McPherson and Traystman 1988) and clinical studies (Olsen et al. 1994) indicate that cerebral autoregulation is intact at 1 MAC isoflurane, but defective at 2 MAC isoflurane. In this context, the end-expiratory concentrations of isoflurane in the present study, ranging between 0.2% and 1.5%, seem too low to have any influence on cerebral autoregulation.

References

Asgeirsson B, Grände P, Nordström C et al (1994) A new therapy of posttrauma brain oedema based on haemodynamic principles of brain volume regulation. Intensive Care Med 20:260–267

Asgeirsson B, Grände P, Nordström C et al (1995) Cerebral haemodynamic effect of dihydroergotamine in patients with severe traumatic brain lesions. Acta Anaesthesiol Scand 39:922–930

Bedford RF, Persing JA, Pobereskin L et al (1980) Lidocaine or thiopental for rapid control of intracranial hypertension? Anesth Analg 59:435–437

Bundgaard H, Jensen K, Cold GE et al (1996) Effects of perioperative indomethacin in intracranial pressure, cerebral blood flow, and cerebral metabolism in patients subjected to craniotomy for cerebral tumours. J Neurosurg Anesthesiol 8:273–279

Bundgaard H, von Oettingen G, Jørgensen H et al (2001) Effects of dihydroergotamine on intracranial pressure, cerebral blood flow, and cerebral metabolism in patients undergoing craniotomy for brain tumours. J Neurosurg Anesthesiol 3:195–201

Cenic A, Craen RA, Lee TY et al (2000) Cerebral blood volume and blood flow responses to hyperventilation in brain tumours during isoflurane or propofol anesthesia. Anesth Analg 90:1376–1383

Cold GE (1989) Does acute hyperventilation provoke cerebral oligaemia in comatose patients after acute head injury? Acta Neurochir 96:100–106

Glusa E, Markwandt F (1984) Studies of 5-hydroxytryptamine receptors on isolated human femoral veins and arteries and the influence of dihydroergotamine. Pharmacology 29:336–342

Grände P (1989) The effects of dihydroergotamine in patients with head injury and raised intracranial pressure. Intensive Care Med 15:523–527

Kaufmann AM, Cardoso ER (1992) Aggravation of vasogenic cerebral edema by multiple-dose mannitol. J Neurosurg 77:584–589

Mellander S, Johansson B (1968) Control of resistance, exchange and capacitance functions in the peripheral circulation. Pharmacol Rev 20:96–117

McPherson RW, Traystman RJ (1988) Effects of isoflurane on cerebral autoregulation in dogs. Anesthesiology 69:493–499

Mellander S, Nordenfelt I (1970) Comparative effects of dihydroergotamine and noradrenaline on resistance, exchange and capacitance function in the peripheral circulation. Clin Sci 39:183–201

Miller JD, Leech P (1975) Effects of mannitol and steroid therapy on intracranial volume-pressure relationship in patients. J Neurosurg 42:274–275

Muizelaar JP, Marmarou A, Ward JD et al (1991) Adverse effects of prolonged hyperventilation in patients with severe head injury: a randomized clinical trial. J Neurosurg 75:731–739

Müller H, Glusa E, Markwandt F (1988) Dual effect of dihydroergotamine at vascular 5-hydroxytryptamine receptors in pithed rats. Pharmacology 37:248–253

Müller-Scheweinitzer E (1984) What is known about the action of dihydroergotamine on the vasculature in man? Int J Clin Pharmacol Ther Toxicol 22:677–682

Müller-Scheweinitzer E, Rosenthaler J (1987) Dihydroergotamine: pharmacokinetics, pharmacodynamics, and mechanism of venoconstrictor action in beagle dogs. J Cardiovasc Pharmacol 9:686–693

Nilsson F, Messeter K, Grände P et al (1995) Effects of dihydroergotamine on central circulation and systemic circulation during experimental intracranial hypertension. Acta Anaesthesiol Scand 39:916–921

Nilsson F, Nilsson T, Edvinsson L et al (1997) Effects of dihydroergotamine and sumatriptan on isolated human cerebral and peripheral arteries and veins. Acta Anaesthesiol Scand 41:1257–1262

Olsen KS, Henriksen L, Owen-Falkenberg A et al (1994) Effect of 1 or 2 MAC isoflurane with or without ketanserin on cerebral blood flow autoregulation in man. Br J Anaesth 72:66–71

Raichle ME, Plum F (1972) Hyperventilation and cerebral blood flow. Stroke 3:566–575

Tankisi A, Rolighed Larsen J, Rasmussen M et al (2002) The effects of 10 degrees reverse Trendelenburg position on ICP and CPP in prone positioned patients subjected to craniotomy for occipital or cerebellar tumours. Acta Nerochir 144:665–670

Todd MM, Drummond JCA (1984) A comparison of the cerebrovascular and metabolic effects of halothane and isoflurane in the cat Anesthesiology 60:276–282

van Aken H, Puchstein C, Fitch W et al (1984) Haemodynamic and cerebral effects of ATP-induced hypertension. Br J Anaesth 56:1409–1416

Chapter 13
Effect of a Bolus Dose of an Analgetic on Subdural Intracranial Pressure and Cerebral Haemodynamics During General Anaesthesia for Craniotomy in Patients with Supratentorial Cerebral Tumours

Karsten Skovgaard Olsen and Georg Emil Cold

Abstract

Many studies regarding the effects of synthetic opioids on ICP, arterio-venous oxygen difference, mean arterial blood pressure and the CO_2 reactivity have been carried out. Contradictory results have been obtained. This, however, is most likely due to different study designs and to different patient populations studied. The overall result seems to be that these opioids depress the blood pressure in a dose-related way. This blood pressure decrease may affect the cerebral parameters depending on whether cerebral autoregulation is intact or not.

In this chapter three studies regarding analgetic boluses and the influence on the cerebral haemodynamics are presented. A bolus dose of alfentanil during propofol-fentanyl maintenance, a bolus dose of remifentanil during propofol-remifentanil anaesthesia and a bolus dose of fentanyl during propofol-fentanyl anaesthesia were studied.

The opioids fentanyl, alfentanil, sufentanil and remifentanil are all used for induction as well as for maintenance of anaesthesia in patients with space-occupying lesions. In the patient with spontaneous breathing these drugs may increase ICP dangerously due to a depressing effect on the respiratory drive and consequently lead to an increasing $PaCO_2$.

Clinical studies comprising artificially ventilated patients gave contradictory results with regard to changes in ICP, while decreases in MABP and CPP are found to be relatively constant. The magnitude of these effects is related to the choice of opioid and the dose used.

Several synthetic opioids, for example alfentanil, are administered for maintenance of anaesthesia either as a continuous infusion and/or as bolus doses to depress sympathetic stimulation. Studies on the effect on ICP of alfentanil administered during craniotomy have, however, given somewhat contradictory results. Thus, in a study comparing the effect on ICP of fentanyl, sufentanil and alfentanil administered to patients with supratentorial tumours, fentanyl did not change lumbar CSF pressure, while administration of sufentanil and most markedly alfentanil was followed by an increase in lumbar CSF pressure and a decrease in MABP and CPP (Marx et al. 1989). In another human study comprising patients with brain tumour, CSF pressure remained unchanged in patients who received nitrous oxide whether or not fentanyl was administered for maintenance of anaesthesia. However, in the patients who received alfentanil, a gradual increase in ICP was found (Jung et al. 1990). This is consistent with the observation by Mayberg et al. (1993) who found a small ICP increase after an alfentanil dose of 50 µg/kg and with the observation by Moss (1992) who found that alfentanil increased ICP in patients with suspected normal pressure hydrocephalus. The increase in ICP occurred immediately after alfentanil administration and was accompanied by a fall in blood pressure. It was presumed that cerebral autoregulatory mechanisms, leading to vasodilation and hence to an increase in ICP, were activated by the decrease in arterial pressure. In contrast to this result, alfentanil did not change ICP in children undergoing shunt revision (Marcovitz et al. 1990). Neither did alfentanil change ICP from pre-anaesthetic levels in a study on patients with supratentorial tumours, where thiopentone was used for induction of anaesthesia (Hung et al. 1992). In artificially ventilated patients with closed head injury, injection of alfentanil before suction of the airways did not change ICP. In that study, however, decreases in blood pressure and CPP were observed (Hanowell et al. 1993). These findings are also in accordance with studies using transcranial Doppler sonography, where no change in vessel diameter in the middle cerebral artery was found, indicating that alfentanil did not alter the vessel tonus (Schregel et al. 1992). In a study comprising patients subjected to craniotomy for supratentorial tumours the effects of remifentanil 0.5 µg/kg and alfentanil 1.0 µg/kg, respectively, on ICP and MABP were compared. Neither of these opioids caused significant changes in ICP, but both drugs were associated with a dosage-dependent decrease in MABP (Warner et al. 1996).

Four clinical studies on the effect of remifentanil administered to patients undergoing craniotomy for cerebral tumours are available:

1. In a clinical study of patients undergoing supratentorial craniotomy a dose-dependent decrease in CPP was observed. ICP, however, did not change, and the effect of remifentanil did not differ from those of equipotent doses of alfentanil (Hindman et al. 1994).
2. In another study of patients subjected to craniotomy for supratentorial tumours the effect of remifentanil 0.5 µg/kg and alfentanil 1.0 µg/kg on ICP and MABP were compared. Neither of these opioids caused significant changes in ICP, but both drugs were associated with a dosage-dependent decrease in MABP (Warner et al. 1996).
3. Continuous infusion of either remifentanil 0.03 µg/kg/min or fentanyl 0.2 µg/kg/min was compared. The anaesthesia was induced with thiopental

and maintained with nitrous oxide supplemented with one of the opioids. ICP and CPP were identical in the two groups. MABP was highest in the fentanyl group (Guy et al. 1997).

4. Anaesthesia supplemented with remifentanil 0.2 µg/kg/min, alfentanil 20 µg/kg/h or fentanyl 2 µg/kg/h was compared in patients undergoing craniotomy. There were no differences among the groups as regards heart rate and MABP. ICP was not monitored (Coles et al. 2000).

Compared with fentanyl, emergence is more rapid with remifentanil (Balakrishnan et al. 2000). To our knowledge, the effect of a bolus dose of remifentanil on subdural ICP and cerebral haemodynamics in patients undergoing craniotomy in propofol-remifentanil anaesthesia has not so far been studied.

In patients with space-occupying lesions fentanyl may increase ICP (Miller et al. 1975). In many cases the increase in ICP is caused by hypercapnia due to pulmonary hypoventilation. However, an increase in CSF pressure has also been observed in normocapnic volunteers (Benzer et al. 1992). In contrast, some studies indicate that ICP is unchanged during induction of anaesthesia with thiopentone and fentanyl and controlled hyperventilation (Moss et al. 1978). On the other hand in newer studies comprising patients with severe head injury administration of fentanyl in doses of 2 µg/kg was accompanied by a moderate increase in ICP and a fall in MABP and CPP, but no change in $AVDO_2$ (de Nadal et al. 1998, 2000). Thus, due to the inconsistency in the above-mentioned results three studies were carried out. The first study is a blinded and randomized dose-response study which has been presented by Olsen et al. in Acta Anaesthesiol Scand (2005) 49:445–452. The other two studies are non-randomized and both based on the database.

Study 1: Effect of Alfentanil on Subdural Intracranial Pressure, Cerebral Haemodynamics and CO_2 Reactivity During Propofol-Fentanyl Anaesthesia in Patients Subjected to Craniotomy for Supratentorial Cerebral Tumours

Aim To investigate the effect of intravenous bolus doses of alfentanil on subdural ICP and cerebral haemodynamics during propofol-fentanyl anaesthesia in patients subjected to craniotomy for supratentorial cerebral tumours.

Method The study was designed as a randomized and controlled dose-response study and comprised 31 patients with supratentorial cerebral tumours undergoing craniotomy. Maintenance of anaesthesia was obtained with administration of propofol and fentanyl. After removal of the bone flap a bolus dose of alfentanil 10 µg/kg (group 1), 20 µg/kg (group 2) or 30 µg/kg (group 3) was administered followed by an infusion of 10, 20 or 30 µg/kg/h to the patients in groups 1, 2 and 3, respectively. A control group received no alfentanil. Subdural ICP, JBP and cerebral haemodynamics, including CPP and gas analysis from jugular and arterial blood, were monitored during a 5-min observation period. $AVDO_2$ was calculated as the difference between oxygen content in arterial blood and jugular bulb blood. After the 5-min observation period, the effect of hyperventilation was tested. The CO_2 reactivity was calculated as the $\Delta AVDO_2$ (%)/$\Delta PaCO_2$ (kPa).

The CVR was calculated before and after 5 min of hyperventilation as $CPP \times AVDO_2 \times$ a constant. Percentage change in CVR was calculated as (CVR (before hyperventilation) – CVR (during hyperventilation))/CVR (before hyperventilation).

The degree of dural tension and the degree of brain swelling were evaluated by the surgeon. For details concerning histopathology, neuroradiological findings, anaesthetic maintenance doses, intravenous fluid management and monitoring, see Chapter 3.

Statistical analysis One-way analysis of variance was used when tests for normality and equal variance were passed. If not, the non-parametric Kruskal-Wallis one-way analysis of variance by ranks was used. Tukey's test and Dunn's method were used for multiple comparisons. For analysis within groups, one-way repeated measures analysis of variance was used. If the normality test failed, Friedman's repeated analysis of variance on ranks was used. For pair-wise multiple comparison procedures Dunnett's method was used. A t-test was used for analysis between groups, when only two groups were compared. If the normality test failed the Wilcoxon signed rank test was used. $P<0.05$ signifies statistical significance.

Results Two neuroanaesthesiological departments participated in the study. Twenty patients were included from one of the clinics and 11 from the other.

Table 13.1 Demographic data, preoperative variables and neuroradiological findings. Mean±SD are indicated

	Control	Group 1	Group 2	Group 3
Age (years)	42.0±14.0	50.0±10.0	54.0±10.0	45.0±16.0
Weight (kg)	76.0±16.0	71.0±11.0	81.0±11.0	81.0±12.0
Height (cm)	174.0±8.0	174.0±8.0	177.0±9.0	179.0±6.0
Men/women	5/4	5/2	4/3	8/1
MABP (mmHg) before induction	95.0±16.0	99.0±15.0	97.0±14.0	108.0±11.0
Steroid (+/−)	2/7	6/1	4/3	4/5
Glioblastoma	0	3	3	2
Meningioma	0	1	1	0
Metastasis	0	0	1	1
Glioma	4	1	1	4
Other	4	2	1	2
Tumour area (cm^2)	10.0±8.0	18.0±7.0	17.0±10.0	8.0±6.0
Midline shift (mm)	2.7±3.4	6.1±3.5	5.4±4.0	2.8±3.9
Propofol (mg/h)	661.0±141.0	586.0±94.0	642.0±181.0	687.0±160.0
Fentanyl (µg/h)	133.0±43.0	157.0±45.0	169.0±60.0	194.0±71.0
Temperature (°C)	35.6±0.4	35.9±0.7	35.8±0.5	36.0±0.3

Eight patients were allocated to the control group, seven to group 1, seven to group 2 and nine to group 3. Table 13.1 indicates demographic data, anaesthetic maintenance doses before alfentanil administration and histopathology. No statistically significant intergroup differences were disclosed. Following the administration of alfentanil, MABP and CPP decreased in all groups. However, the values of subdural ICP and JBP did not change in any of the groups.

After hyperventilation (from time 5 min to time 10 min) decreases in $PaCO_2$ were found in all groups. A decrease in subdural ICP was found in all groups. No significant intergroup differences in CO_2 reactivity or percentage change in CVR was found (Table 13.2). No intergroup differences were disclosed as regards the degree of dural tension and the degree of brain swelling after opening of dura.

Table 13.2 Change in subdural ICP, MABP, CPP, SjO_2 and $AVDO_2$ in the control group and in groups 1–3 with increasing doses of alfentanil. Time zero to 5 min indicates changes in the 5-min observation period after alfentanil administration. From time 5 to 10 min hyperventilation was applied. The CO_2 reactivity and percentage change in CVR before and after hyperventilation are indicated

	Control	Group 1	Group 2	Group 3
$PaCO_2$ (kPa)				
Time zero	4.6±0.4	4.5±0.4	4.4±0.4	4.8±0.5
Time 10 min	4.0±0.4**	3.7±0.3**	3.9±0.5**	4.2±0.2**
ICP (mmHg)				
Time zero	4.3±2.5	11.7±6.3	9.7±7.9	6.8±3.6
1 min	4.6±2.2	11.1±6.1	9.9±7.9	7.0±3.6
2 min	4.4±1.6	10.9±5.7	9.6±6.4	6.7±3.7
3 min	4.1±2.0	11.4±5.6	9.9±6.7	6.6±3.7
4 min	4.0±1.9	11.7±5.7	9.9±6.5	7.0±3.8
5 min	4.1±2.0	11.7±6.1	9.6±6.7	6.9±3.7
10 min	2.6±2.0**	9.0±5.3**	8.0±6.5**	5.3±4.5**
MABP (mmHg)				
Time zero	89.0±7.0	75.0±10.0	83.0±9.0	85.0±13.0
1 min	90.0±7.0	75.0±9.0	79.0±8.0	76.0±11.0
2 min	89.0±7.0	75.0±8.0	77.0±8.0	69.0±10.0*
3 min	89.0±8.0	72.0±8.0	75.0±9.0	68.0±10.0*
4 min	88.0±7.0	72.0±8.0	75.0±8.0	67.0±10.0*
5 min	88.0±8.0	72.0±9.0	75.0±9.0	69.0±8.0*
10 min	87.0±6.0	74.0±10.0	76.0±8.0	70.0±8.0
CPP (mmHg)				
Time zero	86.0±8.0	64.0±9.0	73.0±8.0	78.0±13.0
1 min	86.0±7.0	64.0±9.0	70.0±9.0	69.0±13.0
2 min	84.0±8.0	64.0±7.0	67.0±7.0	63.0±11.0*
3 min	85.0±9.0	61.0±7.0	65.0±8.0	61.0±11.0*
4 min	84.0±8.0	60.0±9.0	65.0±8.0	60.0±10.0*
5 min	84.0±8.0	60.0±9.0	66.0±10.0	62.0±8.0*
10 min	84.0±6.0	65.0±10.0	68.0±9.0	65.0±8.0

Table 13.2 *(continued)*

	Control	Group 1	Group 2	Group 3
SjO_2 (%)				
Time zero	54.0±15.0	56.0±9.0	50.0±9.0	60.0±9.0
1 min	51.0±9.0	56.0±8.0	50.0±10.0	59.0±12.0
2 min	51.0±9.0	55.0±9.0	47.0±11.0	58.0±12.0
3 min	51.0±8.0	53.0±12.0	50.0±9.0	58.0±12.0
4 min	51.0±8.0	54.0±11.0	49.0±10.0	57.0±14.0
5 min	51.0±9.0	52.0±11.0	49.0±10.0	59.0±12.0
10 min	45.0±9.0**	49.0±8.0	46.0±9.0	55.0±11.0
$AVDO_2$ (mmol/L)				
Time zero	3.6±0.6	3.2±0.9	3.8±0.9	3.3±0.7
1 min	3.6±0.6	3.2±0.7	3.8±1.0	3.2±1.0
2 min	3.6±0.5	3.4±0.9	4.0±1.1	3.4±1.0
3 min	3.6±0.4	3.4±1.2	4.0±1.1	3.3±1.1
4 min	3.6±0.5	3.4±1.1	3.9±1.0	3.4±1.1
5 min	3.6±0.5	3.5±1.1	3.8±1.0	3.3±1.1
10 min	4.0±0.6**	3.8±0.9	4.1±1.0	3.5±1.0
CO_2 reactivity	16.3±6.3	12.6±11.3	15.5±9.9	17.1±17.3
$\%AVDO_2/\Delta PaCO_2$ (kPa)				
% change CVR	12.0±9.0	23.0±20.0	12.0±8.0	15.0±17.0

*$P<0.05$ intergroup differences
**$P<0.05$ after hyperventilation

Conclusion Administration of iv alfentanil to propofol-fentanyl-anaes-thetized patients with supratentorial cerebral tumours decreases MABP and CPP in a dose-related way, but does not influence subdural ICP, $AVDO_2$, the CO_2 reactivity or the percentage change in CVR.

Study 2: Effect of a Bolus Dose of Remifentanil on Cerebral Haemodynamics During Propofol-Remifentanil Anaesthesia in Patients Subjected to Craniotomy for Supratentorial Cerebral Tumours

Aim To investigate the effect of an intravenous dose of remifentanil on sub-dural ICP and cerebral haemodynamics.

Method Two groups of 15 patients each were studied. One of the groups was a control group and received only a maintenance dose of remifentanil. Patients in the other group received 10% of the remifentanil maintenance dose per hour as a bolus dose. All patients in both groups were scheduled for craniotomy for supratentorial cerebral tumours and propofol-remifentanil was used for maintenance of anaesthesia. Subdural ICP, MABP and CPP were monitored every minute for 5 min after the bolus dose of remifentanil.

$PaCO_2$, SjO_2 and $AVDO_2$ were measured at time zero and after 5 min (for details concerning histopathology, neuroradiological findings, anaesthesia, intravenous fluid management and monitoring, see Chapter 3).

Statistical analysis One-way analysis of variance was used when tests for normality and equal variance were passed. If not, the non-parametric Kruskal-Wallis one-way analysis of variance by ranks was used. Tukey's test and Dunn's method were used for multiple comparisons. For analysis within groups, one-way repeated measures analysis of variance was used. If the normality test failed, Friedman's repeated analysis of variance on ranks was used. For pair-wise multiple comparison procedures Dunnett's method was used. A t-test was used for analysis between groups, when only two groups were compared. If the normality test failed the Wilcoxon signed rank test was used. $P<0.05$ signifies statistical significance.

Results No differences in demographic data, preoperative blood pressure, $PaCO_2$, rectal temperature, neurological data (tumour size, midline shift, localization of tumour) or pathohistology of the tumours were disclosed (see Tables 13.3 and 13.4). The remifentanil bolus dose (averaging 188 µg) induced a statistically significant fall in MABP and CPP for 4 min. No falls werefound in the control group (Table 13.5). The remifentanil administration did not change ICP. In both groups $PaCO_2$, SjO_2 and $AVDO_2$ were unchanged during the 5-min study period (Table 13.6).

Table 13.3 Preoperative demographic data, neuroradiological data, maintenance dose of anaesthesia and parameters related to cerebral haemodynamics in a control group and in a group where 10% of the remifentanil maintenance dose per hour was given intravenously. Data were obtained before the administration of remifentanil bolus. No significant differences were disclosed between groups

	Control group	Remifentanil group
Men/women	6/9	7/8
Weight (kg)	79.0±17.0	74.0±16.0
Preoperative MABP (mmHg)	96.0±6.0	94.0±11.0
Maximal tumour area (cm^2)	11.0±7.0	8.0±6.0
Midline shift (mm)	4.2±0.6	2.0±4.0
Propofol (mg/h)	460.0±135.0	386.0±52.0
Remifentanil (ml/h)	23.5±9.1	18.9±3.4
$PaCO_2$ (kPa)	4.5±0.3	4.6±0.2
Temperature (°C)	35.7±0.4	35.8±0.3
MABP (mmHg)	77.0±15.0	75.0±10.0
ICP (mmHg)	9.5±6.2	7.2±4.6
CPP (mmHg)	68.0±15.0	68.0±12.0
SjO_2 (%)	50.0±8.7	52.0±12.0
$AVDO_2$ (mmol/L)	3.6±0.8	3.6±1.1

Table 13.4 Localization and pathology of the tumours in the control group and in a group where 10% of the remifentanil maintenance dose per hour was given intravenously

	Control group	Remifentanil group
Localization of tumour		
Frontal	2	4
Parietal	4	2
Temporal	4	5
Occipital	1	0
Basal	3	3
Central	1	1
Pathology		
Glioblastoma	3	4
Meningioma	4	1
Metastasis	0	4
Glioma	4	4
Other	4	2

Table 13.5 MABP, ICP and CPP in the control group and in the remifentanil bolus group. Mean values are indicated

Minutes	Control			Remifentanil		
	MABP (mmHg)	ICP (mmHg)	CPP (mmHg)	MABP (mmHg)	ICP (mmHg)	CPP (mmHg)
0	77.3	9.5	67.8	74.6	7.2	68.3
1	77.3	9.3	68.1	73.2*	7.2	66.0*
2	77.1	9.3	67.7	71.7*	7.3	64.7*
3	76.5	9.5	67.0	71.0*	7.3	63.9*
4	77.2	9.3	67.8	70.9*	7.3	63.4*
5	77.7	9.4	67.6	71.5*	7.3	64.3

*$P \leq 0.01$ significant difference from 0 min

Table 13.6 SjO_2, $AVDO_2$ and $PaCO_2$ in the control group and the remifentanil bolus group. No significant differences were disclosed within the groups

Minutes	Control			Remifentanil		
	S_jO_2 (%)	$AVDO_2$ (mmol/L)	$PaCO_2$ (kPa)	S_jO_2 (%)	$AVDO_2$ (mmol/L)	$PaCO_2$ (kPa)
0	49.8±8.7	3.6±0.8	4.4±0.3	52.4±12	3.6±1.1	4.6±0.3
5	49.7±8.4	3.6±0.8	4.5±0.4	51.8±13	3.6±1.1	4.5±0.3

Conclusion   A bolus dose of remifentanil administered during propofol-remifentanil anaesthesia does not change ICP, SjO_2 or $AVDO_2$, but reduces blood pressure and CPP.

Study 3: Effect of a Bolus Dose of Fentanyl on Cerebral Haemodynamics During Propofol-Fentanyl Anaesthesia in Patients Subjected to Craniotomy for Supratentorial Cerebral Tumours

Aim   To investigate the effect of an intravenous dose of fentanyl on subdural ICP and cerebral haemodynamics.

Method   Two groups of 15 patients each were studied, a control group receiving no fentanyl and a group in which intravenous fentanyl (1 µg/kg) was administered. All patients were scheduled for craniotomy for supratentorial cerebral tumours, and propofol-fentanyl was used for maintenance of anaesthesia. Subdural ICP, MABP and CPP were monitored every minute for 5 min after a bolus dose of fentanyl. $PaCO_2$, SjO_2 and $AVDO_2$ were measured at time zero and after 5 min (for details concerning histopathology, neuroradiological findings, anaesthesia, intravenous fluid management and monitoring, see Chapter 3).

Statistical analysis   One-way analysis of variance was used when tests for normality and equal variance were passed. If not, the non-parametric Kruskal-Wallis one-way analysis of variance by ranks was used. Tukey's test and Dunn's method were used for multiple comparisons. For analysis within groups, one-way repeated measures analysis of variance was used. If the normality test failed, Friedman's repeated analysis of variance on ranks was used.

Table 13.7   Preoperative demographic data, neuroradiological data, maintenance dose of anaesthesia and parameters related to cerebral haemodynamics in a control group and in a group where fentanyl (1 µg/kg) was given intravenously. Data were obtained before the administration of a fentanyl bolus. No significant differences were disclosed between groups

	Control group	Fentanyl group
Men/women	7/8	8/7
Weight (kg)	76.0±16.0	74.0±15.0
Preoperative MABP (mmHg)	95.0±7.0	94.0±10.0
Maximal tumour area (cm^2)	12.0±8.0	10.0±6.0
Midline shift (mm)	3.1±5.4	2.9±3.5
Propofol (mg/kg/h)	8.8±1.7	9.2±2.2
Fentanyl (µg/kg/h)	2.1±0.5	2.4±0.3
$PaCO_2$ (kPa)	4.6±0.2	4.6±0.2
Temperature (°C)	35.6±0.3	35.7±0.3
MABP (mmHg)	84.0±13.0	87.0±11.0
ICP (mmHg)	9.0±5.8	8.5±5.6
CPP (mmHg)	75.0±15.0	78.0±11.0
SjO_2 (%)	52.0±7.6	53.0±7.4
$AVDO_2$ (mmol/L)	3.5±0.7	3.4±0.8

Table 13.8 Localization and pathology of the tumours in the control group and in the group where fentanyl was administered as a bolus dose

	Control group	Fentanyl group
Localization of tumour		
Frontal	4	4
Parietal	3	2
Temporal	5	4
Occipital	2	2
Basal	0	1
Central	1	2
Pathology		
Glioblastoma	6	5
Meningioma	3	3
Metastasis	2	2
Glioma	2	3
Other	2	2

For pair-wise multiple comparison procedures Dunnett's method was used. A t-test was used for analysis between groups, when only two groups were compared. If the normality test failed the Wilcoxon signed rank test was used. $P<0.05$ signifies statistical significance.

Results No difference in demographic data, preoperative blood pressure, $PaCO_2$, rectal temperature, neurological data (tumour size, midline shift, localization of tumour) or pathohistology of the tumours were disclosed (see Tables 13.7 and 13.8). During the 5-min observation period fentanyl induced a significant fall in MABP and CPP lasting 4 min, but ICP was unchanged. MABP, ICP and CPP were unchanged in the control group (Table 13.9). In both groups $PaCO_2$, SjO_2 and $AVDO_2$ were unchanged during the 5-min study period (Table 13.10).

Table 13.9 MABP, ICP and CPP in the control group and the fentanyl bolus group. Mean values are indicated

Minutes	Control			Fentanyl		
	MABP (mmHg)	ICP (mmHg)	CPP (mmHg)	MABP (mmHg)	ICP (mmHg)	CPP (mmHg)
0	84.3	9.0	75.4	86.8	8.5	78.2
1	83.2	8.8	74.4	86.5	8.5	78.1
2	83.8	9.1	74.2	85.2	8.1	77.1
3	84.4	9.2	75.3	82.2	8.3	73.9
4	84.2	9.0	75.4	81.3	8.4	73.0
5	84.0	8.9	75.2	77.2*	8.2	69.0*

*$P\leq0.01$ significant difference from 0 min

Table 13.10 SjO_2, $AVDO_2$ and $PaCO_2$ in the control group and the fentanyl bolus group. No significant difference was disclosed within the groups

Minutes	Control			Fentanyl		
	S_jO_2 (%)	AVDO$_2$ (mmol/L)	PaCO$_2$ (kPa)	S_jO_2 (%)	AVDO$_2$ (mmol/L)	PaCO$_2$ (kPa)
0	52.1±7.6	3.5±0.7	4.6±0.2	53.4±7.4	3.4±0.8	4.6±0.2
5	50.2±7.9	3.6±0.9	4.6±0.3	52.9±8.8	3.5±0.7	4.6±0.2

Conclusion A bolus dose of fentanyl administered during propofol-fentanyl anaesthesia does not change ICP, SjO_2 or $AVDO_2$, but reduces blood pressure and CPP significantly.

Discussion

The three studies presented in this chapter show identical patterns as regards changes in subdural ICP and cerebral haemodynamics. Bolus injections of the three analgetics (alfentanil, remifentanil and fentanyl) were accompanied by a decrease in blood pressure and CPP, while subdural ICP was unchanged. A dose-response relationship was found with alfentanil as regards the decrease in MABP and CPP. The cerebral haemodynamics, indirectly registered by monitoring the $AVDO_2$ and the SjO_2, were unchanged for all three analgetics during the observation period, and the CO_2 reactivity or changes in CVR were not influenced by increasing doses of alfentanil. The decreases in CPP found after bolus injections of the three analgetics were not accompanied by changes in SjO_2 or $AVDO_2$, indicating that these analgetic drugs did not jeopardize cerebral oxygen delivery (or provoke potential cerebral ischaemia) in spite of the decrease in CPP.

The results of the experimental and clinical studies of the effects of analgetics on CBF and $CMRO_2$ are complex. In cats, fentanyl induces an increase in CBF and $CMRO_2$ (Nilsson and Ingvar 1965; Freeman and Ingvar 1967). In comparison, studies of venous outflow in dogs during nitrous oxide anaesthesia indicate an 18% decrease in $CMRO_2$ and a 47% decrease in CBF after fentanyl 0.006 mg/kg (Michenfelder and Theye 1971). Milde et al. (1989) studied the effect of fentanyl 50 and 100 mg/kg, respectively, on CBF and $CMRO_2$ in dogs, and found that these doses had minimal effect on CBF, oxygen uptake and the energy state of the brain. In studies of pigs, subjected to fentanyl-nitrous oxide anaesthesia and pancuronium relaxation, CBF, $CMRO_2$, CO_2 reactivity and EEG were stable throughout a 100-min period (Åkeson et al. 1993). Studies with a Doppler technique indicate that fentanyl during normocapnia increases flow velocity (Trindle et al. 1993). This effect is abolished during hypocapnia (Kolbitsch et al. 1997). During induction of anaesthesia with fentanyl 100 mg/kg and diazepam 0.4 mg/kg for cardiac surgery a 25% decrease in CBF was observed, while $CMRO_2$ was unchanged. Administration of fentanyl during controlled ventilation, however, might be accompanied by an increase in ICP and a decrease in blood pressure (Knüttgen et al. 1989). In dogs, alfentanil induces a dose-related decrease in CBF, the CO_2 reactivity is preserved and the upper autoregulatory threshold is shifted to the right (McPherson et al. 1982). Healthy volunteers were subjected to remifentanil infusion (0.1 µg/kg/min) and cerebral parameters were measured with a magnetic resonance (MR) technique. Remifentanil increased rCBF and rCBV in white and grey matter (striatal, thalamic, occipital, parietal, frontal) regions with a parallel decrease in transit time in these regions with the exception of the occipital grey matter. Regional CVR was decreased in all regions studied. The authors concluded that these findings were consistent with cerebral excitement and/or disinhibition (Lorenz et al. 2000). In volunteers remifentanil induces dose-dependent changes in relative rCBF in areas involved in pain processing. Furthermore, at moderate doses of remifentanil rCBF responses were detected in structures known to participate in modulation of vigilance and alertness (Wagner et al. 2001). Using contrast-enhanced MR perfusion measurement in human volunteers, a comparative study of nitrous oxide (50%) and remifentanil (0.1 µg/kg/min) indicated that nitrous oxide produced a greater increase in rCBV in all grey matter regions than did remifentanil. However, the increase in rCBF, especially in the basal ganglia, was less pronounced than during infusion of remifentanil (Lorenz et al. 2002). In patients with head trauma, who were sedated with propofol and sufentanil, a bolus dose of remifentanil (0.5 µg/kg) followed by continuous infusion (0.25 µg/kg/min for 20 min) did not change flow velocity, ICP or CPP (Engelhard et al. 2004). In patients subjected to coronary by-pass graft surgery remifentanil (3 µg/kg/min) reduced flow velocity by 31%. The flow velocity was not changed by 1 µg/kg/min remifentanil (Paris et al. 1998). Thus, based on the cited experimental and clinical studies of CBF and $CMRO_2$, it seems as if a bolus dose of one of the three analgetics administered under maintenance anaesthesia as described either leaves CBF unchanged or reduces CBF and $CMRO_2$. Consequently, a decrease in ICP or an unchanged ICP should be the most reliable finding.

The decrease in blood pressure and CPP, as well as the unchanged ICP found in the three studies presented in this chapter, are in agreement with other studies. Thus, a decrease in MABP and CPP was found in patients with severe head injury, where fentanyl in doses of 2 mg/kg resulted in a fall in MABP and CPP, but did not change $AVDO_2$ (de Nadal et al. 1998, 2000). In another study of patients subjected to craniotomy for supratentorial tumours the effects of remifentanil 0.5 µg/kg and alfentanil 1.0 µg/kg on ICP and MABP were compared. Neither opioid caused significant changes in ICP, but both drugs were associated with a dosage-dependent decrease in MABP (Warner et al. 1996). Alfentanil did not change ICP in children undergoing shunt revision (Marcovitz et al. 1990). In another study alfentanil and thiopentone were used for induction of anaesthesia in patients with supratentorial tumours and ICP remained stable without significant difference from pre-anaesthetic levels (Hung et al. 1992). In artificially ventilated patients with closed head injury, pretreatment with alfentanil before suction did not change ICP. In this study a decrease in blood pressure and in CPP were observed (Hanowell et al. 1993). These findings are in accordance with studies of transcranial Doppler sonography, indicating that alfentanil does not alter the vessel diameter in the middle cerebral artery (Schregel et al. 1992). However, the unchanged subdural ICP found in the present study is in conflict with some other studies. Thus, in a comparative study in patients with supratentorial tumours fentanyl did not change lumbar CSF pressure, while administration of sufentanil and especially alfentanil was followed by an increase in lumbar CSF pressure, and a decrease in MABP and CPP (Marx et al. 1989). In propofol-sedated patients with head injury the decrease in MABP was accompanied by an increase in ICP after alfentanil administration (Albanese et al. 1999). In another human study of brain tumour patients the CSF pressure remained unchanged in patients who received nitrous oxide with or without fentanyl for maintenance of anaesthesia. In contrast, in the patients who received alfentanil, a gradual increase in lumbar CSF pressure was found (Jung et al. 1990). This is consistent with the result of a study by Mayberg et al. (1993), who found a small ICP increase with an alfentanil dose of 50 µg/kg, and also with the observation by Moss (1992), who found that alfentanil increased ICP in patients with suspected normal pressure hydrocephalus.

Compensatory cerebral vasodilatation has been observed during alfentanil-induced decrease in MABP in orthopaedic patients (Mayberg et al. 1993). This mechanism implies that the cerebral autoregulation is intact. Thus, theoretically, the decrease in CPP should be accompanied by an increase in CBV and ICP, which could explain the increase in ICP found in some studies. In contrast, an increase in CPP should be followed by a decrease in ICP, if cerebral autoregulation is intact. However, cerebral autoregulation is easily disturbed in patients with mass-expanding lesions, such as a brain tumour (Palvölgyi 1969; Endo et al. 1977), and in patients with severe head injury (Fieschi et al. 1974; Enevoldsen et al. 1976; Muizalaar et al. 1989; Jünger et al. 1997). Nevertheless, deliberate blood pressure increase induced by vasopressors is used in the treatment of intracranial hypertension in patients with severe head injury, and this treatment is often accompanied by a decrease in ICP (Rosner and Coley 1986). Another confounding factor is that in several studies where an increase in ICP has been observed after administration of analgetics, anaesthetics disturbing cerebral autoregulation (such as isoflurane or nitrous oxide) have been used (Strebel et al. 1995; Matta et al. 1999; Summors et al. 1999). Most intravenous anaesthetics, for example propofol, do not disturb cerebral autoregulation (Harrison et al. 1999).

In some of the cited studies showing increasing CSF pressure, a lumbar approach was used (Jung et al. 1990). The subdural method used in the studies presented in this chapter seems to be a more relevant method, as cerebral mass-expanding processes probably affect the subdural ICP more than lumbar CSF pressure, and obliterations of the CSF flow from the brain to the spinal canal may invalidate the lumbar approach as a reliable method. In the study by Warner et al. (1996) and in the present studies of alfentanil, remifentanil and fentanyl only patients with cerebral tumours were included, and maintenance of anaesthesia was provided with either inhalation agents or propofol supplemented with one of the analgetics. Generally speaking, the results as regards subdural ICP, CPP and $AVDO_2$ were identical. None of the analgetics changed ICP or $AVDO_2$, but decreased CPP in a dose-dependent manner. Based on these studies we find that moderate bolus doses of all three analgetics can be used safely during craniotomy for space-occupying processes. High doses, however, may decrease blood pressure and thereby CPP to levels which, in some patients, may be inappropriate.

References

Åkeson J, Messeter K, Rosén I et al (1993) Cerebral haemodynamic and electrocortical CO_2 reactivity in pigs anaesthetized with fentanyl, nitrous oxide and pancuronium. Acta Anaesthesiol Scand 37:85–91

Albanese J, Viviand X, Potie F et al (1999) Sufentanil, fentanyl, and alfentanil in head trauma patients: a study on cerebral hemodynamics. Crit Care Med 27:407–411

Balakrishnan G, Raudzens P, Samra SK et al (2000) A comparison of remifentanil and fentanyl in patients undergoing surgery for intracranial mass lesions. Anesth Analg 91:163–169

Benzer A, Gottardis M, Russigger L et al (1992) Fentanyl increases cerebrospinal fluid pressure in normocapnic volunteers. Eur J Anesthesiol 9:473–477

Coles JP, Leary TS, Monteiro JN et al (2000) Propofol anesthesia for craniotomy: a double-blind comparison of remifentanil, alfentanil, and fentanyl. J Neurosurg Anesthesiol 12:15–20

de Nadal M, Austina A, Sahuquillo J et al (1998) Effects on intracranial pressure of fentanyl in severe head injured patients. Acta Neurochir 71(suppl):10–12

de Nadal M, Munar F, Poca MA et al (2000) Cerebral hemodynamic effects of morphine and fentanyl in patients with severe head injury. Anesthesiology 92:11–19

Endo H, Larsen B, Lassen NA (1977) Regional cerebral blood flow alterations remote from the site of intracranial tumours. J Neurosurg 46:271–281

Enevoldsen EM, Cold GE, Jensen FT (1976) Dynamic changes in regional CBF, intraventricular pressure, CSF-pH and lactate levels during the acute phase of head injury. J Neurosurg 44:191–214

Engelhard K, Reeker W, Kochs E et al (2004) Effect of remifentanil on intracranial pressure and cerebral blood flow velocity in patients with head trauma. Acta Anaesthesiol Scand 48:396–399

Fieschi C, Battistini N, Beduschi A et al (1974) Regional cerebral blood flow and intraventricular pressure in acute head injuries. J Neurol Neurosurg Psychiatry 37:1378–1388

Freeman J, Ingvar DH (1967) Effects of fentanyl on cerebral cortical blood flow and EEG in the cat. Acta Anaesthesiol Scand 11:381–391

Guy J, Hindman BJ, Baker KZ et al (1997) Comparison of remifentanil and fentanyl in patients undergoing craniotomy for supratentorial space-occupying lesions. Anesthesiology 86:514–524

Hanowell LH, Thurston JD, Behrman KH et al (1993) Alfentanil administered prior to endotracheal suctioning reduces cerebral perfusion pressure. J Neurosurg Anesthesiol 5:31–35

Harrison JM, Girling KJ, Mahajan RP (1999) Effects of target-controlled infusion of propofol on the transient hyperaemic response and carbon dioxide reactivity in the middle cerebral artery. Br J Anaesth 83:839–844

Hindman B, Warner D, Todd M et al (1994) ICP and CPP effects of remifentanil and alfentanil. J Neurosurg Anesthesiol 6:304

Hung OR, Hope CE, Laney G et al (1992) The effect of alfentanil on intracranial dynamics and hemodynamics in patients with brain tumours undergoing craniotomy. Can J Anesth A4

Jung R, Shah N, Reinsel R et al (1990) Cerebrospinal fluid pressure in patients with brain tumours: impact of fentanyl versus alfentanil during nitrous oxide-oxygen anesthesia. Anesth Analg 71:419–422

Jünger EC, Newell DW, Grant GA et al (1997) Cerebral autoregulation following minor head injury. J Neurosurg 86:425–432

Kolbitsch C, Hörmann C, Schmidauer C et al (1997) Hypocapnia reverses the fentanyl-induced increase in cerebral blood flow velocity in awake humans. J Neurosurg Anesthesiol 9:313–315

Knüttgen D, Doehn M, Eymer D et al (1989) Hirndrucksteigerung nach fentanyl. Anaesthesist 38:73–75

Lorenz IH, Kolbitsch C, Schocke M et al (2000). Low-dose remifentanil increases regional cerebral blood flow and regional cerebral blood volume, but decreases regional mean transit time and regional cerebrovascular resistance in volunteers. Br J Anaesth 85:199–204

Lorenz IH, Kolbitsch C, Hörmann C et al (2002) The influence of nitrous oxide and remifentanil on cerebral hemodynamics in conscious human volunteers. Neuroimage 17:1056–1064

Markovitz PB, Cohen DE, Duhaime A et al (1990) Effects of alfentanil in intracranial pressure in children undergoing ventriculo-periodoneal shunt revision. Anesthesiology 73:A213

Marx W, Shah N, Long C et al (1989) Sufentanil, alfentanil, and fentanyl: impact on cerebrospinal fluid pressure in patients with brain tumours. J Neurosurg Anesthesiol 1:3–7

Matta BF, Heath KJ, Tipping K et al (1999) Direct cerebral vasodilatory effects of sevoflurane and isoflurane. Anesthesiology 91:677–680

Mayberg TS, Lam AM, Eng CC et al (1993) The effect of alfentanil on cerebral blood flow velocity and intracranial pressure during isoflurane-nitrous oxide anesthesia in humans. Anesthesiology 78:288–294

McPherson RW, Johnson RM, Traystman RJ (1982) The effects of alfentanil on the cerebral vasculature. Anesthesiology 57:A354

Michenfelder JD, Theye RA (1971) Effects of fentanyl, droperidol, and Innovar on canine cerebral metabolism and blood flow. Br J Anaesth 43:630–636

Milde LN, Milde JH, Gallagher WJ (1989) Cerebral effects of fentanyl in dogs. Br J Anaesth 63:710–715

Miller R, Tausk HC, Stark DCC (1975) Effect of Innovar, fentanyl and droperidol on the cerebrospinal fluid pressure in neurosurgical patients. Can Anaesth Soc J 22:502–508

Moss E (1992) Alfentanil increases intracranial pressure when intracranial compliance is low. Anaesthesia 47:134–136

Moss E, Powell D, Gibson RM et al (1978) Effects of fentanyl on intracranial pressure and cerebral perfusion pressure during hypocapnia. Br J Anaesth 50:779–784

Muizelaar JP, Ward JD, Marmarou A (1989) Cerebral blood flow and metabolism in severely head-injured children. Part 2: autoregulation. J Neurosurg 71:72–76

Nilsson E, Ingvar DH (1965) Cerebral blood flow during neuroleptanalgesia in the cat. Acta Anaesth Scand 10:47–54

Olsen KS, Juul N, Cold GE (2005) Effect of alfentanil on intracranial pressure during propofol-fentanyl anesthesia for craniotomy. A randomized prospective dose-response study. Acta Anaesthesiol Scand 49:445–452

Palvölgyi R (1969) Regional cerebral blood flow in patients with intracranial tumours. J Neurosurg 31:149–163

Paris A, Scholz J, von Knobelsdorff G et al (1998) The effect of remifentanil on cerebral blood flow velocity. Anesth Analg 87:569–573

Rosner MJ, Coley IB (1986) Cerebral perfusion pressure, intracranial pressure, and head elevation. J Neurosurg 65:636–641

Schregel W, Schäfermeyer H, Müller C et al (1992) Einfluss von halothan, alfentanil und propofol auf der flussgeschwindigkeiten, „gefässquerschnitt" und „volumenfluss" in der a. cerebri media. Anaesthesist 41:21–26

Strebel S, Lam AM, Matta B et al (1995) Dynamic and static cerebral autoregulation during isoflurane, desflurane and propofol anesthesia. Anesthesiology 83:66–76

Summors AC, Gupta AK, Matta BF (1999) Dynamic cerebral autoregulation during sevoflurane anesthesia: a comparison with isoflurane. Anesth Analg 88:341–345

Trindle MR, Dodson BA, Rampil IJ (1993) Effects of fentanyl versus sufentanil in equianesthetic doses on middle cerebral artery blood flow velocity. Anesthesiology 78:454–460

Wagner KJ, Willoch F, Kochs EF et al (2001) Dose-dependent regional cerebral blood flow changes during remifentanil infusion in humans. Anesthesiology 94:732–739

Warner DS, Hindman BJ, Todd MM et al (1996) Intracranial pressure and hemodynamic effects of remifentanil versus alfentanil in patients undergoing supratentorial craniotomy. Anesth Analg 83:348–353

Chapter 14
Effect of a Propofol Bolus Dose on Subdural Intracranial Pressure and Cerebral Haemodynamics During General Anaesthesia for Craniotomy in Patients with Supratentorial Cerebral Tumours

Georg Emil Cold and Niels Juul

Abstract

Like barbiturates, propofol suppresses cerebral blood flow and cerebral metabolic rate of oxygen. As a consequence, a decrease in ICP is also expected. Rapid intraoperative reduction of ICP with thiopental has been demonstrated. In patients with head injury, propofol decreases both ICP and mean arterial blood pressure. Cerebral perfusion pressure, however, decreases as well, making the use of propofol in patients with head injury controversial. In patients subjected to craniotomy for space-occupying lesions in propofol-fentanyl or propofol-remifentanil anaesthesia, the effect of a bolus dose of propofol are poorly studied.

In this chapter the effect of a propofol bolus during maintenance of anaesthesia with either propofol-remifentanil or propofol-fentanyl is studied, and differences in cerebral haemodynamic parameters are discussed.

Like barbiturates, propofol suppresses CBF and $CMRO_2$. As a consequence, a decrease in ICP is also expected. Rapid intraoperative reduction of ICP with thiopental has been demonstrated (Shapiro et al. 1973). In a study of rabbits subjected to intracranial hypertension by an extradural balloon, propofol had a greater effect on ICP than hyperventilation, and the effect of the two treatments was additive (Watts et al. 1998). In patients with head injury, propofol decreases both ICP and MABP. CPP, however, decreases as well, making the use of propofol in patients with head injury controversial (Hartung 1987). In another study it was concluded that propofol 1–2 mg/kg decreased ICP, that the hypotensive effect on blood pressure was mild and that no inadvertent CPP changes were observed (Weinstabl et al. 1990). In patients subjected to craniotomy for space-occupying lesions in propofol-fentanyl or propofol-remifentanil anaesthesia, the effect of a bolus dose of propofol are poorly studied.

Study 1: Effect of a Propofol Bolus Dose on Subdural Intracranial Pressure and Cerebral Haemodynamics in Patients Subjected to Craniotomy for Supratentorial Cerebral Tumours in Propofol-Remifentanil Anaesthesia

Aim   We tested the hypothesis that a bolus dose of propofol or remifentanil decreases ICP in patients scheduled for craniotomy during propofol-remifentanil anaesthesia.

Method   Two groups of 15 patients each were studied: a control group and a group where 10% of the maintenance dose per hour of propofol was given as a bolus dose. All patients were scheduled for craniotomy for supratentorial

Table 14.1 Preoperative demographic data, neuroradiological data, perioperative data concerning maintenance of anaesthesia and data related to measurement of subdural ICP and cerebral haemodynamics in a control group and a group where propofol was administered as a bolus dose. The perioperative data are obtained before the administration of propofol bolus dose. No significant differences were disclosed between groups

	Control group	Propofol group
Men/women	6/9	7/8
Weight (kg)	79.0±17.0	75.0±15.0
Preoperative MABP (mmHg)	96.0±6.0	94.0±10.0
Maximal area of tumour (cm^2)	11.0±7.0	15.0±15.0
Midline shift (mm)	4.2±6.6	4.2±6.1
Propofol (mg/h)	460.0±135.0	473.0±101.0
Remifentanil (mg/h)	23.5±9.1	23.6±7.3
Temperature (°C)	35.7±0.4	35.9±0.3
$PaCO_2$ (kPa)	4.5±0.3	4.7±0.5
MABP (mmHg)	77.0±15.0	72.0±11.0
ICP (mmHg)	9.5±6.2	5.9±4.8
CPP (mmHg)	68.0±15.0	66.0±10.0
SjO_2 (%)	50.0±8.7	50.0±8.1
$AVDO_2$ (mmol/L)	3.6±0.8	3.3±0.5

Table 14.2   Localization of the tumours in a control group and a group where propofol was administered as a bolus dose. Number of patients is indicated

Localization	Control group	Propofol group
Frontal	2	7
Parietal	4	3
Temporal	4	3
Occipital	1	0
Basal	3	1
Central	1	1

cerebral tumours. Subdural ICP, MABP and CPP were monitored every minute for 5 min after a bolus dose of propofol. $PaCO_2$, SjO_2 and $AVDO_2$ were measured at time zero and after 5 min.

Statistical analysis Within groups the paired *t*-test was used for the analyses of normally distributed data. Between groups, analysis of variance was used. The chi-square test was used to estimate the difference in proportion. Mean±SD are indicated. $P<0.05$ was considered significant.

Results No differences in demographic data, preoperative blood pressure, $PaCO_2$, rectal temperature, neurological data (tumour size, midline shift, localization of tumour) or pathohistology of the tumours were disclosed (Tables 14.1–14.3). Propofol (average dose 47 mg) induced a significant fall in MABP and CPP lasting from 1 min after administration and for the following

Table 14.3 Histopathology in a control group and a group where propofol was administered as a bolus dose

Pathology	Control group	Propofol group
Glioblastoma	3	3
Meningioma	4	5
Metastasis	0	2
Glioma	4	3
Other	4	2

Table 14.4 MABP, ICP and CPP in the control group ($n=15$) and the propofol bolus group ($n=15$). Mean values are indicated

Minutes	Control			Propofol		
	MABP (mmHg)	ICP (mmHg)	CPP (mmHg)	MABP (mmHg)	ICP (mmHg)	CPP (mmHg)
0	77.3	9.5	67.8	72.3	5.9	66.5
1	77.3	9.3	68.1	67.9*	6.0	62.1*
2	77.1	9.3	67.7	67.8*	6.5	62.1*
3	76.5	9.5	67.0	69.5*	5.7	63.7*
4	77.2	9.3	67.8	69.8*	5.8	63.3*
5	77.7	9.4	67.6	70.1	5.9	64.2

*$P\leq0.01$ significant difference from 0 min

Table 14.5 SjO_2, $AVDO_2$ and $PaCO_2$ before and at 5 min in the control group and the propofol bolus group. No significant difference was disclosed within the groups

Minutes	Control			Propofol		
	$PaCO_2$ (kPa)	SjO_2 (%)	$AVDO_2$ (mmol/L)	$PaCO_2$ (kPa)	SjO_2 (%)	$AVDO_2$ (mmol/L)
0	4.4±0.3	49.8±8.7	3.6±0.8	4.7±0.5	49.9±8.1	3.3±0.5
5	4.5±0.4	49.7±8.4	3.6±0.8	4.6±0.4	49.6±8.3	3.3±0.5

4 min, but subdural ICP was unchanged. In the control group subdural ICP, MABP and CPP were unchanged (Table 14.4). In both groups $PaCO_2$, SjO_2 and $AVDO_2$ were unchanged during the 5-min study period (Table 14.5).

Conclusion A bolus dose of propofol administered during propofol-remifentanil anaesthesia does not change ICP, SjO_2 or $AVDO_2$ but reduces blood pressure and CPP significantly.

Study 2: Effect of a Propofol Bolus Dose on Subdural Intracranial Pressure and Cerebral Haemodynamics in Patients Subjected to Craniotomy for Supratentorial Cerebral Tumours in Propofol-Fentanyl Anaesthesia

Aim We tested the hypothesis that a propofol bolus dose decreases ICP in patients scheduled for craniotomy during propofol-fentanyl anaesthesia.

Method In 11 patients scheduled for craniotomy for cerebral tumours subdural ICP, MABP and CPP were monitored every minute for 5 min after a bolus dose of propofol (10% of maintenance dose per hour). SjO_2 and $AVDO_2$ were measured at time zero and 5 min after propofol injection. Fifteen patients served as control.

Statistical analysis Within groups the paired t-test was used for the analysis of normally distributed data. Between groups, analysis of variance was used. The chi-square test was used to estimate the difference in proportion. Mean±SD are indicated. $P<0.05$ was considered significant.

Table 14.6 Preoperative demographic data, neuroradiological data, perioperative data concerning maintenance of anaesthesia and data related to measurement of subdural ICP and cerebral haemodynamics in a control group and a group where propofol was administered as a bolus dose. The perioperative data are obtained before the administration of propofol bolus dose. No significant differences were disclosed between groups

	Control group	Propofol group
Women/Men	7/8	2/9
Weight (kg)	74.0±12.0	77.0±12.0
Maximal tumour area (cm^2)	13.0±10.0	13.0±8.0
Midline shift (mm)	4.8±6.6	3.7±4.2
Propofol maintenance (mg/h)	677.0±190.0	509.0±83.0
Fentanyl maintenance (µg/h)	137.0±40.0	136.0±23.0
$PaCO_2$ (kPa)	4.6±0.4	4.5±0.3
Temperature (°C)	35.7±0.5	35.8±0.4
MABP (mmHg)	90.0±11.0	93.0±11.0
ICP (mmHg)	5.3±3.1	6.7±2.1
CPP (mmHg)	86.0±13.0	86.0±11.0
SjO_2 (%)	55.8±14.1	55.4±6.9

Table 14.7 Localization of the tumours in a control group and a group where propofol was administered as a bolus dose

Localization	Control group	Propofol group
Frontal	7	4
Parietal	2	2
Temporal	4	2
Occipital	0	1
Basal	1	0
Central	1	2

Table 14.8 Histopathology in a control group and a group where propofol was administered as a bolus dose

Pathology	Control group	Propofol group
Glioblastoma	2	4
Meningioma	1	1
Metastasis	2	4
Glioma	9	2
Other	1	0

Table 14.9 MABP, ICP and CPP in the control group and the propofol bolus group. Mean values are indicated

Minutes	Control			Propofol		
	MABP (mmHg)	ICP (mmHg)	CPP (mmHg)	MABP (mmHg)	ICP (mmHg)	CPP (mmHg)
0	90.1	5.3	85.5	93.2	6.7	86.2
1	89.9	5.5	84.8	90.4	6.8	83.5
2	89.0	5.6	83.4	86.3*	6.8	79.5*
3	89.5	5.4	84.1	86.7*	6.8	79.9*
4	89.6	5.3	83.3	87.6*	7.0	80.6*
5	89.2	5.3	84.2	88.2*	7.0	81.2*

*$P \leq 0.002$ significant difference from 0 min

Results No differences in demographic data, preoperative blood pressure, $PaCO_2$, rectal temperature, neurological data (tumour size, midline shift, localization of tumour) or pathohistology of the tumours were disclosed (Tables 14.6–14.8). The propofol dose (averaging 51 mg, induced a significant fall in MABP and CPP lasting from 1 min after administration and for the following 5 min. The maximum fall in MABP and CPP averaged 6.9 and 6.8 mmHg, respectively. ICP did not change significantly. In the control group MABP, ICP and CPP were unchanged (Table 14.9). In both groups SjO_2 and $AVDO_2$ were unchanged (Table 14.10).

Table 14.10 $PaCO_2$, SjO_2 and $AVDO_2$ before, and at 5 min in the control group and the propofol bolus group

Minutes	Control			Propofol		
	$PaCO_2$ (kPa)	SjO_2 (%)	$AVDO_2$ (mmol/L)	$PaCO_2$ (kPa)	SjO_2 (%)	$AVDO_2$ (mmol/L)
0	4.6±0.4	55.8±14.1	3.4±0.7	4.5±0.3	55.4±6.9	3.3±0.4
5	4.6±0.4	53.5±10.8	3.5±0.8	4.5±0.3	54.8±7.6	3.3±0.4

Conclusion A bolus dose of propofol administered during propofol-fentanyl anaesthesia does not change ICP, SjO_2 or $AVDO_2$ but reduces CPP significantly.

Discussion

The principal findings in the presented studies are as follows: During maintenance anaesthesia with propofol-fentanyl or propofol-remifentanil a bolus dose of propofol decreases blood pressure and CPP, but leaves ICP unchanged. In contrast, in experimental studies (Watts et al. 1998) and in clinical studies in patients with head injury (Hartung 1987; Weinstabl et al. 1990), a decrease in ICP, eventually accompanied by a decrease in CPP, was found. A decrease in blood pressure and CPP was also observed after a propofol bolus dose of 2.5 mg/kg (Hemelrijck et al. 1992). As cerebral metabolism, cerebral autoregulation and the CO_2 reactivity are influenced by changes in CPP, these factors should be discussed as a reason for the unchanged ICP found in the present studies.

In experimental studies propofol is known to reduce both CBF and $CMRO_2$ (Vandesteene et al. 1988; Werner et al. 1992). A dose-related decrease in CBF and $CMRO_2$ under conditions where blood pressure is maintained has been found (Ramani et al. 1992). In dogs low and moderate doses of propofol decrease the EEG activity and $CMRO_2$, causing an associated decrease of CBF and CSF pressure. Cerebral autoregulation and CO_2 reactivity were found to be preserved. In contrast, high-dose propofol decreases CPP below the lower point of cerebral autoregulation (Artru et al. 1992). In rabbits cerebrovascular reactivity of blood flow and CBV are markedly decreased during hypocapnia, but are maintained during hypercapnia (Cenic et al. 2000). In the rat and pig autoregulation is present during propofol anaesthesia (Werner et al. 1990; Lagerkranser et al. 1997).

In humans propofol, given as a bolus injection, suppresses CBF and $CMRO_2$ (Stephan et al. 1987, 1988). Similar changes in CBF and $CMRO_2$ have been observed during continuous infusion with propofol (Vandesteene et al. 1988), and in a clinical study $CMRO_2$ was reduced about 50% compared with values obtained in awake healthy humans (Madsen et al. 1989). In healthy volunteers $AVDO_2$ is unchanged during continuous propofol induction, suggesting parallel changes in CBF and $CMRO_2$. The decrease in flow velocity, measured with transcranial Doppler, reaches a minimum value of 40% of baseline within 5 min, and the bispectral index (BIS) decreases to a minimum value at around 7 min from the onset of propofol administration (Ludbrook et al. 2002). Several studies have suggested that during propofol anaesthesia, the reduction of CBF is larger than the reduction of $CMRO_2$, resulting in a decrease of the $CBF/CMRO_2$ ratio (Manohar 1986; Scheller et al. 1988, 1990; Mielck et al. 1999). Likewise, other studies indicate that the SjO_2 is low or the $AVDO_2$ is high during propofol anaesthesia (Jansen et al. 1999; Munoz et al. 2002; Petersen et al. 2003), at least when compared with isoflurane anaesthesia (Jansen et al. 1999; Petersen et al. 2003) or sevoflurane anaesthesia (Munoz et al. 2002; Petersen et al. 2003; Kawano et al. 2004). On the other hand, Iwata et al. (2006) found that increasing the dose of propofol did not affect SjO_2. Both during sevoflurane, isoflurane and propofol anaesthesia, hyperventilation aggravates the changes in $AVDO_2$ and SjO_2 (Petersen et al. 2003; Kawano et al. 2004). These findings suggest that maintenance of normocarbia may be critical to maintenance of adequate cerebral perfusion. Kaisti et al. (2002) studied rCBF with positron emission tomography (PET) in volunteers when they were awake and during increasing propofol concentrations of 1, 1.5 and $2 EC_{50}$. They found that rCBF during EC_{50} was reduced by 62–70% with minor additional effect when the concentration was further increased. In a similar study they found that at a BIS value of 40 propofol reduced rCBF and $rCMRO_2$ comparably (Kaisti et al. 2003). After propofol bolus injection the CO_2 reactivity was preserved (Stephan et al. 1987). This finding was also confirmed in studies with a Doppler technique (Jansen and Kagenaar 1993; Strebel et al. 1994; Ederberg et al. 1998). In a study including healthy adults the slope of the CBF versus $PaCO_2$ was 1.56 ml/100 g/min/mmHg $PaCO_2$ (Fox et al. 1992). During continuous propofol infusion in patients without brain disorders the CO_2 reactivity was also found to be intact (Craen et al. 1992; Harrison et al. 1999). In other studies the CO_2 reactivity based on flow velocity was attenuated (Mirzai et al. 2004). Hyperventilation during propofol anaesthesia to end-tidal CO_2 values less than 30 mmHg is without effect on CBF because flow velocity is unchanged below this level (Karsli et al. 2004). In a randomized study, including patients with supratentorial cerebral tumours, the CO_2 reactivity was significantly lower during propofol anaesthesia compared with the reactivates obtained during isoflurane and sevoflurane (Petersen et al. 2003). In comparison with sevoflurane (Conti et al. 2006) or 1.5 MAC isoflurane and desflurane anaesthesia cerebral autoregulation is preserved with propofol (Matta et al. 1995; Strebel et al. 1995). In healthy subjects the effect of graded hypercapnia on cerebral autoregulation was tested during sevoflurane and propofol anaesthesia. The threshold of $PaCO_2$ to significantly impair cerebral autoregulation averaged 56 mmHg during sevoflurane anaesthesia and 61 mmHg during propofol anaesthesia (McCulloch et al. 2000).

From the cited studies it seems likely that cerebral autoregulation did not influence the results. If cerebral autoregulation is intact a decrease in CPP should elicit an increase in ICP, while a decrease in ICP was expected if cerebral autoregulation was intact. Furthermore, changes in $PaCO_2$ were not observed in either study and therefore could be excluded as a factor influencing ICP. A substantial decrease in $CMRO_2$ and CBF during maintenance of anaesthesia, however, seems to be a reasonable explanation why ICP was unchanged. A 50% decrease in $CMRO_2$ has been observed during propofol-fentanyl anaesthesia, and very low values of SjO_2 have been observed as well. Under such circumstances it is unlikely that a bolus dose of propofol might suppress $CMRO_2$ and CBF further, and thereby elicit a fall in CBV and ICP.

References

Artru AA, Shapira Y, Bowdle A (1992) Electroencephalogram, cerebral metabolism, and vascular responses to propofol anesthesia in dogs. J Neurosurg Anesthesiol 4:99–109

Cenic A, Craen RA, Howard-Lech VL et al (2000) Cerebral blood volume and blood flow at varying arterial carbon dioxide tension levels in rabbits during propofol anaesthesia. Anesth Analg 90:1376–1383

Conti A, Iacopino DG, Fodale V et al (2006) Cerebral haemodynamic changes during propofol-remifentanil or sevoflurane anaesthesia: transcranial Doppler study under bispectral index monitoring. Br J Anaesth 97:333–339

Craen RA, Gelb AW, Murkin JM et al (1992) CO_2 responsiveness of cerebral blood flow is maintained during propofol anaesthesia. Can J Anaesth A7

Ederberg S, Westerlind A, Houltz E et al (1998) The effects of propofol on cerebral blood flow velocity and cerebral oxygen extraction during cardiopulmonary bypass. Anest Analg 86:1201–1206

Fox J, Gelb AW, Enns J et al (1992) The responsiveness of cerebral blood flow to changes in arterial carbon dioxide is maintained during propofol-nitrous oxide anesthesia in humans. Anesthesiology 77:453–456

Harrison JM, Girling KJ, Mahajan RP (1999) Effects of target-controlled infusion of propofol on the transient hyperaemic response and carbon dioxide reactivity in the middle cerebral artery. Br J Anaesth 83:839–844

Hartung HJ (1987) Beeinflussung des Intrakraniellen Druckes durch Propofol (disoprivan). Anaesthesist 36:66–68

Hemelrijck JV, Tempelhoff R, White PF et al (1992) EEG-assisted titration of propofol infusion during neuroanesthesia: effect of nitrous oxide. J Neurosurg Anesthesiol 4:11–20

Iwata M, Kawaguchi M, Inoue S et al (2006) Effects of increasing concentrations of propofol on jugular venous bulb oxygen saturation in neurosurgical patients under normothermic and mildly hypothermic conditions. Anesthesiology 104:33–38

Jansen GF, Kagenaar D (1993) Effects of propofol in the relation between CO_2 and cerebral blood flow velocity. Anesth Analg 76:S163

Jansen GF, van Praagh BH, Kedaria MB et al (1999) Jugular bulb oxygen saturation during propofol and isoflurane/nitrous oxide anesthesia in patients undergoing brain tumour surgery. Anesth Analg 9:358–363

Kaisti KK, Metsähonkala L, Teräs M et al (2002) Effects of surgical levels of propofol and sevoflurane anesthesia on cerebral blood flow in healthy subjects studied with positron emission tomography. Anesthesiology 96:1358–1370

Kaisti KK, Långsjö JW, Aalto S et al (2003) Effects of sevoflurane, propofol, and adjunct nitrous oxide on regional cerebral blood flow, oxygen consumption, and blood volume in humans. Anesthesiology 99:603–613

Karsli C, Luginbuehl I, Bissonnette B (2004) The cerebrovascular response to hypocapnia in children receiving propofol. Anesth Analg 99:1049–1052

Kawano Y, Kawaguchi M, Inoue S et al (2004) Jugular bulb oxygen saturation under propofol or sevoflurane/nitrous oxide anesthesia during deliberate mild hypothermia in neurosurgical patients. J Neurosurg Anesthesiol 16:6–10

Lagerkranser M, Stånge K, Sollevi A (1997) Effects of propofol on cerebral blood flow, metabolism, and cerebral autoregulation in the anesthetized pig. J Neurosurg Anesthesiol 9:188–193

Ludbrook GL, Visco E, Lam AM (2002) Relation between brain concentrations, electroencephalogram, middle cerebral artery blood flow velocity, and cerebral oxygen extraction during induction of anesthesia. Anesthesiology 97:1363–1370

Madsen JB, Guldager H, Jensen FM (1989) CBF and $CMRO_2$ during neuroanaesthesia with continuous infusion of propofol. Acta Anaesthesiol Scand Suppl 91:33:143

Manohar M (1986) Regional brain blood flow and cerebral cortical O_2 consumption during sevoflurane anesthesia in healthy isocapnic swine. J Cardiovasc Pharmacol 8:1268–1275

Matta BF, Lam AM, Strebel S, Mayberg TS (1995) Cerebral pressure autoregulation and carbon dioxide reactivity during propofol-induced EEG suppression. Br J Anaesth 74:159–163

McCulloch TJ, Visco E, Lam AM (2000) Graded hypercapnia and cerebral autoregulation during sevoflurane or porpofol anaesthesia. Anesthesiology 93:1205–1209

Mielck F, Stephan H, Weyland A et al (1999) Effects of one minimum alveolar anesthetic concentration sevoflurane on cerebral metabolism, blood flow, and CO_2 reactivity in cardiac patients. Anesth Analg 89:364–369

Mirzai H, Tekin I, Tarhan S et al (2004) Effect of propofol and clonidine on cerebral blood flow velocity and carbon dioxide reactivity in the middle cerebral artery. J Neurosurg Anesthesiol 16:1–5

Munoz HR, Nunez GE, de la Fuente JE et al (2002) The effect of nitrous oxide on jugular bulb saturation during remifentanil plus target-controlled infusion propofol or sevoflurane in patients with brain tumours. Anesth Analg 94:389–392

Petersen KD, Landsfeldt U, Cold GE et al (2003). Intracranial pressure and cerebral hemodynamic in patients with cerebral tumours. A randomized prospective study of patients subjected to craniotomy in propofol/fentanyl, isoflurane/fentanyl or sevoflurane/fentanyl anesthesia. Anesthesiology 98:329–336

Ramani R, Todd MM, Warner DS (1992) A dose-response study of the influence of propofol on cerebral blood flow, metabolism and the electroencephalogram in the rabbit. J Neurosurg Anesthesiol 4:110–119

Scheller MS, Tateichi A, Drummond JC et al (1988) The effects of sevoflurane on cerebral blood flow, cerebral metabolic rate of oxygen, intracranial pressure, and the electroencephalogram are similar to those of isoflurane in the rabbits. Anesthesiology 68:548–551

Scheller MS, Nakakimura K, Fleischer JE et al (1990) Cerebral effects of sevoflurane in the dog: comparison with isoflurane and enflurane. Br J Anaesth 65:388–392

Shapiro HM, Galindo A, Wyte SR et al (1973) Rapid intraoperative reduction of ICP with thiopental. Br J Anaesth 45:1057–1061

Stephan H, Sonntag H, Schenk HD et al (1987) Einfluss von Disoprivan (Propofol) auf die Durchblutung und Sauerstoffverbrauch des Gehirns and die CO_2 Reaktivität der Hirngefässe beim Menschen. Anaesthesist 36:60–65

Stephan H, Sonntag H, Seyde WC et al (1988) Energy and amino acid metabolism in the human brain under Disoprivan anesthesia with various $PaCO_2$ values. Anaesthetist 37:297–304

Strebel S, Kaufmann M, Guardiola P-M et al (1994) Cerebral vasomotor responsiveness to carbon dioxide is preserved during propofol and midazolam anaesthesia in humans. Anaesth Analg 78:884–888

Strebel S, Lam AM, Matta B et al (1995) Dynamic and static cerebral autoregulation during isoflurane, desflurane, and propofol anesthesia. Anesthesiology 83:66–76

Vandesteene A, Trempont V, Engelman E et al (1988) Effect of propofol on cerebral blood flow and metabolism in man. Anaesthesia 43(suppl):42–43

Watts ADJ, Eliasziw M, Gelb AW (1998) Propofol and hyperventilation for the treatment of increased intracranial pressure in rabbits. Anesth Analg 87:564–568

Weinstabl C, Mayer N, Hammerle AF et al (1990) Effekte von Propofolbolusgaben auf das Intrakranielle Druckverhalten beim Schädel-Hirn-Trauma. Anaesthesist 39:521–524
Werner C, Hoffman WE, Segil LJ et al (1990) Effects of propofol on cerebral and spinal cord blood flow autoregulation in rats. Anesthesiology 73:No 3A, A694
Werner C, Hoffman WE, Kochs E et al (1992) The effects of propofol on cerebral blood flow in correlation to cerebral blood flow velocity in dogs. J Neurosurg Anesthesiol 4:41–46

Chapter 15
Effect of Reverse Trendelenburg Position on Subdural Intracranial Pressure and Cerebral Haemodynamics During General Anaesthesia for Craniotomy in Patients with Supratentorial Cerebral Tumours

Alp Tankisi and Georg Emil Cold

Abstract

The effects of head and trunk elevation on cerebral haemodynamics have been investigated in intensive care patients. In most of these studies, head and trunk elevation resulted in decreased ICP. The effect of head elevation on ICP and cerebral haemodynamics during general anaesthesia for craniotomy in patients with cerebral tumours has only been sparsely investigated.

In this chapter data on four studies concerning the reverse Trendelenburg position in patients with significant space-occupying lesions as well as patients with cerebral aneurysms are presented and discussed. The ICP-lowering effect of 10 degrees reverse Trendelenburg position in two groups of prone- and supine-positioned patients are presented. The optimal reverse position is disclosed and the influence of the anaesthetic regime discussed.

The effects of head and trunk elevation (flexion with the hips in a sitting and semi-sitting position) on cerebral haemodynamics have been investigated in intensive care patients. In patients with severe head injury the head-up position reduced ICP in the intensive care setting (Durwald et al. 1983; Rosner and Coley 1986; Porchet et al. 1998; Moraine et al. 2000). In contrast, the head-down position increases ICP compared to the neutral position (Lee 1989; Hung et al. 2000). The effect of head elevation on ICP in anaesthetized patients has only sparsely been investigated. The effect of head elevation on lumbar spinal pressure in anaesthetized patients was studied by Mavrocordatos et al. (2000) who investigated lumbar cerebrospinal pressure and found an increase of around 1 mmHg with a 30° head-up position, depending on the position of the neck. Rolighed

Larsen et al. (2002) studied subdural ICP during craniotomy before and 1 min after a change in position from supine to 10° rTp and found that subdural ICP and MABP decreased significantly, but CPP remained unchanged. In this chapter we present further studies in prone-positioned patients, patients with cerebral aneurysm and in supine-positioned patients of changes in subdural ICP and CPP with the patients in the neutral position and in 5°, 10° and 15° rTp.

This chapter is based on three published studies and one unpublished study: study 1 has been presented by Haure et al. in J Neurosurg Anesthesiol (2003) 15:297–301, study 2 has been presented by Tankisi et al. in Acta Neurochir (2002) 144:665–670 and study 3 has been presented by Tankisi and Cold in J Neurosurg (2007) 106:239–244; study 4 is unpublished.

Study 1: The Intracranial Pressure-Lowering Effect of 10 Degrees Reverse Trendelenburg Position During Craniotomy is Stable During a 10-Minute Period

Aim To study the effect of 10° rTp on subdural ICP, CPP and JBP during a 10-min period during craniotomy.

Method Fifteen adult patients scheduled for craniotomy for supratentorial cerebral tumours were included in the study. After exposure of dura, subdural ICP, MABP, CPP and JBP were monitored continuously before and 10 min after change in position from supine to 10° rTp. The degree of dural tension was evaluated by the surgeon as well. End tidal CO_2 was monitored during the study period, and arterial and jugular venous blood were analysed for PaO_2, $PaCO_2$, oxygen content and oxygen saturation. $AVDO_2$ was calculated as the difference in oxygen content between arterial and venous blood. (For details concerning methods, see Chapter 3.)

Statistical analysis Mean values, SD and standard error of mean (SE) were calculated. One-way repeated measures of variance was performed. If the test for normality failed, Friedman's repeated measures of analysis on ranks was used to analyse paired data. Dunnett's method was used for pair-wise multiple comparison. $P<0.05$ was considered significant.

Results No significant changes as regards $PaCO_2$, PaO_2, arterial oxygen saturation, SjO_2, $AVDO_2$ or end-tidal CO_2 were disclosed when values before and 10 min after change in position were compared. One minute after change in position, subdural ICP decreased from 10.9 (5.7) mmHg to 7.3 (5.2) mmHg, $P<0.05$, and remained stable during the next 9 min (Fig. 15.1). A significant decrease in MABP was also disclosed after 1 min after change in position from 81 (15) mmHg to 77 (15) mmHg, $P<0.05$, but for the following 9 min MABP remained constant. JBP decreased significantly from 7.7 (1.7) mmHg to 5.5 (2.0) mmHg after 1 min. CPP did not change during the study period being 70 (16) mmHg before and 70 (17) mmHg after change in position (Fig. 15.2).

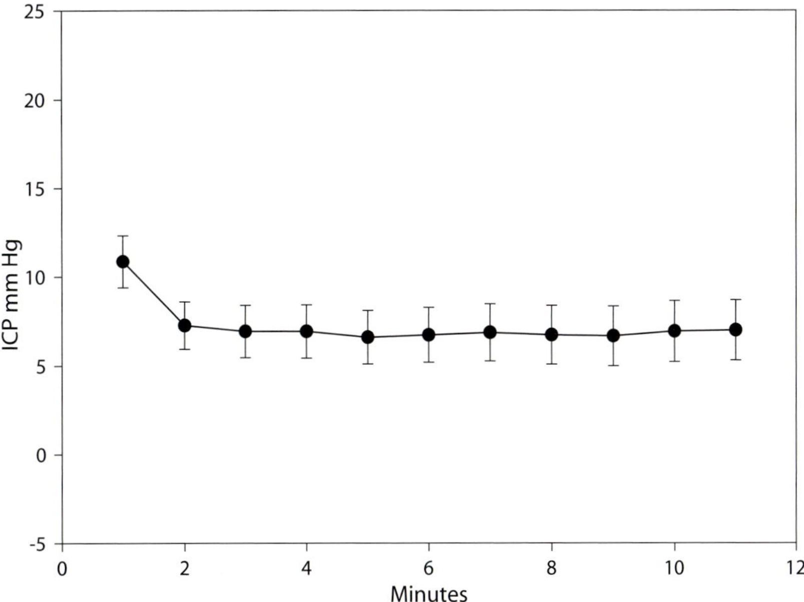

Fig. 15.1 Changes in subdural ICP in the supine position and during a 10-min period of 10° rTp. Means and SE are indicated

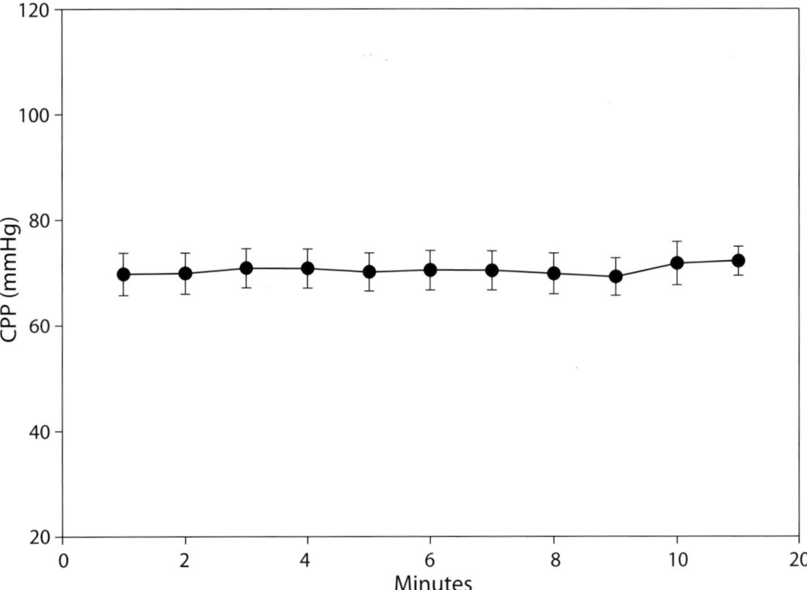

Fig. 15.2 Changes in CPP in the supine position and during a 10-min period of 10° rTp. Means and SE are indicated

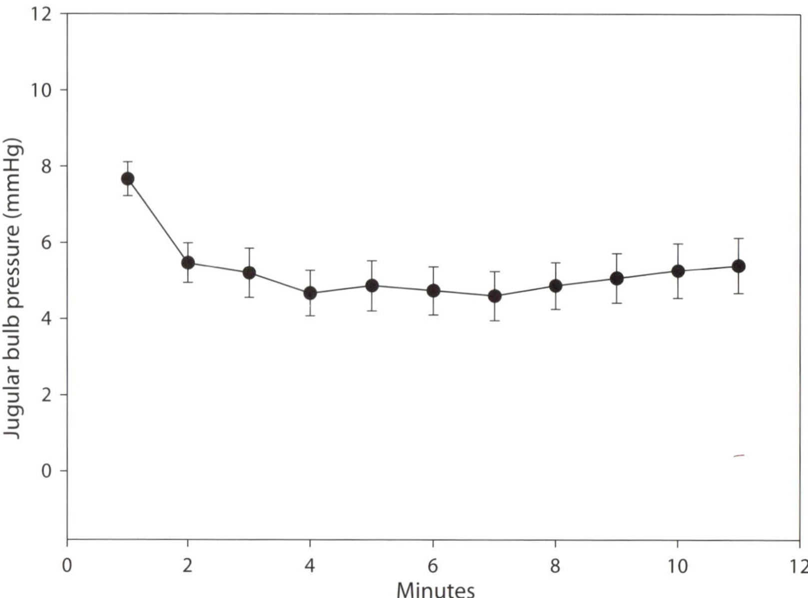

Fig. 15.3 Changes in JBP in the supine position and during a 10-min period of 10° rTp. Means and SE are indicated

Table 15.1 Degrees of dural tension in 15 patients evaluated before and repeatedly up to 10 min after change in position form supine to 10° rTp. Number of patients is indicated

	Dura very slack	Normal tension of dura	Increased tension of dura	Pronounced increased tension
Before tilting	1	5	8	1
One minute after tilting	3	8	4	0
Five minutes after tilting	3	9	3	0
Ten minutes after tilting	3	9	3	0

A significant decrease in JBP was also demonstrated (Fig. 15.3). The degree of dural tension as estimated by the neurosurgeon is indicated in Table 15.1. One minute after change in position the tension of dura decreased significantly, $P<0.05$. The degree of dural tension thereafter remained unchanged. Neither the correlation between subdural ICP and JBP, nor the correlation between change in subdural ICP and change in JBP following tilting of the table were significant.

Conclusion During craniotomy 10° rTp reduces subdural ICP and MABP significantly, while CPP is unchanged. These changes occur within 1 min after change in position, and during the next 9 min subdural ICP and CPP remain stable. The change in position is accompanied by a decrease in dural tension.

Study 2: Effect of 10 Degrees Reverse Trendelenburg Position on Intracranial Pressure and Cerebral Perfusion Pressure in Prone-Positioned Patients Subjected to Craniotomy for Occipital or Cerebellar Tumours

Aim   The aim of the study is to evaluate the effect of 10° rTp on subdural ICP, CPP, MABP and JBP in prone-positioned patients subjected to craniotomy for occipital or cerebellar tumours.

Method   Twelve patients with occipital tumour and 14 patients with cerebellar tumour underwent propofol-fentanyl anaesthesia in the prone position. The patients were moderately hyperventilated, with attempted $PaCO_2$ levels between 4.0 and 5.0 kPa, and PaO_2 > 13 kPa. After induction of anaesthesia 500 ml of 6% hydroxyethyl starch was infused. Catheters were inserted in the radial artery and jugular vein. MABP, subdural ICP and JBP were measured in the neutral position and in 10° rTp. CPP was calculated as MABP − subdural ICP. Measurements were performed in the neutral position and after change in position to 10° rTp. Changes in subdural ICP and JBP were calculated. Tension of dura was estimated in the neutral position and again at 10° rTp by the neurosurgeon. Dural tension was graded as: normal, increased tension and pronounced increased tension (for details, see Chapter 3).

Statistical analysis   Mean±SD were calculated. Between groups and within groups Student's *t*-test and paired *t*-test were used for analyses, respectively. When the normality test failed the Mann-Whitney rank sum test and the Wilcoxon test were used.

Results   In patients with occipital tumours subdural ICP decreased from 21.0 to 15.6 mmHg ($P<0.05$) after change in position. In 7 of 12 patients the decrease in ICP was ≥ 5 mmHg. MABP and JBP also decreased significantly from 87.9 to 83.3 mmHg and from 14.3 to 7.7 mmHg, respectively. CPP did not change significantly (Table 15.2). In patients with cerebellar tumours a significant decrease in subdural ICP from 18.3 to 14.2 mmHg was found. In 6 of 14 patients the decrease in ICP was ≥ 5 mmHg. MABP and JBP decreased significantly as well, but CPP did not change significantly (Table 15.3). In Table 15.4 the tactile estimations of dural tension are indicated before and after change in position. Both occipital and cerebellar tumours are included. The

Table 15.2   MABP, subdural ICP, CPP and JBP in the neutral position and after change in position to 10° rTp. Twelve patients with occipital tumours are included. Mean±SD are indicated

Position	MABP (mmHg)	ICP (mmHg)	CPP (mmHg)	JBP(mmHg)
Neutral	87.9±16.4	21.0±4.6	66.9±16.9	14.3±5.5
10° rTp	83.3±16.0*	15.6±5.6*	67.7±16.5	7.7±5.3*

*$P<0.05$

Table 15.3 MABP, subdural ICP, CPP and JBP in the neutral position and after change in position to 10° rTp. Fourteen patients with cerebellar tumours are included. Mean±SD are indicated

Position	MABP (mmHg)	ICP (mmHg)	CPP (mmHg)	JBP (mmHg)
Neutral	93.8±13.4	18.3±6.1	75.5±14.3	12.1±6.3
10° rTp	90.5±13.7*	14.2±5.9*	76.4±15.2	5.0±4.6*

*$P<0.05$

Table 15.4 Estimation of tension of dura in prone-positioned patients with the operating table in the neutral position and after change to 10° rTp. Numbers of patients are indicated

Tension of dura	Neutral position	10° rTp
Normal	1	7
Increased	15	10
Pronounced increased	10	9

number of patients with normal tension of dura increased from 1 to 7. When patients with cerebellar and occipital tumours were compared, no significant differences between MABP, subdural ICP, CPP and JBP were disclosed. Neither did the changes in subdural ICP, MABP, CPP and JBP differ between occipital and cerebellar tumours.

Conclusion   In prone-positioned patients 10° rTp significantly decreases subdural ICP, MABP and JBP, while CPP is unchanged.

Study 3: Optimal Reverse Trendelenburg Position in Patients Undergoing Craniotomy for Cerebral Tumours

Aims 1: Investigation of the effects of the neutral position and 5°, 10° and 15° rTp on subdural pressure, MABP, CPP and JBP in supine-positioned patients undergoing craniotomy for cerebral tumour. 2: To determine the optimal rTp, defined as the position at which subdural ICP is as low as possible and CPP ≥ 60 mmHg. 3: On the basis of subdural ICP measurements during neutral position and 5°, 10° and 15° rTp, to define risk groups for development of cerebral swelling.

Method Fifty-three patients underwent craniotomy in propofol-fentanyl anaesthesia in the supine position. The patients were moderately hyperventilated, the aim being a $PaCO_2$ level between 4.0 and 5.0 kPa and $PaO_2 \geq 13$ kPa. After induction of anaesthesia 500 ml of 6% hydroxyethyl starch was infused. Catheters were inserted in the radial artery and jugular vein. MABP, subdural ICP and JBP were measured in the neutral position. These measurements were repeated after change in position to 5°, 10° and 15° rTp. The pressure measurements were performed about 1 min after change in position, immediately after readjustment of the transducer position, the reference point being the horizontal level of dura perforation for subdural ICP measurement. CPP was calculated as MABP – subdural ICP. Measurements were performed in the neutral position and after change in position to 10° rTp. Changes in subdural ICP, MABP, CPP and JBP were calculated for each 5° step in position. Tension of dura was estimated at the neutral position and again at 10° rTp by the neurosurgeon. Dural tension was graded as: normal, increased tension and pronounced increased tension. The optimal position was defined as the position at which subdural ICP was as low as possible and CPP ≥ 60 mmHg. Tension of dura was estimated by the surgeon as slack, normal tension, increased tension, and pronounced increased tension (for details, see Chapter 3). The distribution of optimal positions was divided into three groups of patients at the neutral position. Group 1 consisted of 15 patients with subdural ICP < 5 mmHg, group 2 included 29 patients with subdural ICP ranging from 5 to 13 mmHg and group 3 contained 9 patients with subdural ICP > 13 mmHg.

Statistical analysis Mean±SD are presented. Comparisons of pressure within the group were performed using analysis of variance for repeated studies. Comparisons between groups were performed using an independent t-test. The chi-square test was used for comparisons of demographic data, the degree of dural tension and distributions of optimal positions. $P<0.05$ was considered significant.

Results Subdural ICP, MABP and JBP decreased significantly after each 5° change in position compared with the preceding position. In contrast CPP remained unchanged at 5° rTp, but decreased significantly at 10° and 15° rTp compared with the neutral position (Table 15.5). At the neutral position, 9 patients were at high risk of cerebral swelling, defined as subdural ICP > 13 mmHg, compared with only 1 patient at 15° rTp. The number of patients with low risk of cerebral swelling (subdural ICP < 5 mmHg) increased from 15 to 39 at 10° rTp, and from 39 to 42 when the position was changed from 10° to 15° rTp (Table 15.6).

The optimal position was the neutral position in 5 patients, 5° rTp in 5 patients, 10° rTp in 10 patients and 15° rTp in 33 patients (Table 15.7). No significant intergroup differences as regards the distribution of the optimal posi-

Table 15.5 Subdural ICP, MABP, CPP and JBP in the neutral position and after 5°, 10° and 15° rTp. Fifty-three supine-positioned patients with cerebral tumours were included

Variable	Neutral position	5° rTp	10° rTp	15° rTp
MABP (mmHg)	82.9±15.8	79.9±15.6*	76.9±15.2*	73.6±15.4*
ICP (mmHg)	7.6±5.1	5.1±5.3*	3.2±5.1*	1.8±5.0*
CPP (mmHg)	75.3±15.5	74.7±15.3	73.7±14.8*	71.8±15.2*
JBP (mmHg)	2.5±3.1	0.6±2.8*	−1.3±2.7*	−2.9±2.7*

*Significant change compared with the preceding position

Table 15.6 Distribution of number of patients in three risk groups related to the occurrence of brain swelling after opening of dura

ICP risk group	Neutral position	5° rTp	10° rTp	15° rTp
Group 1 (ICP < 5 mmHg)	15	26	39	42
Group 2 (ICP 5–13 mm Hg)	29	22	12	10
Group 3 (ICP > 13 mmHg)	9	5	2	1

Table 15.7 Number (%) of patients with optimal position related to risk groups for the occurrence of cerebral swelling after opening of the dura: group 1 (subdural ICP < 5 mmHg), group 2 (subdural ICP 5–13 mmHg) and group 3 (subdural ICP > 13 mmHg). The distributions of patients into the optimal position are independent of the level of ICP measured in the neutral position

Optimal position	All patients (n=53)	Group 1 (n=15)	Group 2 (n=29)	Group 3 (n=9)
Neutral position	5 (9.4%)	1 (6.7%)	3 (10.3%)	1 (11.1%)
5° rTp	5 (9.4%)	2 (13.3%)	2 (6.9%)	1 (11.1%)
10° rTp	10 (18.9%)	4 (26.7%)	5 (17.2%)	1 (11.1%)
15° rTp	33 (62.3%)	8 (53.3%)	19 (65.5%)	6 (66.7%)

tion were found. At the neutral position, 23 patients had increased tension of dura. The number of patients with increased tension of dura decreased to 17 at 5° rTp, to 10 at 10° rTp and to 9 patients at 15° rTp. Compared with the neutral position the degree of dural tension decreased significantly at 5° and 10° rTp, but the changes in tension from 10° to 15° rTp were not significant.

Conclusion Before opening the dura mater for craniotomy, repeated measurements of ICP and CPP in the neutral position and at 5°, 10° and 15° rTp provide valuable information regarding the optimal level of ICP and CPP.

Study 4: Effect of Reverse Trendelenburg Position on Intracranial Pressure and Cerebral Perfusion Pressure in Patients with Cerebral Tumours. A Comparative Study of Propofol-Fentanyl and Propofol-Remifentanil Anaesthesia

Aim To investigate whether the effect of 10° rTp on ICP, CPP and JBP differed in propofol-fentanyl- and propofol-remifentanil-anaesthetized patients.

Method Patients scheduled for elective craniotomy for supratentorial cerebral tumours were included. Fifty-eight patients were anaesthetized with propofol-fentanyl and 52 patients with propofol-remifentanil. As regards principles for monitoring and anaesthetic procedures, see Chapter 3. Subdural ICP, MABP and JBP were measured in the neutral position and thereafter during tilting of the table to 5°, 10° and 15° rTp. CPP was calculated as MABP – subdural ICP. Optimal position was defined as the position where

CPP was ≥ 60 mmHg, or as high as possible, and ICP was as low as possible. The level of ICP and CPP and the distributions of optimal positions were compared.

Statistical analysis   With data from another study, including patients with cerebral tumours, and where SD of ICP was 5 mmHg (Petersen et al. 2003), the sample size was calculated to be 44 and it provided a minimum detectable difference of 3 mmHg, power 0.8 and a significance level of $P<0.05$. Data were tested with normality and equal variance tests. One-way analysis of variance was used when these tests were passed and the Tukey test was used for pair-wise multiple comparison. Otherwise the Kruskall-Wallis test of variance on ranks was used. The Bonferroni test was applied. The chi-square test was used for analysis of demographics. For correlation studies Pearson's product moment correlation was performed. Mean±SD are indicated for normal distributions and median (range) for non-normal distributions. $P<0.05$ was considered significant.

Results   No significant difference was found in the neuroradiological data and histopathology. The ages of the patients were significantly higher in the propofol-fentanyl group. Likewise, the propofol maintenance doses were significantly higher in the propofol-fentanyl group (8.0±2.2 mg/kg/h) compared with the propofol-remifentanil group (5.6±1.4 mg/kg/h) (Table 15.8). In the neutral position ICP averaged 7.5±5.0 and 7.8±5.3 mmHg in the propofol-fentanyl- and propofol-remifentanil-anaesthetized patients, respectively. At each 5° step of rTp, subdural ICP decreased significantly in both groups. In the neutral position and at all steps of rTp, MABP and CPP were significantly lower in the propofol-remifentanil group. In both groups CPP was unchanged during 5° rTp, but a significant decrease was disclosed in each group when tilting of the table was forced to 10° and 15° rTp (Table 15.9). The medians of JBP decreased significantly during each step of rTp (Table 15.10). Although the median values were highest in the propofol-fentanyl group, the difference in JBP never reached significant levels. In all positions, the correlation coefficients r between JBP and subdural ICP were significant in the propofol-fentanyl group, but not in the propofol-remifentanil group (Table 15.11). No significant differences as regards the distribution of number of patients in positions at which ICP and CPP were optimal were found. In the majority of patients the optimal position was 15° rTp in both groups (Table 15.12). In this position, however, the operation could not proceed because the steepness of the table prevented surgical access.

Conclusion   In this non-randomized study, rTp reduces subdural ICP to the same level whether propofol-fentanyl or propofol-remifentanil were used for anaesthesia. Although CPP is significantly lower during propofol-remifentanil compared with propofol-fentanyl anaesthesia, the distribution of optimal position as defined in this study was independent of choice of anaesthesia. A randomized study seems justified to verify these findings.

Table 15.8 Demographics, neuroradiological data, histopathology, maintenance dose of anaesthesia and data obtained immediately before subdural ICP measurements with the patients in the neutral position

	Propofol-fentanyl	Propofol-remifentanil
Preoperative values		
Number	58	52
Men/women	26/32	28/24
Age (years)	56.0±12.0	49.0±15.0*
Weight (kg)	76.0±17.0	74.0±17.0
Steriods (+/−)	31.0/27.0	29.0/23.0
Serum Na$^+$ (mmol/L)	137.0±5.0	138.0±4.0
MABP before anaesthesia (mmHg)	103.0±16.0	103.0±12.0
Tumour area (cm^2)	15.0±12.0	15.0±17.0
Midline shift	7.5±7.2	5.9±6.6
Localization of tumour		
Frontal	20	17
Parietal	15	6
Temporal	14	13
Occipital	2	7
Hemispheric	4	4
Basal	3	5
Histopathology		
Glioblastoma	15	12
Meningioma	14	14
Metastasis	12	5
Glioma	15	13
Other	2	8
Maintenance of anaesthesia		
Propofol (mg/kg/h)	8.0±2.2	5.6±1.4*
Fentanyl (µg/kg/h)	1.8±0.4	0
Remifentanil (µg/kg/h)	0	29.0±10.0
Data in neutral position		
Temperature (°C)	35.8±0.5	35.8±0.4
PaCO$_2$ (kPa)	4.6±0.5	4.6±0.5
PaO$_2$ (kPa)	27.0±9.6	24.0±7.9
SjO$_2$ (%)	53.0±9.3	51.0±9.6
AVDO$_2$ (mmol/L)	3.4±0.7	3.5±0.7

*$P<0.01$

Table 15.9 MABP, subdural ICP and CPP in propofol-fentanyl (P/F)- and propofol-remifentanil (P/R)-anaesthetized patients. Mean±SD is indicated in the neutral position and during 5°, 10° and 15° rTp position

	Neutral	5° rTp	10° rTp	15° rTp
MABP (P/F) (mmHg)	83.0±15.0	79.0±14.0*	77.0±15.0*	74.0±15.0*
MABP (P/R) (mmHg)	75.0±13.0**	71.0±13.0*,**	68.0±12.0*,**	66.0±12.0*,**
ICP (P/F) (mmHg)	7.5±5.0	5.0±5.2*	3.0±5.0*	1.6±5.0*
ICP (P/R) (mmHg)	7.8±5.3	5.4±5.2*	3.1±5.0*	1.3±5.4*
CPP (P/F) (mmHg)	75.0±14.0	75.0±14.0	74.0±14.0*	72.0±15.0*
CPP (P/R) (mmHg)	67.0±14.0**	66.0±13.0**	65.0±12.0*,**	64.0±12.0*,**

*$P<0.05$ intragroup difference
**$P<0.05$ intergroup difference

Table 15.10 Median and range of JBP in propofol-fentanyl (P/F)- and propofol-remifentanil (P/R)-anaesthetized patients. The measurements were performed in the neutral position and during 5°, 10° and 15° rTp

	Neutral	5° rTp	10° rTp	15° rTp
JBP (P/F) (mmHg)	3 (−4 to 13)	1 (−5 to 7)*	−1 (−7 to 4)*	−3 (−8 to 3)*
JBP (P/R) (mmHg)	2 (−2 to 13)	0 (−6 to 10)*	−2 (−8 to 8)*	−4 (−7 to 6)*

*$P<0.05$ significant difference from the preceding value

Table 15.11 Correlation coefficient (r) for the relationship between JBP and subdural ICP in the neutral position and during 5°, 10° and 15° rTp. The patients were anaesthetized with propofol-fentanyl (P/F) or propofol-remifentanil (P/R)

	Neutral	5° rTp	10° rTp	15° rTp
Correlation coefficient(r) for JBP related to ICP (P/F)	0.2878	0.1304	0.1746	0.3176
Correlation coefficient(r) for JBP related to ICP (P/R)	0.4044*	0.4512*,#	0.4067*	0.3437*

*$P<0.05$
#Power > 0.8

Table 15.12 Number of patients at which optimal position was found. Optimal position had the following criteria: CPP ≥ 60 mmHg, or as high as possible, and subdural ICP as low as possible. The patients were anaesthetized with propofol-fentanyl or propofol-remifentanil, and the measurement of subdural ICP and CPP was performed in the neutral position and during 5°, 10° and 15° rTp. The distribution did not differ significantly. Chi-square ($P=0.526$)

	Neutral	5° rTp	10° rTp	15° rTp
Propofol-fentanyl (n)	4	5	8	41
Propofol-remifentanil (n)	8	3	7	34

Discussion

Intracranial pressure is not the only important physiological factor during elevation of the head and trunk. A decrease in MABP and CPP can have important consequences, partly because of a decline in CBF, if cerebral autoregulation is impaired or CPP is below the lower point of autoregulation, and partly because a fall in CPP provokes an increase in ICP if cerebral autoregulation is intact (Rosner and Coley 1986). Therefore, either the neutral position (Rosner and Coley 1986; Schwarz et al. 2002) or 15–30° head-trunk elevation are recommended to optimize the therapy of increased ICP (Davenport et al. 1990; Feldman et al. 1992; Schneider et al. 1993; Meixensberger et al. 1997).

In patients with severe head injury, routine nursing at 30° semi-sitting position has been recommended. A decrease in ICP and unchanged CPP, SjO_2, and partial tissue oxygen tension ($PtiO_2$) were reported during 30° elevation (Ng et al. 2004). Moraine et al. recommended that, when the ICP is high and CBF is normal, the head-up position should not exceed 30° because greater head elevation increased ICP (Moraine et al. 2000). Meixensberger et al. (1997) reported a decrease in ICP and unchanged cerebral brain tissue-PaO_2 during 30° head-trunk elevation in patients with acute brain injury. In patients with fulminant hepatic-renal failure after acetaminophen self-poisoning, ICP decreased and CPP was unchanged during 20° semi-sitting position. Elevations to 40–60° increased ICP in some patients (Davenport et al. 1990). In awake patients with cerebral tumours, 20° head-trunk elevation reduced ICP (Hung et al. 2000). In summary, in the clinical setting it is possible to define an "optimal position" at which the ICP-reducing effect is pronounced or maximal (Kenning et al. 1981; Ropper et al. 1982) without compromising CPP and CBF (Yoshida et al. 1993; Schneider et al. 1993).

In one study, the effects of supine, prone and sitting positions on epidural ICP were investigated during posterior fossa procedures in patients anaesthetized with fentanyl, thiopental and nitrous oxide/oxygen. ICP, measured by means of an epidural sensor, was lowest at the lateral 45° sitting position, with only minimal change in CPP compared to the neutral position. Furthermore, MABP, mean pulmonary artery/wedge pressure, cardiac output, CVP and lung compliance did not change in this position (Calliauw et al. 1987).

In propofol-fentanyl-anaesthetized patients with intracranial tumours or cerebral aneurysms, a decrease in lumbar cerebrospinal pressure averaging 1.8 mmHg and unchanged MABP/CPP with 30° table head-up position has been demonstrated during craniotomy. A non-significant decrease in CVP averaging 1 mmHg was also apparent in this position. In contrast, during 30° head-down position, mean ICP increased significantly from 8.8±2.5 to 13.3±2.9 mmHg and mean CVP increased from 3.9±2.3 to 8.4±2.4 mmHg ($P<0.05$) (Mavrocordatos et al. 2000). In nitrous oxide/oxygen isoflurane-alfentanil-anaesthetized patients with cerebral tumours, a decrease in ICP (Camino fiberoptic monitor) averaging 5.0±5.9 mmHg was reported during 20° head-up position combined with flexion at the hips (Hung et al. 2000).

Rolighed Larsen et al. (2002) studied the effect of 10° rTp on ICP and CPP in 40 supine-positioned patients with space-occupying lesions. The subdural ICP decreased significantly from 9.5 to 6.0 mmHg within 1 min after change in position, and CPP was unchanged. The number of patients with increased tension of the dura, as estimated by the neurosurgeon, decreased from 24 to 8 at 10° rTp. The correlation between the ICP at the neutral position and the decrease in ICP (ΔICP) at 10° rTp was positive and significant. In another study including supine-positioned patients with cerebral tumours, the effect of 10° rTp were analysed during a 10-min period. One minute after change in position subdural ICP, JBP and MABP decreased but remained stable during the subsequent 9 min. The subdural ICP was 10.9±5.7 mmHg at the neutral position and decreased to 7.3±5.2 mm Hg at 10° rTp (Fig 15.1). During the 10-min study period, CPP, heart rate, $AVDO_2$ and arterial and venous oxygen saturation did not change. The degree of dural tension as estimated by the neurosurgeon also decreased within 1 min after assumption of the rTp position (Haure et al. 2003).

In a recent study ICP was the strongest predicting factor of cerebral swelling after opening of dura during craniotomy (Rasmussen et al. 2004). However, maintenance of CPP is essential during intracranial surgery because falling CPP may decrease CBF below the ischaemic threshold. Furthermore, in patients with intact cerebral autoregulation, a fall in CPP may precipitate an increase in ICP (Rosner and Coley 1986). Consequently, measurements of both ICP and MABP (CPP) have been performed at the neutral position and again at 5°, 10° and 15° rTp in a series of 53 supine-positioned patients anaesthetized with propofol-fentanyl-air during operation for cerebral tumours. The optimal position was defined as the position at which subdural ICP was as low as possible, with CPP remaining greater than 60 mmHg, or as high as possible. There was considerable individual variation in the optimal position, which was the neutral position in 5 patients (9.4%), 5° rTp in 5 patients (9.4%), 10° rTp in 10 patients (18.9%) and 15° rTp in 33 patients (62.3%). The lowest ICP was disclosed in 1 patient (2%) in the neutral position, 2 patients (4%) in 5° rTp, 10 patients (19%) in 10° rTp and 40 patients (75%) in 15° rTp. The number of the patients with increased dural tension decreased from 23 to 10 during 10° rTp and 9 during 15° rTp. During 5° and 10° rTp, the tension of dura decreased significantly compared to the neutral position. There was no significant change in the tension of dura when the position was changed from 10° to 15° rTp (Tankisi and Cold 2007).

Anaesthetic agents have different effects on cardiovascular and cerebrovascular physiology. In study 4, the effect of rTp on subdural ICP, CPP and JBP were analysed in supine-positioned patients with supratentorial cerebral tumours. The patients were anaesthetized with either propofol-fentanyl ($n=58$) or propofol-remifentanil-air ($n=52$). The distribution of optimal positions was analysed in positions extending from neutral up to 15° rTp. In patients scheduled for propofol-fentanyl anaesthesia, a significantly higher maintenance dose of propofol was disclosed. A significant fall in ICP and JBP during increasing rTp was observed in both groups without significant intergroup ICP differences. At each 5° step of increasing rTp subdural ICP decreased significantly in each group, averaging 1.6 and 1.3 mmHg at 15° rTp in the propofol-fentanyl and propofol-remifentanil groups, respectively. Thus, rTp reduced subdural ICP to the same level, whether anaesthesia was maintained with propofol-fentanyl or propofol-remifentanil. The levels of CPP and MABP, however, were significantly lower during propofol-remifentanil anaesthesia. In both groups, CPP was unchanged during 5° rTp, but there was a significant decrease in CPP when tilting was forced to 10° and 15° rTp. JBP decreased significantly during each successive step of rTp. In the majority of patients, the optimal position was 15° rTp for both types of anaesthesia. No significant intergroup difference in the distribution of optimal position was found. In supine-positioned patients with cerebral aneurysm, 10° rTp reduces the ICP and dural tension significantly compared to the neutral position ($P<0.05$) (for details see Chapter 19 or Tankisi et al. (2006)). In prone-positioned patients, ICP decreased significantly from 21.0 ± 4.6 to 15.6 ± 5.6 mmHg in patients with occipital tumours and from 18.3 ± 6.1 to 14.2 ± 5.9 mmHg in patients with cerebellar tumours ($P<0.05$). CPP remained unchanged during 10° rTp compared to the neutral position. In the neutral position JBP was 14.3 ± 5.5 and 12.1 ± 6.3 mmHg in patients with occipital and cerebellar tumours, respectively (Tankisi et al. 2002).

According to the Monro-Kellie doctrine, the intracranial volume consist of a sphere of bone (rigid cranium) that is exactly filled by its contents (Lundberg 1983):

$$\text{ICP}_{\text{Monro-Kellie Doct}}$$
$$V_{\text{Cerebrum}}\ (80\text{–}85\%) + V_{\text{Blood}}\ (5\text{–}8\%) + V_{\text{CSF}}\ (7\text{–}10\%) + V_{\text{Pathology}}\ (?\%)$$
$$= \text{Constant}\ (100\%)$$

According to the doctrine, a decrease in the volume of one of the intracranial contents decreases ICP. As 70–80% of the CBV is located in cerebral veins, this compartment, together with the CSF volume are the most important volumes, as regards the possibilities for changing the total volume of the intracranial content. This model therefore predicts that, during head elevation, a decrease in CBV and/or CSF displacement from the intracranial compartment to the spinal compartment may decrease ICP. A decrease in CBV during elevation of the head has been reported (Lovell et al. 2000; Pichler et al. 2004). In anaesthetized subjects, the reduction of CBV was less compared to the change found in awake patients, probably because the CBV was already reduced by propofol anaesthesia (Lovell et al. 2000).

In neutral positioned, propofol-anaesthetized patients with unruptured aneurysm, the ICP was 2.9 ± 2.6 mmHg (Tankisi et al. 2006). In contrast, the ICP in supine-positioned, propofol-anaesthetized patients with cerebral tumours averaged between 7.5±5.0 and 7.8±5.3 mmHg. The ICP in awake patients without space-occupying lesions was between 7 and 11 mmHg (Albeck et al. 1991). The difference in ICP is supposed to be caused by propofol, which decreases CBF, CBV and ICP (Lagerkranser et al. 1997; Kaisti et al. 2002; Petersen et al. 2003).

In several studies, a decrease in JBP is accompanied by a decrease in ICP during rTp (Rolighed Larsen et al. 2002; Tankisi et al. 2002, 2006; Haure et al. 2003; Tankisi and Cold 2007), presumably because an increase in cerebral venous outflow reduces ICP (Toole 1968; Marmarou et al. 1975; Magnaes 1976a, b; Davenport et al. 1990; Yoshida et al. 1993). Rotating the head to the right/left and neck flexion increases ICP compared to baseline neutral neck position (Hulme and Cooper 1976; Williams and Coyne 1993; Hung et al. 2000; Mavrocordatos et al. 2000). Furthermore, application of a rigid cervical collar has been associated with elevated ICP due to impaired venous drainage (Craig and Nielsen 1991; Davies et al. 1996; Kolb et al. 1999; Hunt et al. 2001; Ho et al. 2002; Mobbs et al. 2002). In contrast, the elevation of the head above the heart level decreases the increased ICP associated with head position (Hung et al. 2000; Mavrocordatos et al. 2000). A significant correlation between the decrease in JBP (ΔJBP) and the decrease in ICP (ΔICP) was expected in those studies during rTp, but could not be detected.

A Starling resistor is defined as any collapsible vein/vessel surrounded in its middle section by an external pressure that is higher than the outlet pressure (Holt 1941). The cerebral bridging veins, which drain blood from the cerebral cortex into the superior sagittal sinus, may collapse and act as a Starling resistor (Huseby et al. 1981). During intracranial hypertension, for example, the veins connecting cortical veins and the superior sagittal sinus collapse and prevent the superior sagittal sinus pressure from affecting the pressure and volume in cortical veins (Huseby et al. 1981; Luce et al. 1982a, b). In dogs, the decrease in dorsal sagittal sinus pressure is small when the superior vena cava pressure decreases during adoption of the upright position, and maintenance of CBV caused by a decrease in venous outflow (or increased arterial flow) is the "key factor" in increasing ICP in this model (Luce et al. 1982a, b). Thus, studies in experimental animals may explain the observation that JBP decreases but ICP is unaffected in some patients during rTp (Tankisi et al. 2002, 2006; Tankisi and Cold 2007). Furthermore, during rTp the collapse of cerebral bridging veins may explain the insignificant correlation between ΔJBP and ΔICP.

Another potential resistor for cerebral venous outflow is the jugular veins. Postural changes lead to a gradual collapse of the internal jugular veins, caused mainly by the external pressure. Postural dependency of the cerebral venous outflow was evaluated in 23 young healthy adults by colour-coded duplex sonography. The measurements were performed with the body at 0°, 15°, 30°, 45° and 90° elevation. During body elevation internal jugular vein flow decreased from 700±270 ml/min at the neutral position to 70 ml/min at 90° body elevation, whereas the vertebral venous blood flow increased from

40±20 ml/min at the neutral position to 210±120 ml/min. The largest decrease in internal jugular venous flow, from 700±270 to 150±130 ml/min, was observed between 0° and 15° elevation of the body. Results of this study indicate that an increase in vertebral venous blood flow was not sufficient to compensate for the drop in jugular flow. The spinal epidural veins are the most probable additional drainage pathway in the upright position (Valdueza et al. 2000). The above findings from colour-coded duplex sonography studies are supported by studies of cerebral venous blood flow measurements using MR technology (Alperin 2004). In healthy upright-positioned volunteers venous drainage shifted from the jugular vein to the epidural and the deep neck veins. An increase in intracranial compliance and a decrease in ICP were also documented (Alperin 2004).

In another study cerebral venous drainage patterns were studied in healthy adult volunteers. Three types of venous drainage patterns were defined as follows: A total jugular flow of more than 2/3, between 1/3 and 2/3 and less than 1/3 of the global arterial blood flow. In 72% of the individuals jugular venous drainage was predominant in the supine position, whereas the jugular drainage was equal to extrajugular drainage in 22% (Doepp et al. 2004). Extrajugular pathways of cerebral venous blood drainage were also investigated. Total venous blood flow at rest was 766±226 ml/min (internal jugular vein 720±232 ml/min; vertebral vein 47±33 ml/min) in supine-positioned volunteers. During circular neck compression, vertebral vein flow increased to 186±70 ml/min. However, this flow increase did not compensate for the fall in internal jugular vein flow, and the authors concluded the existence of additional alternative drainage pathways, including the intraspinal epidural veins and the deep cervical veins (Schreiber et al. 2003).

The existence of a Starling resistor-type mechanism in the jugular veins has also been investigated during positive end-expiratory pressure (PEEP) application in human. An increase in PEEP did not increase cerebral venous pressure when the head was elevated in dogs (Toung et al. 2000). In sitting and standing humans, the veins above the heart level collapse. However, this collapse can be prevented with sufficiently high positive pressure breathing (Cirovic et al. 2003), and a marked increase in CVP in the standing position completely re-opens the jugular vein (Gisolf et al. 2004). Moreover, venous collapse prevents venous pressure variations inside the cranium during head elevation (Asgeirsson and Grände 1996; Kongstad and Grände 1999). Our results are in agreement with the existence of venous outflow Starling resistors. During rTp the jugular veins collapse due to a decrease in JBP, and the collapse of the jugular veins prevents a large decreases in ICP. As a consequence the correlation between ΔICP and ΔJBP is insignificant (Tankisi et al. 2002, 2006; Tankisi and Cold 2007). Thus, extra jugular pathways influence changes in JBP during rTp (Doepp et al. 2004).

According to Moraine et al. (2000) the difference between arterial blood pressure at the level of the foramen of Monro and JBP is the major determinant of CBF during head elevation. In a recent study it was documented that a siphon mechanism in human does not support CBF in the standing position (Dawson et al. 2004). During 10° rTp the decrease in MABP in counteracted by the decrease in jugular venous pressure, leaving CPP unchanged in the majority of patients (Tankisi et al. 2002, 2006; Tankisi and Cold 2007) and CBF is therefore unchanged.

In experimental (Halverson et al. 1998; Rosenthal et al. 1998a, b) and human studies (Hering et al. 2001), the prone position increases intraabdominal pressure, and ICP is higher in prone-positioned patients (Calliauw et al. 1987; Lee 1989; Tankisi et al. 2002). An increase in intraabdominal pressure causes a significant rise in ICP in head trauma patients with ICP less than 20 mmHg. Any rise in intraabdominal pressure causes a concomitant and rapid significant increase in CVP from 6.2±2.4 to 10.4±2.9 mmHg, while internal jugular pressure increases from 11.9±3.2 to 14.3±2.4 mmHg, and ICP increases from 12.0±4.2 to 15.5±4.4 mmHg (Citerio et al. 2001). In prone-positioned patients undergoing to craniotomy (Tankisi et al. 2002) the ICP at the neutral position averaged 21.0 mmHg in occipital tumours and 18.3 mmHg in cerebellar tumours, while the JBP averaged 14.3 mmHg in occipital tumours and 12.1 mmHg in cerebellar tumours. These values were significantly higher than those reported in supine-positioned patients (Rolighed Larsen 2002; Haure et al. 2003; Tankisi and Cold 2007), where mean ICP and JBP levels below 10 mmHg were recorded. Thus, an elevated ICP is more likely to occur in prone-positioned patients, due in part to the occurrence of increased jugular venous pressure. The Monro-Kellie doctrine predicts that any reduction in volume of the intracranial compartment should decrease ICP. Hydrodynamic forces in CSF pressure may decrease ICP during elevation of the head by displacement of CSF into the spinal segment. Displacement of relatively small volumes of intracranial CSF produces a prompt decrease in ICP, provided that the volumetric limit of the spinal sac capacity is not exceeded (Kenning et al. 1981). Studies of CSF volume and dislocation of CSF to the spinal compartment during rTp are not available and so the part they play in reducing ICP during head elevation or rTp is unanswered.

References

Albeck MJ, Børgesen SE, Gjerris F et al (1991) Intracranial pressure and cerebrospinal fluid outflow conductance in healthy subjects. J Neurosurg 74:597–600

Alperin N (2004) MR-intracranial compliance and pressure: a method for noninvasive measurement of important neurophysiologic parameters. Methods Enzymol 386:323–349

Asgeirsson B, Grände PO (1996) Local vascular responses to elevation of an organ above the heart. Acta Physiol Scand 156:9–18

Calliauw L, Van Aken J, Rolly G et al (1987) The position of the patient during neurosurgical procedures on the posterior fossa. Acta Neurochir 85:154–158

Cirovic S, Walsh C, Fraser WD et al (2003) The effect of posture and positive pressure breathing on the hemodynamics of the internal jugular vein. Aviat Space Environ Med 74:125–131

Citerio G, Vascotto E, Villa F et al (2001) Induced abdominal compartment syndrome increases intracranial pressure in neurotrauma patients: a prospective study. Crit Care Med 29:1466–1471

Craig GR, Nielsen MS (1991) Rigid cervical collars and intracranial pressure. Intensive Care Med 17:504–505

Davenport A, Will EJ, Davison AM (1990) Effect of posture on intracranial pressure and cerebral perfusion pressure in patients with fulminant hepatic and renal failure after acetaminophen self-poisoning. Crit Care Med 18:286–289

Davies G, Deakin C, Wilson A (1996) The effect of a rigid collar on intracranial pressure. Injury 27:647–649

Dawson EA, Secher NH, Dalsgaard MK et al (2004) Standing up to the challenge of standing: a siphon does not support cerebral blood flow in humans. Am J Physiol Regul Integr Comp Physiol 287:R911–R914

Doepp F, Schreiber SJ, Von Munster T et al (2004) How does the blood leave the brain? A systematic ultrasound analysis of cerebral venous drainage patterns. Neuroradiology 46:565–570

Durward QJ, Amacher AL, Del Maestro RF et al (1983) Cerebral and cardiovascular responses to changes in head elevation in patients with intracranial hypertension. J Neurosurg 59:938–944

Feldman Z, Kanter MJ, Robertson CS et al (1992) Effect of head elevation on intracranial pressure, cerebral perfusion pressure, and cerebral blood flow in head-injured patients. J Neurosurg 76:207–211

Gisolf J, van Lieshout JJ, van Heusden K et al (2004) Human cerebral venous outflow pathway depends on posture and central venous pressure. J Physiol 560:317–327

Halverson A, Buchanan R, Jacobs L et al (1998) Evaluation of mechanism of increased intracranial pressure with insufflation. Surg Endosc 12:266–269

Haure P, Cold GE, Hansen TM et al (2003) The ICP-lowering effect of 10 degrees reverse Trendelenburg position during craniotomy is stable during a 10-minute period. J Neurosurg Anesthesiol 15:297–301

Hering R, Wrigge H, Vorwerk R et al (2001). The effects of prone positioning on intraabdominal pressure and cardiovascular and renal function in patients with acute lung injury. Anesth Analg 92:1226–1231

Ho AM, Fung KY, Joynt GM et al (2002) Rigid cervical collar and intracranial pressure of patients with severe head injury. J Trauma 53:1185–1188

Holt JP (1941) The collapse factors in the measurement of venous pressure. Am J Physiol 134:292–299

Hulme A, Cooper R (1976) The effects of head position and jugular vein compression (JVC) on intracranial pressure. A clinical study. In: Beks JWF, Bosch DA, Brock M (eds) Intracranial pressure III. Springer, Berlin, pp 259–263

Hung OR, Hare GM, Brien S (2000) Head elevation reduces head-rotation associated increased ICP in patients with intracranial tumours. Can J Anaesth 47:415–420

Hunt K, Hallworth S, Smith M (2001) The effects of rigid collar placement on intracranial and cerebral perfusion pressures. Anaesthesia 56:511–513

Huseby JS, Luce JM, Cary JM et al (1981) Effects of positive end-expiratory pressure on intracranial pressure in dogs with intracranial hypertension. J Neurosurg 55:704–705

Kaisti KK, Metsahonkala L, Teras M et al (2002) Effects of surgical levels of propofol and sevoflurane anesthesia on cerebral blood flow in healthy subjects studied with positron emission tomography. Anesthesiology 96:1358–1370

Kenning JA, Toutant SM, Saunders RL (1981) Upright patient positioning in the management of intracranial hypertension. Surg Neurol 15:148–152

Kolb JC, Summers RL, Galli RL (1999) Cervical collar-induced changes in intracranial pressure. Am J Emerg Med 17:135–137

Kongstad L, Gründe PO (1999) Local vascular response during organ elevation. A model for cerebral effects of upright position and dural puncture. Acta Anaesthesiol Scand 43:438–446

Lagerkranser M, Stange K, Sollevi A (1997) Effects of propofol on cerebral blood flow, metabolism, and cerebral autoregulation in the anesthetized pig. J Neurosurg Anesthesiol 9:188–193

Lee ST (1989) Intracranial pressure changes during positioning of patients with severe head injury. Heart Lung 18:411–414

Lovell AT, Marshall AC, Elwell CE et al (2000) Changes in cerebral blood volume with changes in position in awake and anesthetized subjects. Anesth Analg 90:372–376

Luce JM, Huseby JS, Kirk W et al (1982a) A Starling resistor regulates cerebral venous outflow in dogs. J Appl Physiol 53:1496–1503

Luce JM, Huseby JS, Kirk W (1982b) Mechanism by which positive end-expiratory pressure increases cerebrospinal fluid pressure in dogs. J Appl Physiol 52:231–235

Lundberg N (1983) The saga of the Monro-Kellie doctrine. In: Ishii S, Nagai H, Brock M (eds) Intracranial pressure V. Springer, Berlin, pp 68–76

Magnaes B (1976a) Body position and cerebrospinal fluid pressure. Part 1: clinical studies on the effect of rapid postural changes. J Neurosurg 44:687–697

Magnaes B (1976b) Body position and cerebrospinal fluid pressure. Part 2: clinical studies on orthostatic pressure and the hydrostatic indifferent point. J Neurosurg 44:698–705

Marmarou A, Shulman K, LaMorgese J (1975) Compartmental analysis of compliance and outflow resistance of the cerebrospinal fluid system. J Neurosurg 43:523–534

Mavrocordatos P, Bissonnette B, Ravussin P (2000) Effects of neck position and head elevation on intracranial pressure in anaesthetized neurosurgical patients: preliminary results. J Neurosurg Anesthesiol 12:10–14

Meixensberger J, Baunach S, Amschler J et al (1997) Influence of body position on tissue-pO_2, cerebral perfusion pressure and intracranial pressure in patients with acute brain injury. Neurol Res 19:249–253

Mobbs RJ, Stoodley MA, Fuller J (2002) Effect of cervical hard collar on intracranial pressure after head injury. ANZ J Surg 72:389–391

Moraine JJ, Berre J, Melot C (2000) Is cerebral perfusion pressure a major determinant of cerebral blood flow during head elevation in comatose patients with severe intracranial lesions? J Neurosurg 92:606–614

Ng I, Lim J, Wong HB (2004) Effects of head posture on cerebral hemodynamics: its influences on intracranial pressure, cerebral perfusion pressure, and cerebral oxygenation. Neurosurgery 54:593–597

Petersen KD, Landsfeldt U, Cold GE et al (2003) Intracranial pressure and cerebral hemodynamic in patients with cerebral tumours: a randomized prospective study of patients subjected to craniotomy in propofol-fentanyl, isoflurane-fentanyl, or sevoflurane-fentanyl anesthesia. Anesthesiology 98:329–336

Pichler G, Urlesberger B, Schmolzer G et al (2004) Effect of tilting on cerebral haemodynamics in preterm infants with periventricular leucencephalomalacia. Acta Paediatr 93:70–75

Porchet F, Bruder N, Boulard G et al (1998) The effect of position on intracranial pressure. Ann Fr Anesth Reanim 17:149–156

Rasmussen M, Bundgaard H, Cold GE (2004) Craniotomy for supratentorial brain tumors: risk for brain swelling after opening the dura mater. J Neurosurg 101:621–626

Rolighed Larsen JK, Haure P, Cold GE (2002) Reverse Trendelenburg position reduces intracranial pressure during craniotomy. J Neurosurg Anesthesiol 14:16–21

Ropper AH, O'Rourke D, Kennedy SK (1982) Head position, intracranial pressure, and compliance. Neurology 32:1288–1291

Rosenthal RJ, Friedman RL, Chidambaram A et al (1998a) Effects of hyperventilation and hypoventilation on $PaCO_2$ and intracranial pressure during acute elevations of intra-abominal pressure with CO_2 pneumoperitoneum: large animal observations. J Am Coll Surg 187:32–38

Rosenthal RJ, Friedman RL, Kahn AM et al (1998b) Reasons for intracranial hypertension and hemodynamic instability during acute elevations of intra-abdominal pressure: observations in a large animal model. J Gastrointest Surg 2:415–425

Rosner MJ, Coley IB (1986) Cerebral perfusion pressure, intracranial pressure, and head elevation. J Neurosurg 65:636–641

Schneider GH, von Helden GH, Franke R et al (1993) Influence of body position on jugular venous oxygen saturation, intracranial pressure and cerebral perfusion pressure. Acta Neurochir Suppl 59:107–112

Schreiber SJ, Lurtzing F, Gotze R et al (2003) Extrajugular pathways of human cerebral venous blood drainage assessed by duplex ultrasound. J Appl Physiol 94:1802–1805

Schwarz S, Georgiadis D, Aschoff A (2002) Effects of body position on intracranial pressure and cerebral perfusion in patients with large hemispheric stroke. Stroke 33:497–501

Tankisi A, Cold GE (2007) Optimal reverse Trendelenburg position in patients undergoing craniotomy for cerebral tumours. J Neurosurg 106:239–244

Tankisi A, Rolighed Larsen J, Rasmussen M et al (2002)The effects of 10 degrees reverse Trendelenburg position on ICP and CPP in prone positioned patients subjected to craniotomy for occipital or cerebellar tumours. Acta Neurochir 144:665–670

Tankisi A, Rasmussen M, Juul N et al (2006) The effects of 10° reverse Trendelenburg position (rTp) on subdural intracranial pressure and cerebral perfusion pressure in patients subjected to craniotomy for cerebral aneurysm. J Neurosurg Anesthesiol 18:11–17

Toole JF (1968) Effects of change of head, limb and body position on cephalic circulation. N Engl J Med 279:307–311

Toung TJ, Aizawa H, Traystman RJ (2000) Effects of positive end-expiratory pressure ventilation on cerebral venous pressure with head elevation in dogs. J Appl Physiol 88:655–661

Valdueza JM, von Munster T, Hoffman O et al (2000) Postural dependency of the cerebral venous outflow. Lancet 355:200–201

Williams A, Coyne SM (1993) Effects of neck position on intracranial pressure. Am J Crit Care 2:68–71

Yoshida A, Shima T, Okada Y et al (1993) Effects of postural changes on epidural pressure and cerebral perfusion pressure in patients with serious intracranial lesions. In: Avezaat CJJ, van Eijndhoven JHM, Maas AIR, Tans JTJ (eds) Intracranial pressure VIII. Springer, Berlin, pp 433–436

Chapter 16
Effect of Evacuation of Cerebral Cysts on Subdural Intracranial Pressure and Cerebral Perfusion Pressure

Niels Juul and Georg Emil Cold

Abstract
Patients with intracerebral cysts are frequently presented to the neuro-surgical team. Cerebral cysts can either be part of a tumour process or a parasitic disease, such as neurocysticercosis, or present as an arachnoid cyst. The presence of a cerebral cyst can give rise to classic symptoms of increased ICP, and during intracranial surgery a cyst can jeopardize surgical access to deep brain structures and increase the risk of cerebral ischaemia with possible worsening of the outcome. When fluid is removed from a cystic process in the cranial vault the pressure in the cyst will decrease. We have not found any literature addressing this subject. In this chapter unpublished data concerning subdural ICP monitoring in patients with intercerebral cysts and the pressure/volume relationship during emptying are discussed.

Patients with intracerebral cysts are frequently presented to the neurosurgical team. Cerebral cysts can either be part of a tumour process or a parasitic disease, such as neurocysticercosis, or present itself as an arachnoid cyst. Arachnoid cysts are CSF-filled sacs localized either in the brain or the spinal cord. They are divided into primary cysts, present at birth and the result of development abnormalities that arise in the early weeks of gestation, and secondary cysts, which are not as common as primary cysts and developed as a result of head injury, meningitis or as a complication to previous brain surgery. The presence of a cerebral cyst can give rise to classic symptoms of increased ICP, and during intracranial surgery a cyst can jeopardize surgical access to deep brain structures and increase the risk of cerebral ischaemia with possible worsening of the outcome.

When fluid is removed from a cystic process in the cranial vault the pressure in the cyst will decrease. We have not found any literature addressing this subject. In this chapter unpublished data concerning subdural ICP monitoring in patients with intercerebral cysts and the pressure/volume relationship during emptying are discussed.

Study Outline

Aim To study the changes in subdural pressure and CPP after evacuation of cerebral cysts.

Method Data from the perioperative ICP database were used (Chapter 2). Thirty-eight patients, 26 with supratentorial and 12 with infratentorial cysts, were included. Subdural ICP and CPP were measured before opening of dura and immediately after evacuation of the cystic process. In 4 patients with supratentorial cysts and 5 patients with infratentorial cysts the volume of drainage from the cysts was correlated to changes in subdural ICP. The degree of dural tension and degree of cerebral swelling after opening of dura was evaluated by the surgeon.

Statistical analysis Mann-Whitney's test and Wilcoxon's test were used to compare data within and between groups. Median and range are indicated. $P<0.05$ was considered significant.

Results In patients with supratentorial cerebral cysts subdural ICP decreased from 14 to 0 mmHg ($P<0.05$). MABP was unchanged, while CPP increased from 61 to 75 mmHg ($P<0.05$). In patients with infratentorial cysts the subdural ICP decreased from 20 to 1 mmHg ($P<0.05$). MABP was unchanged, while CPP increased from 67 to 86 mmHg (Tables 16.1 and 16.2). The amounts of removed fluid were registered in 13 patients. This volume was plotted against the reduction in ICP (Fig. 16.1). With a Z of −1.266 (Wilcoxon's signed ranks test) we did not find any correlation between volume of fluid removed and reduction in ICP. The relationship between volume of drained fluid and decrease in subdural ICP are indicated for supra- and infratentorial cysts in Figs. 16.2 and 16.3. The slope of the individual curves differed considerably in both groups without any significant differences between the two groups. In both groups the decrease in subdural ICP was accompanied by a significant decrease in dural tension. Cerebral swelling after opening of dura was not registered in any of the patients (Table 16.2).

Conclusion Perioperative evacuation of cerebral cystic processes before opening of dura reduces subdural ICP substantially, and reduces the tactile estimation of dural tension considerably.

Table 16.1 Demographic data, level of $PaCO_2$ and drainage volume. Median and range are indicated

	Localization of cysts	
	Supratentorial	Infratentorial
Age (years)	45 (9–71)	52 (3–68)
Men/women	14/12	5/7
$PaCO_2$ (kPa)	4.2 (3–6)	4.3 (3.7–5.4)
Drainage volume (ml)	20 (9–30)	11 (5–27)

Table 16.2 Values of MABP, subdural ICP and CPP before and immediately after evacuation of cystic processes in patients with supratentorial and infratentorial tumours. Median and range are indicated

Localization of cysts	Supratentorial		Infratentorial	
	Before evacuation	After evacuation	Before evacuation	After evacuation
MABP (mmHg)	79 (60–122)	77 (52–122)	90 (65–123)	91 (65–120)
ICP (mmHg)	14 (4–32)	0 (−2 to 5)*	20 (13–33)	1 (0–11)*
CPP (mmHg)	61 (38–112)	75 (52–122)*	67 (46–108)	86 (65–118)*

*$P<0.05$ significant intragroup difference

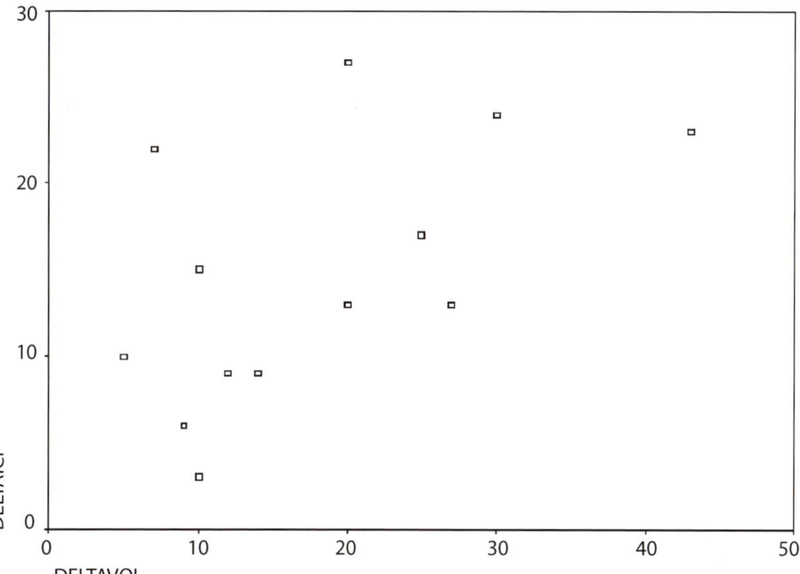

Fig. 16.1 Relationship between reduction in volume and reduction in ICP in 13 patients (deltavol in ml, deltaICP in mmHg)

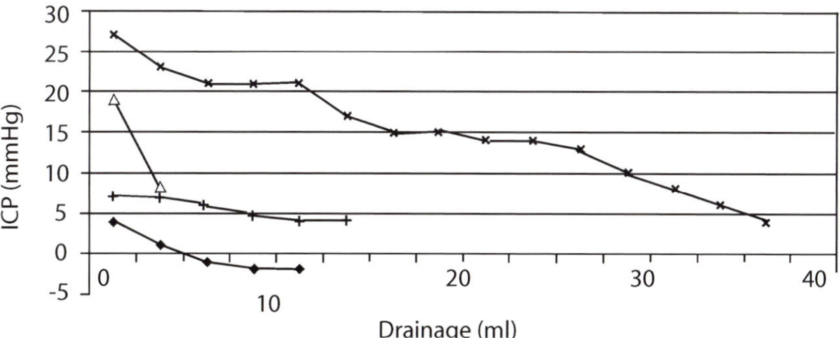

Fig. 16.2 Relationship between drainage volume and subdural ICP before and during gradual evacuation of cystic supratentorial processes in four patients

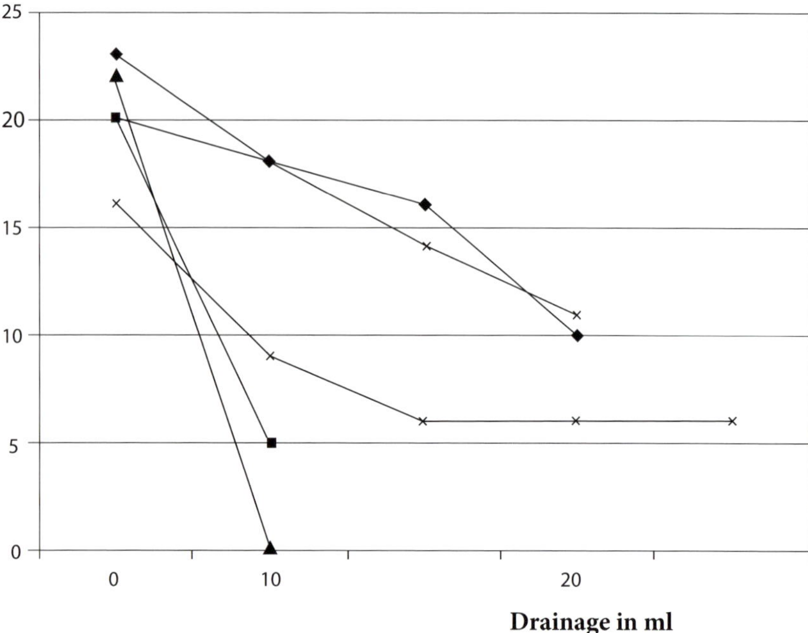

Fig. 16.3 Relationship between drainage volume and subdural ICP before and during gradual evacuation of cystic infratentorial processes in five patients

Discussion

Cystic processes in the cranial vault result in either direct pressure on adjacent structures or universally increased ICP. The net result will eventually be pressure on brain structures, where the clinical impact depends on the speed of growth of the process and its anatomical localization. One must assume that when you subtract fluid from a cystic process in a vault with limited volume, the pressure will decrease, but we were not able to find any correlation between the amount of fluid removed and the reduction in subdural pressure recorded.

Intercerebral cysts can be treated in different ways depending on the anatomical localization, size of the cyst, rate of growth, age of the patient and last but not least the patients symptoms. Treatment can be craniotomy (Yan and Yu 2004), ventriculoperitoneal shunting (Boltshauser et al. 2002) or endoscopic opening of the process to the normal CSF-containing system (Tirakotai et al. 2004). Outcome after treatment varies depending on age of the patient, anatomical localization of the process and chosen treatment (Colli et al. 1994).

We have not been able to identify any studies in the literature which have addressed the issue of volume reduction of cerebral cysts during continuous

ICP monitoring. In a study of prolonged ICP monitoring of Sylvian arachnoid cysts, Di Rocco et al. (2003) found patients with increased ICP but without any clinical symptoms. In contrast, normal ICP recordings were found in three children, despite the fact that two of them were apparently symptomatic; one complained of recurrent headaches and one had epileptic seizures. It was not possible in this study to elucidate any correlation between cystic volume, anatomical localization and ICP.

A graphic evaluation of cyst reduction in millilitres of fluid removed and reduction in ICP is presented in Fig. 16.1. It was not possible to define a significant correlation between the ICP reduction and volume reduction, in the group. When you consider each patient the ICP reduction concurrently with the volume reduction is evident, but we only had data on volume reduction in 13 patients, and that could explain the lack of statistical significance. In 4 patients with supratentorial (Fig. 16.2) and 5 patients with infratentorial cysts (Fig. 16.3) we measured the gradual pressure reduction when fluid was removed from the intracranial cysts. As with the overall fluid removal, it was impossible to find a regression line that in any way connected the amount of removed fluid with the reduction in pressure measured. The missing statistical significance in our material may have several reasons. One reason may be a small sample size; 38 patients might seem sufficient, but the ages of the patients spanned over 68 years, from 3 to 71 years. It is reasonable to assume that the pressure/volume relationship is dependent on the size of the cranial vault. Different anatomical localizations of cysts may also influence the pressure/volume relationship. A small cystic process in the posterior fossa might exert more pressure on adjacent structures and cause hydrocephalus and an increase in ICP. In comparison, a similar-sized cystic process in the supratentorial compartment might be asymptomatic or show symptoms not directly related to high ICP.

In recent studies of patients subjected to craniotomy in the prone position ICP averaged 18.3 mmHg for patients with occipital tumours and 21.0 mmHg for infratentorial tumours (Tankisi et al. 2002). These levels of ICP were identical with the ICP levels observed in another study of infratentorial tumours (Jørgensen et al. 1999). Concerning the difference in pressure in the different cranial compartments, a previous study (Chapter 5) indicates that between compartments of the neuroaxis differences in pressure exist, with the smallest differences within the supratentorial compartment and higher differences between the supra- and infratentorial compartments. In addition, there might be a difference in the pressure/volume relationship when a cystic process with a thin wall is evacuated compared to a process with a thicker wall, since the thin-walled structure will be more collapsible and hence the pressure/volume curve will be much steeper. Moreover, will there be differences in the pressure/volume relationship between patients with slowly growing processes with a thick wall and faster-growing cystic processes with a thin wall. The pathology of the cyst may play an important role since different pathologies will give rise to different macroscopic structures of the cyst and thus a variation in the pressure/volume relationship.

Volume changes in the cranial vault are being used as a novel way to describe the pressure/volume relationship. Intracranial compliance is defined as the pressure reaction to a change in intracranial volume ($\Delta V/\Delta P$). The exponential nature of the pressure/volume curve indicates that a similar volume increment at different points of the curve results in different pressure responses. The pressure/volume index is defined as the volume necessary to raise the ICP by a factor of 10. The pressure/volume relationship in the cranial vault has been investigated in recent years by use of the Spiegelberg intracranial compliance monitor which calculates intracranial compliance ($C = \Delta V/\Delta P$) from a moving average of small ICP perturbations (ΔP) resulting from a sequence of up to 200 pulses of added volume ($\Delta V = 0.1$ ml, total $V = 0.2$ ml) made into a double lumen intraventricular balloon catheter (Abdullah et al. 2005). This method has been used to monitor intracranial compliance in different patient categories. In a study of patients with severe head injury it was found that at ICP > 20 mmHg compliance was linearly correlated to CPP suggesting failure of autoregulatory mechanisms (Portella et al. 2000). In another study of patients with closed head injury it was found that at similar values of ICP, intracranial compliance depends on the age of the patient (Kiening et al. 2000).

References

Abdullah J, Zamzuri I, Awang S et al (2005) Preliminary report on Spiegelberg pre- and post-operative monitoring of severe head-injured patients who received decompressive craniectomy. Acta Neurochir Suppl 95:311–314

Boltshauser E, Martin F, Altermatt S (2002) Outcome of children with space-occupying posterior fossa arachnoid cysts. Neuropediatrics 33:118–121

Colli BO, Martenelli N, Assirati JJA et al (1994) Cysticercosis of the central nervous system. I. Surgical treatment of cerebral cysticercosis; a 23 years experience in the Hospital das Clinicas of Ribeirao Preto Medical School. Arq Neuropsiquiatr 52:166–186

Di Rocco C, Tamburrini G, Caldarelli M et al (2003) Prolonged ICP monitoring in Sylvian arachnoid cysts. Surg Neurol 60:211–218

Jørgensen HA, Bundgaard H, Cold GE (1999) Subdural pressure measurement during posterior fossa surgery. Correlation studies of brain swelling/herniation after dural incision with measurement of subdural pressure and tactile estimation of dural tension. Br J Neurosurg 13:449–453

Kiening KL, Schoening WN, Unterberg AW et al (2000) Intracranial compliance as bedside monitoring technique in severely head-injured patients. Proceeding XI ICP symposium, Cambridge 01-05, p 30

Portella G, Cormino M, Cierio G (2000) Continuous cerebral compliance monitoring in severe head injury. Relationship with intracranial pressure and cerebral perfusion pressure. Proceeding XI ICP symposium, Cambridge 01-03, p 28

Tankisi A, Rolighed Larsen J, Rasmussen M et al (2002) The effects of 10° reverse Trendelenburg position of ICP and CPP in prone positioned patients subjected to craniotomy for occipital and cerebellar tumours. Acta Neurochir 144:665–670

Tirakotai W, Schulte DM, Bauer BL et al (2004) Neuroendoscopic surgery of intracranial cysts in adults. Childs Nerv Syst 20:842–851

Yan PX, Yu CI (2004) Minicraniotomy treatment of an intracerebral epidermoid cyst. Minim Invasive Neurosurg 47:45–48

Chapter 17
Comparative Studies of Therapeutic Measures to Reduce Subdural Intracranial Pressure During Craniotomy

Mads Rasmussen and Georg Emil Cold

Abstract

The level of ICP is of importance in the surgical management of space-occupying cerebral lesions. For many years hyperventilation-induced reduction of cerebral blood volume and mannitol treatment based on osmotic withdrawal of brain tissue water have been used to reduce dural tension before opening of dura mater. Other therapeutic measures to reduce ICP during craniotomy include intravenous administration of indomethacin, placing the patient in the reverse Trendelenburg position and decompression by puncture of cystic tumours.

In this chapter three studies are presented. The ICP-reducing effects of hyperventilation, 10 degrees reverse Trendelenburg position, mannitol treatment, indomethacin or surgical decompression in patients subjected to craniotomy in the supine and prone positions in either propofol-fentanyl or propofol-remifentanil anaesthesia are discussed.

The level of ICP is of importance in the surgical management of space-occupying cerebral lesions. At high ICP surgical access to deep cerebral structures is impeded, and pressure by self-retaining specula may decrease cerebral perfusion regionally (Hongo et al. 1987; Rosenørn 1987). Likewise, swelling/herniation of cerebral tissue through the opening of dura mater may be deleterious by preventing venous outflow from the affected brain tissue. A vicious circle may develop with increasing cerebral oedema and ischaemia. Surgical decompression by ventricular drainage reduces ICP effectively, but insertion of a ventricular catheter can be difficult during surgery, either because of the position of the patient or because the ventricular system is compressed. For decades, hyperventilation-induced reduction of CBV and mannitol treatment based on osmotic withdrawal of brain tissue water have been used to reduce dural tension before opening of dura mater. Other therapeutic measures to reduce ICP during craniotomy include intravenous administration of indomethacin

(Bundgaard et al. 1996), placing the patient in rTp (Rolighed Larsen et al. 2002; Tankisi et al. 2002, 2006; Haure et al. 2003; Tankisi and Cold 2007) and decompression by puncture of cystic tumours. Comparable clinical studies of ICP-reducing management are not available in patients subjected to craniotomy for supratentorial cerebral tumours. Both hyperventilation (Petersen et al. 2003) and rTp (Rolighed Larsen 2002; Tankisi et al. 2002; Haure et al. 2003) reduce ICP during craniotomy. To our knowledge studies comparing the effects on ICP and CPP of hyperventilation or rTp are not available.

In this chapter three studies are presented which compare the various treatments for ICP reduction under various conditions.

Study 1: A Comparative Study of the Intracranial Pressure-Reducing Effect of Hyperventilation, 10 Degrees Reverse Trendelenburg Position, Mannitol Treatment, Indomethacin or Surgical Decompression in Patients with Intracranial Hypertension Subjected to Craniotomy for Supratentorial Cerebral Tumours in Propofol-Fentanyl Anaesthesia

Aim To compare the ICP-reducing effect of hyperventilation, 10° rTp, mannitol treatment, indomethacin or surgical decompression in patients with intracranial hypertension undergoing craniotomy for supratentorial cerebral tumours in propofol-fentanyl anaesthesia.

Method We included 93 patients undergoing craniotomy for supratentorial tumours in propofol-fentanyl anaesthesia. All patients had a subdural ICP ≥ 10 mmHg. Data were consecutively collected between 1997 and 2005 and subjected to a retrospective analysis. The following ICP-reducing managements were analysed: 5 min of hyperventilation ($n=30$), 10° rTp ($n=16$), mannitol treatment 0.5–1.0 g/kg ($n=19$), surgical decompression 17±9 ml ($n=13$) and indomethacin 0.5 mg/kg ($n=15$). Subdural ICP was measured before opening of dura. The changes in ICP, MABP and CPP were calculated. The effect of mannitol on ICP was measured 5 min after termination of the infusion. The effects on ICP of rTp, drainage and indomethacin were recorded after 1 min. Concerning methodological data, maintenance doses of anaesthesia and neuroradiological data, see Chapter 3.

Statistical analysis Data within groups were tested for normal distribution. The normality test and equal variance test were applied. One-way ANOVA was used for analysis if these tests were passed and the Tukey test was used for pair-wise multiple comparison procedures. The Kruskal-Wallis one-way analysis of variance on ranks and multiple comparisons versus control groups (Dunn's method) were used for statistical analysis when the normality test or equal variance test were not passed. The chi-square test was used for statistical analysis of demographic data, localization, size and histopathological diagnosis of the tumours, preoperative steroid administration and position of the head between the groups. The difference in tension of dura and the degree of cerebral swelling were tested by the chi-square test in 2×4 or 2×3 tables. Mean±SD were calculated. $P<0.05$ was considered statistically significant.

Results No significant differences were disclosed as regards demographic data or data obtained before the ICP-reducing management, including PaO_2, rectal temperature, ICP, MABP or CPP (Table 17.1). The level of $PaCO_2$ was significantly lower in patients treated with mannitol compared with other groups, except drainage (Table 17.1). The maintenance dosages of propofol and fentanyl did not show any significant intergroup difference (Table 17.2). Neither did the neuroradiological findings, including the distribution of localization of tumour, maximal area of the tumours or midline shift differ significantly between the groups (Table 17.1 and 17.2). The average dose of mannitol and indomethacin are indicated in Table 17.2. Indomethacin induced an increase in MABP averaging 9.1 mmHg. This increase was significantly greater that that obtained by hyperventilation (0.3 mmHg), surgical decompression (−0.6 mmHg), 10° rTp (−6.4 mmHg), but not significantly different from mannitol treatment (2.4 mmHg). A significant difference was also found between mannitol treatment and rTp, and between rTp and hyperventilation (Table 17.3). The ICP-reducing effect of surgical decompression averaged 16.2 mmHg. This value was significantly higher than the values obtained by hyperventilation (3.2 mmHg), 10° rTp (5.0 mmHg), mannitol treatment (6.0 mmHg) and indomethacin treatment (6.9 mmHg). Moreover, the ICP-reducing effect of indomethacin treatment was significantly greater than that

Table 17.1 Demographic data, gas analyses, temperature, ICP, MABP, CPP and neuroradiological data in patients subjected to ICP-reducing therapy including hyperventilation, 10° rTp, mannitol treatment, drainage of cystic tumours or indomethacin treatment. Mean±SD are indicated. Data were obtained before the ICP-reducing therapy

	Hyper-ventilation	Reverse Trendelenburg position	Mannitol	Drainage	Indo-methacin
Number	30	16	19	13	15
Men/women	16/14	5/11	11/8	7/6	7/8
Age (years)	52.0±14.0	53.0±10.0	54.0±14.0	50.0±15.0	59.0±14.0
Weight (kg)	77.0±13.0	78.0±20.	76.0±14.0	80.0±19.0	79.0±17.0
$PaCO_2$ (kPa)	4.7±0.5#	4.7±0.6#	4.1±0.4	4.4±0.5	4.6±0.4#
PaO_2 (kPa)	25.0±8.0	27.0±11.0	29.0±10.0	27.0±9.0	21.0±6.0
Temperature (°C)	35.9±0.5	35.9±0.6	36.2±0.4	35.9±0.4	35.9±0.4
Tumour area (cm^2)	16.0±8.0	18.0±9.0	17.0±10.0	23.0±11.0	22.0±13.0
Midline shift (mm)	6.5±7.0	9.3±8.0	9.5±7.8	9.5±6.7	8.5±6.2
ICP (mmHg)	15.1±4.2	14.0±3.8	15.8±4.6	17.5±5.7	16.9±7.2
MABP (mmHg)	85.0±18.0	91.0±15.0	88.0±16.0	79.0±12.0	82.0±13.0
CPP (mmHg)	70.0±17.0	77.0±15.0	72.0±15.0	61.0±14.0	65.0±16.0

#Significantly different from mannitol

Table 17.2 Localization of tumour, histopathology and maintenance doses of propofol and fentanyl in patients with supratentorial tumours undergoing ICP-reducing therapy, including hyperventilation, 10° rTp, mannitol treatment, drainage of cystic tumours or indomethacin treatment. Number±SD are indicated

	Hyper-ventilation	Reverse Trendelen-burg position	Mannitol	Drainage	Indo-methacin
Localization					
Frontal	14	5	8	7	4
Parietal	4	2	3	1	5
Temporal	6	5	3	3	2
Occipital	5	1	4	1	2
Hemispheric	1	2	1	0	0
Basal	0	1	0	1	1
Histopathology					
Glioblastoma	16	5	11	5	7
Meningioma	2	4	0	0	4
Metastasis	6	4	5	3	3
Glioma	5	1	5	4	1
Other	1	2	0	1	0
Anaesthesia					
Propofol (mg/h)	707.0±150.0	706.0±217.0	816.0±212.0	642.0±215.0	700.0±180.0
Fentanyl (µg/h)	166.0±49.0	142.0±270.0	148.0±32.0	138.0±38.0	133.0±26.0
Mannitol (g/kg)			0.8±0.2		
Indomethacin (mg/kg)					0.5±0.0
Drainage (ml)				20.0±8.0	

obtained by hyperventilation (Table 17.3). The increase in CPP during surgical drainage (16.0 mmHg) and indomethacin treatment (16.7 mmHg) was not significantly different, but was significantly greater than that found with hyperventilation (3.4 mmHg), rTp (−1.7 mmHg) or mannitol treatment (8.0 mmHg). Moreover the increase in CPP during mannitol treatment was significantly greater than that obtained by rTp (Table 17.3). In Table 17.4, the changes in $AVDO_2$ and SjO_2 are shown. Hyperventilation, as well as indomethacin, was followed by a significant fall in SjO_2 and an increase in $AVDO_2$. During mannitol treatment no significant changes were observed.

In Table 17.5 the degree of dural tension as estimated by the neurosurgeon is registered. During treatment of intracranial hypertension, the percentage number of patients with increased dural tension decreased in all groups, most pronounced, however, in patients subjected to surgical decompression. In the group of surgical decompression no swelling/herniation of the cerebral tissue was observed after opening of dura. In contrast some degree of cerebral swelling was observed in all other groups. The swelling was most pronounced in

Table 17.3 Differences in $PaCO_2$, ICP, MABP and CPP measured before and after ICP-reducing therapy including hyperventilation, 10° rTp, mannitol treatment, drainage of cystic tumours or indomethacin treatment. Number±SD are indicated

	Hyperventilation	Reverse Trendelenburg position	Mannitol	Drainage	Indomethacin
Decrease in $PaCO_2$ (kPa)	0.8±0.2	0.0±0.0*	0.1±0.1*	0.0±0.0*	0.1±0.1*
Decrease in ICP (mmHg)	3.2±2.2#	5.0±2.2#	6.0±3.9#	16.2±6.1	6.9±3.7*#
Increase in MABP (mmHg)	0.3±3.8	−6.4±4.0*#	2.4±6.3°	−0.6±1.5	9.1±9.4*#°
Increase in CPP (mmHg)	3.4±3.8#	−1.7±3.6#	8.0±7.2°	16.0±6.7	16.7±8.8*°

*Significant difference from hyperventilation
#Significant difference from drainage
°Significant difference from rTp

Table 17.4 SjO_2 and $AVDO_2$ measured before and after treatment with hyperventilation, mannitol or indomethacin, and before rTp and surgical drainage

	Hyperventilation	Reverse Trendelenburg	Mannitol	Drainage	Indomethacin
Number	21	7	7	2	12
Venous saturation before (%)	57.9±9.3	48.8±4.4	66.4±16.0	48.9±4.4	52.8±7.4
Venous saturation after (%)	52.3±9.2*		64.9±		43.4±6.5*
Percent change in venous saturation	−9.7		−2.3		−17.8
$AVDO_2$ (mmol/L) before	3.1±0.8		2.8±0.8		3.5±0.4
$AVDO_2$ (mmol/L) after	3.5±0.8*		2.8±0.5		4.1±0.4*
% change in $AVDO_2$	−12.9		0.0		−17.1

*$P<0.05$ paired comparison

hyperventilated patients (77%) followed by mannitol treatment (68%), indomethacin treatment (60%) and rTp (56%). In patients subjected to surgical decompression swelling did not occur (Table 17.6).

Table 17.5 Degree of dural tension before treatment and after/during treatment with hyperventilation, $10°\,rTp$, mannitol treatment, surgical drainage or indomethacin treatment. Number of patients and percentage of patients are indicated

Dural tension	Before hyper-ventilation	After hyper-ventilation	Before $10°\,rTp$	After $10°\,rTp$	Before mannitol	After mannitol	Before drainage	After drainage	Before indo-methacin	After indo-methacin
No tension	7	11	1	7	0	8	0	13	1	7
Moderate tension	16	14	12	8	16	10	8	0	8	6
Pronounced tension	7	5	3	1	3	1	5	0	6	2
Percentage of patients with increased tension	77	63	94	56	100	58	100	0	93	53

Table 17.6 The degree of brain swelling/herniation after opening of dura in patients subjected to hyperventilation, 10° rTp, mannitol treatment, surgical decompression (drainage of cerebral cysts) or indomethacin treatment. Number of patients and percentage with cerebral swelling are indicated

	Hyper ventilation	Reverse Trendelenburg	Mannitol	Drainage	Indomethacin
No swelling	7 (23)	7 (44)	6 (32)	13(100)	6 (40)
Moderate swelling	17 (57)	8 (50)	9 (47)	0 (0)	8 (53)
Pronounced swelling	6 (20)	1 (6)	4 (21)	0 (0)	1 (7)
Percentage of patients with swelling	77	56	68	0	60

Conclusion The ICP-reducing effect of surgical decompression is superior to hyperventilation, 10° rTp, mannitol treatment or indomethacin, and the effect of indomethacin is superior to 5 min of hyperventilation. The increase in CPP was greater during drainage or indomethacin compared with hyperventilation and rTp.

Study 2: A Comparative Clinical Study of the Intracranial Pressure-Reducing Effect of 10 Degrees Reverse Trendelenburg Position and Hyperventilation in Patients Subjected to Supratentorial Craniotomy for Cerebral Tumours in Propofol-Remifentanil Anaesthesia

Aim Comparative studies of ICP-reducing management are not available in propofol-remifentanil-anaesthetized patients subjected to craniotomy for supratentorial cerebral tumours. In this observational study we analysed the ICP-reducing effect of hyperventilation and 10° rTp in patients with cerebral tumours subjected to propofol-remifentanil anaesthesia.

Method From our database concerning subdural ICP measurement we collected consecutive data from 45 patients subjected to supratentorial tumour surgery in propofol-remifentanil anaesthesia. The following ICP-reducing managements were analysed. Five minutes of hyperventilation ($n=15$) and 10° rTp ($n=15$). Patients, in whom therapeutic intervention was not performed, served as control ($n=15$). Subdural ICP was measured before opening of dura. The changes in ICP (ΔICP), $PaCO_2$ ($\Delta PaCO_2$) and CPP (ΔCPP) were calculated. The effect of hyperventilation were estimated during a 5-min period and the effect of rTp after 1 min. For details concerning methodology including neuroradiological data, histopathology, perioperative fluid management and monitoring and maintenance of anaesthesia, see Chapter 3.

Table 17.7 Demographics, parameters from blood gas analysis, ICP, MABP, CPP, rectal temperature, neuroradiological findings (tumour size, localization), histopathology and maintenance doses of propofol and remifentanil are presented. Three groups were studied including a control group, a group subjected to 5 min of hyperventilation and a group where 10° rTp was applied

	Control group	Hyperventilation	Reverse Trendelenburg
Number	15	15	15
Men/women	9/6	10/5	8/7
Age (years)	44.0±15.0	52.0±16.0	53.0±14.0
Weight (kg)	79.0±17.0	71.0±14.0	73.0±16.0
Height (cm)	174.0±8.0	173.0±8.0	173.0±8.0
$PaCO_2$ (kPa)	4.5±0.3	4.6±0.4	4.6±0.4
PaO_2 (kPa)	25.0±7.0	24.0±9.0	20.0±8.0
Temperature (°C)	35.7±0.4	35.8±0.3	35.8±0.4
ICP (mmHg)	9.5±6.2	7.1±4.0	8.9±5.3
MABP (mmHg)	77.0±15.0	78.0±14.0	72.0±12.0
CPP (mmHg)	68.0±15.0	71.0±14.0	63.0±12.0
Tumour area (cm^2)	11.0±7.0	13.0±9.0	13.0±8.0
Midline shift (mm)	4.2±6.6	5.6±5.9	6.8±7.9
Localization (number)			
Frontal	2	7	7
Parietal	3	2	2
Temporal	4	1	2
Occipital	1	2	2
Hemispheric	1	0	1
Basal	4	3	1
Histopathology			
Glioblastoma	3	4	4
Meningioma	4	4	6
Metastasis	0	2	2
Glioma	5	4	0
Other	3	1	3
Anaesthesia			
Propofol (mg/h)	460.0±115.0	403.0±79.0	383.0±94.0
Remifentanil (ml/h)	48.0±18.0	43.0±12.0	42.0±14.0

Statistical analysis Data within groups were tested for normal distribution. The normality test and equal variance test were applied. One-way ANOVA was used for analysis if these tests were passed, and Tukey's test was used for pair-wise multiple comparison procedures. The Kruskal-Wallis one-way analysis of variance on ranks and multiple comparisons versus control groups (Dunn's method) were used for statistical analysis when the normality test or equal variance test were not passed. The chi-square test was used for statistical analysis of demographic data, tumour localization, size and histopathological diagnosis of the tumours, preoperative steroid administration and position of the head. Difference in tension of dura and the degree of cerebral swelling were tested by the chi-square test. Mean±SD were calculated. $P<0.05$ was considered statistically significant.

Results No significant intergroup differences as regards demographic data, neuroradiological findings (tumour size, tumour volume, midline shift, localization of tumour) or histopathology were found. Neither did parameters of cerebral haemodynamics including ICP, CPP, SjO_2 and $AVDO_2$ show any significant intergroup differences. The same applies to levels of $PaCO_2$, PaO_2 and rectal temperature (Table 17.7).

During the 5-min observation period no significant changes in $PaCO_2$, ICP, MABP or CPP were found in the control group. Hyperventilation and rTp induced a significant decrease in ICP averaging 2.3 and 4.3 mmHg, respectively (Table 17.8). The decrease in ICP was significant after 1 min in the group subjected to rTp, and after 2 min in the hyperventilation group. The ICP-reducing effect of rTp was significantly greater compared with that induced by hyperventilation (Tables 17.8 and 17.9). The rTp induced a significant increase in CPP averaging 2.1 mmHg. CPP was unchanged during hyperventilation (Table 17.8). During hyperventilation SjO_2 decreased significantly from 52.3% to 48.1%, and a significant increase in $AVDO_2$ from 3.3 to 3.7 mmol/L was disclosed. No significant difference in SjO_2 or $AVDO_2$ was found after rTp (Table 17.10).

Table 17.8 Changes in $PaCO_2$ ($\Delta PaCO_2$), MABP ($\Delta MABP$), ICP (ΔICP) and CPP (ΔCPP) in the control group, during 5 min hyperventilation and 1 min after 10° rTp

	Control group	Hyperventilation	Reverse Trendelenburg
$\Delta PaCO_2$ (kPa)	0.0±0.1	0.6±0.2*	0.0±0.1
$\Delta MABP$ (mmHg)	0.0±1.4	1.4±2.0	5.8±2.8°
ΔICP (mmHg)	0.1±0.5	2.3±1.2*	4.3±2.9*#
ΔCPP (mmHg)	−0.5±1.1	−0.2±	2.1±3.8*

*Significant difference from control
#Significant difference from hyperventilation
°Significant difference from the other groups

Table 17.9 MABP, ICP and CPP recorded at time zero and up to 5 min during hyperventilation in 15 patients. Mean values are indicated

	MABP (mmHg)	ICP (mmHg)	CPP (mmHg)
0	78.3	7.1	71.3
1 min	77.6	6.3	71.4
2 min	77.1	5.5*	71.4
3 min	76.6*	5.0*	71.7
4 min	76.4*	4.8*	71.4
5 min	76.2*	4.7*	71.6

$*P \leq 0.01$ significant difference from zero

Table 17.10 SjO_2, $AVDO_2$ and $PaCO_2$ before and at 5 min in the control group and in patients subjected to 5 min of hyperventilation

	Control			Hyperventilation		
	SjO_2 (%)	$AVDO_2$ (mmol/L)	$PaCO_2$ (kPa)	SjO_2 (%)	$AVDO_2$ (mmol/L)	$PaCO_2$ (kPa)
0	49.8±8.7	3.6±0.8	4.4±0.3	52.3±11.6	3.3±0.8	4.6±0.4
5 min	49.7±8.4	3.6±0.8	4.5±0.3	48.1±11.6*	3.7±0.8*	4.0±0.4*

$*P < 0.05$

In comparison with the control group, $10°$ rTp as well as hyperventilation decreased ICP significantly. The decrease in ICP during rTp was more pronounced compared with hyperventilation, and rTp decreased both MABP and CPP significantly.

Conclusion   Compared with the control group rTp and hyperventilation caused a significant decrease in ICP. Reverse Trendelenburg position was associated with a significant increase in CPP.

Study 3: A Comparative Study of the Intracranial Pressure-Reducing Effect of 10 Degrees Reverse Trendelenburg Position, Hyperventilation, Indomethacin and Surgical Drainage in Patients Undergoing Fossa Posterior Surgery in the Prone Position

Aim   To compare the ICP-reducing effect of $10°$ rTp, hyperventilation, surgical draining and indomethacin in patients undergoing fossa posterior surgery in the prone position.

Method   Fifty-three patients with space-occupying processes in the posterior fossa participated in the study. Eleven patients were subjected to $10°$ rTp, 12 patients underwent hyperventilation for 5 min, 12 patients received intravenous indomethacin (0.5 mg/kg) as a bolus and 18 patients were subjected to drainage of cystic processes. Propofol-remifentanil was used for maintenance of anaesthesia. All patients had a subdural ICP ≥ 10 mmHg measured before any intervention to reduce ICP. The effects of rTp, drainage and indomethacin were recorded after 1 min. Concerning methodological data, maintenance doses of anaesthesia and neuroradiological data, see Chapter 3.

Statistical analysis   As study 1; mean±SD are indicated.

Results   No significant differences were disclosed as regards demographic data or data obtained before the ICP-reducing management, including PaO_2, rectal temperature, ICP, MABP, CPP and maintenance dose of anaesthesia. Neither did the neuroradiological findings, including the maximal area of the process, differ significantly between the groups (Table 17.11). In all treatment groups subdural ICP decreased significantly. The decrease in subdural ICP in the drainage group was significantly greater than in the other groups, in which the decrease in ICP did not differ significantly. The increase in CPP was significantly higher in the indomethacin group and in patients subjected to drainage compared with the other two groups (Table 17.12).

Conclusion   In all four groups subdural ICP decreased significantly, but the decrease in ICP was substantially greater in patients subjected to drainage. In the indomethacin and drainage groups an increase in CPP was significantly greater than the changes observed during rTp and during hyperventilation.

Table 17.11   Demographic data, gas analyses, temperature, ICP, MABP, CPP and neuroradiological data in patients subjected to ICP-reducing therapy including 10° rTp, 5 min of hyperventilation, indomethacin bolus (0.5 mg/kg) and drainage of cystic processes. Mean±SD are indicated. Data were obtained before the ICP-reducing therapy. No significant intergroup differences were found

	Reverse Trendelenburg	Hyperventilation	Indomethacin	Drainage
Number	11	12	12	18
Men/women	6/5	5/7	6/6	7/11
Age (years)	42.0±20.0	43.0±19.0	56.0±9.0	48.0±16.0
Weight (kg)	73.0±23.0	74.0±22.0	77.0±17.0	74.0±18.0
$PaCO_2$ (kPa)	4.4±0.4	4.6±0.5	4.5±0.4	4.2±0.5
PaO_2 (kPa)	31.0±5.0	25.0±6.0	24.0±5.0	29.0±9.0
Temperature (°C)	35.9±0.5	35.9±0.6	36.2±0.4	35.9±0.4
ICP (mmHg)	19.9±5.8	19.8±11.1	17.8±5.3	18.8±6.7
MABP (mmHg)	84.0±16.0	78.0±17.0	79.0±20.0	87.0±15.0
CPP (mmHg)	64.0±15.0	51.0±16.0	61.0±20.0	68.0±16.0
Tumour area (cm^2)	7.5±5.3	13.0±6.0	9.0±6.0	10.0±8.0
Midline shift (mm)	0.6±1.6	0.3±0.9	1.4±2.6	0.9±2.1

Table 17.12 Differences in $PaCO_2$, ICP, MABP and CPP measured before and after ICP-reducing therapy including 10° rTp, 5 min hyperventilation, indomethacin treatment (0.5 mg/kg) and drainage of a cystic process. Number±SD are indicated

	Reverse Trendelenburg	Hyper-ventilation	Indomethacin	Drainage
Decrease in $PaCO_2$ (kPa)	0.1±0.1	0.7±0.1*	0.1±0.1	−0.1±0.1
Decrease in ICP (mmHg)	5.6±1.9	2.6±2.6	4.4±2.0	16.6±6.8*
Increase in MABP (mmHg)	−5.1±2.0*	0.0±6.3	13.8±5.1*	1.1±0.5
Increase in CPP (mmHg)	−0.5±2.0	−3.1±4.6	18.0±4.8°	17.7±8.2°

*Significant difference compared with the other groups
°Significant difference from both rTp and hyperventilation

Discussion

In studies 1 and 3 the inclusion criterion was a subdural ICP ≥ 10 mmHg. This threshold is in accordance with recent studies in patients subjected to supratentorial craniotomy where cerebral swelling is rare if ICP is below 5–7 mmHg, while subdural ICP above 10–13 mmHg is accompanied by moderate cerebral swelling and ICP above 15 mmHg is associated with pronounced cerebral swelling (Cold et al. 1996; Bundgaard et al. 1998; Rasmussen et al. 2004). These thresholds are independent of $PaCO_2$ level, choice of anaesthesia and diagnosis (tumour contra aneurysm surgery) (Bundgaard et al. 1998). The tension of dura was not used as an inclusion criterion because it is a based on a subjective evaluation and because the degree of cerebral swelling is better correlated to subdural ICP compared with degree of dural tension (Bundgaard et al. 1998). In the present study, the degree of swelling after opening of dura is semiquantitative and subjective as well. Nevertheless, we used this estimate because the presence of brain swelling increases retractor pressure resulting in low regional perfusion pressure (Hongo et al. 1987; Rosenørn 1987), thereby increasing the risk for development of cerebral ischaemia. Furthermore, brain swelling makes surgical access difficult.

The three studies were based on prospective continuous data collected between the years 1997 and 2005. During that period, subdural ICP monitoring was performed in 289 patients with supratentorial tumours anaesthetized with propofol-fentanyl, indicating that ICP ≥ 10 mmHg occurred in 32% of the patients. Demographic data, histopathological data, neuroradiological data and levels of ICP, MABP and CPP, however, did not show any intergroup difference. A difference in $PaCO_2$ between the mannitol group and the other treatment groups, except patients subjected to surgical decompression, seems of minor importance because the effect of mannitol is based on osmotic activity independent of the level of $PaCO_2$. The ICP-reducing effect used in the present study is elicited by different mechanisms. In the second study the ICP-decreasing effect of rTp was superior to hyperventilation, and in the third study drainage was followed by a substantially greater decrease in subdural ICP compared with rTp, indomethacin treatment and hyperventilation.

Hyperventilation and indomethacin increase cerebrovascular resistance, and thereby decreases CBF and CBV, and as a consequence a decrease in ICP is observed. The decrease in blood volume by hyperventilation is dependent on the change in $PaCO_2$. For the awake normal human the change in CBV is 0.049 ml/100 g/mmHg $PaCO_2$ (Greenberg et al. 1978), meaning that the decrease in blood volume should average 3.8 ml by a 0.8-kPa reduction in $PaCO_2$. Similar studies during indomethacin treatment are not available, but taking the more pronounced decrease in ICP during indomethacin administration into account, the decrease in blood volume must be higher. This is supported by the findings in the present study that the % changes in venous oxygen tension and $AVDO_2$ were higher during indomethacin treatment compared with hyperventilation. At least the decrease in intracranial compartment effected by both hyperventilation and indomethacin is substantially lower compared with the averaged drainage volume of 20 ml found in the group subjected to surgical decompression.

In awake humans a dose-related decrease in CBF has been documented after indomethacin (Jensen et al. 1996). According to previous studies in patients with severe head injury (Jensen et al. 1991; Biestro et al. 1995; Dahl et al. 1996; Imberti et al. 2005) and patients with cerebral tumours (Bundgaard et al. 1996), a 0.5-mg/kg i.v. dose of indomethacin was used in the present study. Although, an experimental study in pigs suggests that indomethacin might cause ischaemic changes (Nilsson et al. 1995), a recent diffusion-weighted MRI study indicates that indomethacin does not cause ischaemic damage in propofol-fentanyl-anaesthetized patients with cerebral tumours (Rasmussen et al. 2004), and in the present study indomethacin did cause unexpected prolonged recovery or neurological changes. In a recent review this issue has been discussed (Rasmussen 2005).

In contrast to hyperventilation and indomethacin the ICP-reducing effect of rTp is based on drainage of CBV primarily from the venous compartment. The decrease in ICP averaging 5.0 mmHg is greater compared with other studies in our clinic where a decrease averaging 3.6 and 3.5 mmHg in supine-positioned patients with cerebral tumours was found (Rolighed Larsen et al. 2002; Haure et al. 2003). The higher level of ICP before intervention in the present study, although not significant, can explain the differences in ICP decrease, because the volume/pressure curves are steeper at the given higher ICP level. According to other studies in our clinic (Rolighed et al. 2002; Tankisi et al. 2002, 2006; Haure et al. 2003) 10° rTp did not change CPP, because the decrease in MABP was similar to the reduction in ICP. According to a recent study a 1-min observation period after the change to 10° rTp, was used. Within this period MABP, ICP and CPP are stabilized (Haure et al. 2003).

In patients with intracranial hypertension, fast intravenous mannitol infusion of 0.5–1 g/kg is followed by a decrease in ICP within 2–5 min. The ICP-reducing effect is of hours duration, dependent on the dose and the infusion rate (James 1980). The faster the concentration difference of mannitol occurs between plasma and extracellular fluid, the stronger and the longer the reduction in ICP (Takagi et al. 1993). The decrease in ICP is correlated to the decrease in the water content in brain tissue (Nath and Galbraith 1986). Following mannitol infusion blood viscosity decreases for at least 2 h, suggesting an enhancement of cerebral microcirculation (Burke et al. 1981). An increase in CBV a few minutes after mannitol infusion has been demonstrated experimentally (Lin et al. 1997) and in human studies (Ravussin et al. 1986a). Accordingly, studies of cerebral circulation indicate an increase in CBF occurring after 10–20 min and lasting for up to 24 h, and a variable increase in $CMRO_2$ (Jafar et al. 1986). The effect of mannitol on ICP has been studied in patients with cerebral tumours and aneurysms. In patients with normal ICP a transient but significant increase in ICP followed by a steady decrease towards values below control were found. In contrast, patients with intracranial hypertension showed no increase in ICP, which decreased immediately after mannitol infusion (Ravussin et al. 1986b). In the present study mannitol (20% solution) was administered in doses ranging from 0.5 to 1.0 g/kg (average 0.8 g/kg). These dosages were given through a fast running i.v. infusion over 5–10 min, and subdural ICP was monitored before and until 5 min after discontinuation of administration. An initial increase in subdural ICP, as demonstrated elsewhere, was not observed (Ravussin et al. 1986b). On the one hand, it can be argued that during the relatively short observation period the maximal ICP-reducing effect was not observed. On the other hand, a prolongation of the observation period, more than 10 min, would produce an unacceptable delay of the surgical procedure.

In the present study all patients were anaesthetized with propofol-fentanyl, which is known to produce a substantial decrease in CBF and cerebral metabolism (Stephan et al. 1987; Vandesteene et al. 1988;). In a randomized study in patients undergoing supratentorial tumour surgery, the level of ICP was lower, the level of $AVDO_2$ higher, and the ICP-reducing effect by hyperventilation was more pronounced in propofol-fentanyl-anaesthetized patients compared with isoflurane-fentanyl- or sevoflurane-fentanyl-anaesthetized patients (Petersen et al. 2003). Although the level of ICP differed from the present study, it cannot be excluded that the ICP-reducing effect of both hyperventilation and indomethacin in patients with intracranial hypertension would be more pronounced if the patients were anaesthetized with one of these volatile agents. This is substantiated in a previous study where indomethacin was highly effective in reducing ICP in isoflurane-anaesthetized patients with a high level of ICP (Bundgaard et al. 1996). A possible explanation is that the CO_2 reactivity is higher during isoflurane-fentanyl or sevoflurane-fentanyl anaesthesia compared with propofol-fentanyl-anaesthetized patients (Petersen et al. 2003), and/or the steeper course of the volume/pressure curve at higher ICP levels.

Limitations of the study include the condition that hyperventilation was only used for a 5-min period. As the ICP-reducing effect during hyperventilation is maximal after 10–15 min, it can be argued that a longer period would elicit a more pronounced decrease in ICP. Nevertheless, the decrease in ICP during hyperventilation starts precipitously, with the greatest fall in ICP within the first few minutes, and the decrease in ICP follows the decrease in end-tidal CO_2, which only decreases little after the first 5 min. Moreover, the decrease in $PaCO_2$ averaged 0.8 kPa, a value which is comparable with other studies where the ICP-reducing effect of hyperventilation has been investigated (Petersen et al. 2003). Another limitation is that ICP was measured 5 min after finishing the mannitol infusion. A prolonged observation period of 15–30 min certainly would reveal a more pronounced decrease in ICP. Nevertheless, the rapid ICP-reducing effects of rTp, indomethacin and surgical decompression, taking place within few minutes, are in sharp contrast to the effects of hyperventilation and mannitol treatment where the maximal effect should be expected after approximately 15 and 45 min, respectively. Accordingly, the operation time would be prolonged and the patience of the neurosurgeon challenged. A randomized study in order to confirm the findings in the present study seems justified. Taking into account that in our clinic data collection spanned over 7 years, such a study should be a designed as a multicentre trial.

Clinical significance The present study demonstrates that surgical decompression, either by withdrawal of CSF via a ventricular catheter or evacuation of cystic processes, is superior in controlling intracranial hypertension and preserving CPP when compared with 5 min of hyperventilation, 10° rTp and mannitol treatment extending 5 min after conclusion of infusion. The ICP-reducing effect of indomethacin is pronounced and is accompanied by a substantial increase in CPP. These observations should be confirmed in a randomized study.

References

Biestro AA, Alberti RA, Soca AE et al (1995) Use of indomethacin in brain-injured patients with cerebral perfusion pressure impairment: preliminary report. J Neurosurg 83:627–630

Bundgaard H, Jensen K, Cold GE et al (1996) Effects of perioperative indomethacin on intracranial pressure, cerebral blood flow, and cerebral metabolism in patients subjected to craniotomy for cerebral tumours. J Neurosurg Anesthesiol 8:273–279

Bundgaard H, Landsfeldt U, Cold GE (1998) Subdural monitoring of ICP during craniotomy: thresholds of cerebral swelling/herniation. Acta Neurochir Suppl 71:276–279

Burke AM, Quest DO, Chien S et al (1981) The effects of mannitol on blood viscosity. J Neurosurg 55:550–553

Cold GE, Tange M, Jensen TM et al (1996) Subdural pressure measurement during craniotomy. Correlation with tactile estimation of dural tension and brain herniation after opening of dura. Br J Neurosurg 10:69–75

Dahl B, Bergholt B, Cold GE et al (1996) CO_2 and indomethacin vasoreactivity in patients with head injury. Acta Neurochir 138:265–273

Greenberg JH, Alavi A, Reivich M et al (1978) Local cerebral blood volume response to carbon dioxide in man. Circ Res 43:324–331

Haure P, Cold GE, Hansen TM et al (2003) The ICP-lowering effect of 10° reverse Trendelenburg position during craniotomy is stable during a 10-minute period. J Neurosurg Anesthesiol 15:297–301

Hongo K, Kabayashi S, Yokoh A (1987) Monitoring retraction pressure in the brain. J Neurosurg 66:270–275

Imberti R, Fuardo M, Bellinzona G (2005) The use of indomethacin in the treatment of plateau waves: effects on cerebral perfusion and oxygenation. J Neurosurg 102:455–459

Jafar JJ, Johns LM, Mullan SF (1986) The effect of mannitol on cerebral blood flow. J Neurosurg 64:754–759

James HE (1980) Methodology for the control of intracranial pressure with hypertonic mannitol. Acta Neurochir (Wien) 51:161–172

Jensen K, Ohrström J, Cold GE et al (1991) The effects of indomethacin on intracranial pressure, cerebral blood flow and cerebral metabolism in patients with severe head injury and intracranial hypertension. Acta Neurchir 108:116–121

Jensen K, Kjærgaard S, Malte E et al (1996) Effect of graduated intravenous and standard rectal doses of indomethacin on cerebral blood flow in healthy volunteers. J Neurosurg Anesthesiol 8:111–116

Lin W, Paczynski RP, Kuppusamy K et al (1997) Quantitative measurements of regional cerebral blood volume using MRI in rats: effects of arterial carbon dioxide tension and mannitol. Magn Reson Med 38:420–428

Nath F, Galbraith S (1986) The effect of mannitol on cerebral white matter water content. J Neurosurg 65:41–43

Nilsson F, Björkman S, Rosen I et al (1995) Cerebral vasoconstriction by indomethacin in intracranial hypertension. Anesthesiology 83:1283–1292

Petersen KD, Landsfeldt U, Cold GE et al (2003) Intracranial pressure and cerebral hemodynamic in patients with cerebral tumours: a randomized prospective study of patients subjected to craniotomy in propofol-fentanyl, isoflurane-fentanyl, or sevoflurane-fentanyl anesthesia. Anesthesiology 98:329–336

Rasmussen M (2005) Treatment of elevated intracranial pressure with indomethacin: friend or foe? Acta Anaesthesiol Scand 49:341–350

Rasmussen M, Bundgaard H, Cold GE (2004) Craniotomy for supratentorial brain tumours: risk factors of brain swelling after opening of the dura. J Neurosurg 101:621–626

Ravussin P, Archer DP, Tyler JL et al (1986a) Effects of rapid mannitol infusion on cerebral blood volume. J Neurosurg 64:104–113

Ravussin P, Chiolero R, Buchser E et al (1986b) CSF pressure changes following mannitol in patients undergoing craniotomy. Anesthesiology 65:A303

Rolighed Larsen JK, Haure P, Cold GE (2002) Reverse Trendelenburg position reduces intracranial pressure during craniotomy. J Neurosurg Anesthesiol 14:16–21

Rosenørn J (1987) Self-retaining brain retractor pressure during intracranial procedures. Acta Neurochir 85:17–22

Stephan H, Sonntag H, Schenk HD et al (1987) Einfluss von Disoprivan (propofol) auf die Durchblutung und Sauerstoffverbrach des Gehirns und die CO_2 Reaktivität der Hirngefässe beim Menschen. Anaesthesist 36:60–65

Takagi H, Tanaka M, Ohwada T et al (1993) Pharmacokinetic analysis of mannitol in relation to the decrease of ICP. In: Avezaat CJJ, van Eijndhoven JHM, Maas AIR, Tans JTJ (eds) Intracranial pressure VIII. Springer, Berlin, pp 596–600

Tankisi A, Cold GE (2007) Optimal reverse Trendelenburg position in patients undergoing craniotomy for cerebral tumours. J Neurosurg 106:239–244

Tankisi A, Rolighed Larsen J, Rasmussen M et al (2002) The effects of 10 degrees reverse Trendelenburg position on ICP and CPP in prone-positioned patients subjected to craniotomy for occipital or cerebellar tumours. Acta Neurochir (Wien) 144:665–670

Tankisi A, Rasmussen M, Juul N et al (2006) The effects of 10° reverse Trendelenburg position (rTp) on subdural intracranial pressure and cerebral perfusion pressure in patients subjected to craniotomy for cerebral aneurysm. J Neurosurg Anesthesiol 18:11–17

Vandesteene A, Trempont V, Engelman E et al (1998) Effect of propofol on cerebral blood flow and metabolism in man. Anaesthesia 43(suppl):42–43

Chapter 18
Effect of Positive End-Expiratory Pressure on Subdural Intracranial Pressure in Patients Undergoing Supratentorial Craniotomy

Birgitte Duch and Georg Emil Cold

Abstract

Adult respiratory distress syndrome develops in up to 20% of patients with severe head injury. Positive end-expiratory pressure (PEEP) is often required to support oxygenation. It is well known that PEEP might increase ICP in intensive care patients through decreased cerebral venous outflow as well as an effect on venous return and subsequent reduced mean arterial blood pressure. The effect of PEEP on ICP have been the focus of several experimental and clinical studies, and the results and their interpretation remain controversial. All studies were performed at intensive care units in trauma patients and patients with subarachnoid haemorrhage, but the effect of PEEP, however, have not been investigated during craniotomy.

In this chapter the effects of 5 and $10\,cmH_2O$ PEEP on subdural ICP, cerebral perfusion pressure and jugular bulb pressure were studied during craniotomy for cerebral tumours or cerebral aneurysms.

Positive end-expiratory pressure has been shown to be an effective means for optimizing alveolar recruitment and improves oxygenation in patients with acute lung injury. However, it may worsen or trigger elevated ICP through decreased cerebral venous outflow as well as have an effect on venous return and subsequently reduce MABP. The effect of PEEP on ICP have been the focus of several experimental and clinical studies, and the results and their interpretation remain controversial. All studies were performed at intensive care units in trauma patients and patients with SAH. Shapiro and Marshall (1978) showed an increase in ICP of up to $10\,mmHg$ after applying 4–$8\,cmH_2O$ of PEEP. A decrease of CPP was also shown. In contrast Frost (1977) did not see any change in ICP after applying up to $40\,cmH_2O$ of PEEP. More recently Mascia et al. (2005) elevated PEEP to 5 and $10\,cmH_2O$ and showed that patients who achieved lung recruitment showed no increase in $PaCO_2$ and ICP remained stable. However, in non-recruiters alveolar hyperinflation occurred, and $PaCO_2$ increased with the consequence of an increase in ICP. It is well known that during anaesthesia lung atelectasis is present in most humans and is the major cause of impaired oxygenation in fragile patients. Hedenstierna and Rothen (2000) showed that by applying PEEP, atelectasis could be avoided.

In neuroanaesthesia PEEP has not routinely been applied to the respirator during operations as controversy exists as to whether a rise in ICP would be the consequence. According to the existing literature obtained in intensive care units, it seems safe to apply PEEP without the risk of raising ICP as long as the PEEP is kept below the ICP and the PEEP results in recruitment and not hyperinflation of the lungs. In this chapter two studies are presented that evaluate the safety of applying PEEP during supratentorial craniotomy.

Study 1: Effect of 5 cmH$_2$O Positive End-Expiratory Pressure on Subdural Intracranial Pressure, Cerebral Perfusion Pressure and Jugular Bulb Pressure

Aim To study the effect of 5 cmH$_2$O PEEP on subdural ICP and CPP during craniotomy.

Method Twenty-five patients without pulmonary disease participated in the study. All patients underwent craniotomy for cerebral tumours (n=22) or cerebral aneurysm (n=3) in the supine position and were anaesthetized with propofol-remifentanil. Before and 3 min after PEEP application subdural ICP and MABP were measured and CPP was calculated. These parameters were recorded every minute for a period of 3 min. In 21 patients a catheter was inserted in the jugular vein and JBP was monitored before and after PEEP application. $PaCO_2$ was measured at time zero, and end-tidal CO_2 was monitored continuously during the study period. As regards perioperative fluid therapy, see Chapter 3.

Statistical analysis Mean±SD are indicated. Intragroup differences were tested with Wilcoxon's test.

Results During 5 cmH$_2$O PEEP the maximal pressure of the respirator increased from 15.6 to 21.8 cmH$_2$O. End-tidal CO_2 remained stable. Three minutes after application of 5 cmH$_2$O PEEP a significant decrease in MABP from 70.9 to 68.2 mmHg was found. Within the same time interval subdural ICP increased significantly from 5.7 to 6.7 mmHg and CPP decreased from 65.4 to 61.5 mmHg (all changes at P<0.001 level). An increase in JBP from 4.6 to 5.5 mmHg was observed following 5 cmH$_2$O PEEP (Table 18.1). At time zero $PaCO_2$ averaged 4.61±0.33 kPa. A significant correlation was found between the changes in subdural ICP and changes in bulb pressure during 5 cmH$_2$O PEEP, ΔICP = 0.0373 + (0.8734 × ΔJBP), r=0.8377, P<0.001.

Conclusion Application of 5 cmH$_2$O PEEP reduces blood pressure and CPP and increases subdural ICP and bulb pressure. A positive significant correla-

Table 18.1 Changes in MABP, subdural ICP, CPP and JBP during a 3-min period, after application of 5 cmH$_2$O PEEP

Minutes	MABP (mmHg)	ICP (mmHg)	CPP (mmHg)	JBP (mmHg)
0	70.9±10.2	5.7±4.0	65.4±10.5	4.6±3.2
1	69.3±10.0	6.2±4.1	63.0±9.8	5.1±3.2
2	68.6±9.5	6.6±4.0	62.0±9.1	5.4±3.0
3	68.2±9.7*	6.7±4.0*	61.5±9.3*	5.5±3.0*
Difference 0–3	2.7±3.0	1.0±1.2	3.9±3.7	1.1±1.1

*$P<0.01$ significant intragroup difference from time 0

tion between change in bulb pressure and change in subdural ICP suggests that the increase in ICP is secondary to an increase in bulb pressure.

Study 2: Effect of 10 cmH$_2$O Positive End-Expiratory Pressure on Subdural Intracranial Pressure, Cerebral Perfusion Pressure and Jugular Bulb Pressure

Aim To study the effect of 10 cmH$_2$O PEEP on subdural ICP and CPP during craniotomy.

Method Twelve patients without pulmonary disease participated in the study. All patients underwent craniotomy for cerebral tumours ($n=11$) or cerebral aneurysm ($n=1$) in the supine position and were anaesthetized with propofol-fentanyl. Before and 3 min after PEEP application subdural ICP and MABP were measured and CPP was calculated. These parameters were recorded every minute for a period of 3 min. A catheter was inserted in the jugular vein and JBP was monitored before and after PEEP application. HAES, as a volume expander, was only used in 4 of 12 patients.

Statistical analysis Mean±SD are indicated. Intragroup differences were tested with Wilcoxon's test, and Mann-Whitney's test was used for intergroup differences (comparison with data from the first study).

Results During PEEP application the respirator pressure increased from 15.8 to 25.0 cmH$_2$O. End-tidal CO$_2$ remained stable. The increase in respirator pressure was significantly greater during 10 cmH$_2$O PEEP compared with 5 cmH$_2$O PEEP (first study). Application of 10 cmH$_2$O resulted in the following changes: MABP decreased from 75.3 to 72.3 mmHg, ICP increased from 5.1 to 8.2 mmHg and CPP decreased from 70.2 to 65.1 mmHg (all changes at $P<0.01$ level). An increase in JBP from −0.8 to 2.4 mmHg followed the application of 10 cmH$_2$O PEEP (Table 18.2). PaCO$_2$ averaged 4.53±0.30 kPa. With 10 cmH$_2$O PEEP the correlation between changes in JBP and changes in subdural ICP was significant: ΔICP = 0.2283 + 0.7913 × ΔJBP, $r=0.9008$, $P<0.001$.

Table 18.2 Changes in MABP, subdural ICP, CPP and JBP during a 3-min period, after application of 10 cmH₂O PEEP

Minutes	MABP (mmHg)	ICP (mmHg)	CPP (mmHg)	JBP (mmHg)
0	85.3±16	5.1±3.0	80.2±16	−0.83±2.4
1	82.8±17	6.2±4.1	75.3±17	1.80±3.9
2	82.8±17	6.6±4.0	75.5±16	2.30±4.0
3	82.3±17*	6.7±4.0*	75.1±16*	2.40±3.9*
Difference 0–3	2.9±3.7	3.3±2.3**	5.1±4.5	3.20±2.1**

*$P<0.01$ significant intragroup difference from time 0
**$P<0.01$ significant intergroup difference compared with the first study

The changes in subdural ICP and changes in JBP were significantly greater in the 10 cmH₂O PEEP study compared with the 5 cmH₂O PEEP study. Thus, the change in ICP averaged 1.0 mmHg during the 5 cmH₂O PEEP study against 3.3 mmHg in the 10 cmH₂O PEEP study ($P<0.01$). Likewise a significant increase in maximal respirator pressure was observed ($P<0.01$) and the increase in JBP from 1.1 to 3.2 mmHg was also disclosed ($P<0.01$).

Conclusion Application of 10 cmH₂O PEEP reduces blood pressure and CPP and increases subdural ICP and bulb pressure. A positive significant correlation between change in bulb pressure and change in subdural ICP suggests that the increase in ICP is secondary to an increase in bulb pressure. Comparison between the two studies with 5 and 10 cmH₂O PEEP suggests a dose relation because the changes in both subdural ICP and JBP were significantly greater during 10 cmH₂O PEEP compared with 5 cmH₂O PEEP.

Discussion

The physiological consequences of the application of PEEP depend on its effects on systemic haemodynamics and gas exchange. The haemodynamic mechanism may alter cerebral circulation both on the arterial side by reducing the arterial pressure and on the venous side by reducing cerebral venous drainage. The gas exchange mechanism may change the cerebral circulation by a CO₂-mediated vasodilatation resulting in an increase in CBV.

A positive significant correlation was disclosed between changes in bulb pressure and changes in subdural ICP, suggesting that the increase in bulb pressure elicits an increase in subdural ICP. This relationship is further strengthened by the fact that the changes in subdural ICP, as well as bulb pressure, were significantly greater during 10 cmH₂O PEEP than during 5 cmH₂O PEEP. In patients McGuier et al. (1997) showed that PEEP increased ICP when the applied PEEP was higher than the baseline ICP, but had less effect if the applied PEEP was lower than the ICP. In our study the baseline ICP was 5.7 and

5.1 mmHg in the two groups. So in the group where $10\,cmH_2O$ PEEP was applied the PEEP was higher than the ICP and this may explain why the change in ICP in this group was more pronounced.

Caricato et al. (2005) investigated the relationship between PEEP and ICP in patients with SAH. The patients were divided into groups based on their respiratory system compliance. ICP was unchanged in both groups with an increase of PEEP from 0 to $12\,cmH_2O$. The haemodynamic effects of PEEP, including a reduced MABP, were only observed in patients with normal respiratory compliance. Those with a reduced compliance were protected.

Mascia et al. (2005) demonstrated in head-injury patients that those who achieved significant alveolar recruitment with PEEP showed no increase in ICP. In contrast, patients who showed no increase in lung volumes had an increase in $PaCO_2$, resulting in a rise in cerebral blood flow and elevated ICP.

In both studies a decrease in both MABP and CPP was seen. Our patients had no lung disease and, therefore, they were expected to have normal compliance. So according to Caricato et al. (2005) the decrease in MABP should be expected. We did not measure the compliance, nor did we measure the lung volumes. At time zero, the $PaCO_2$ in the two studies did not differ significantly, and the end-tidal CO_2 concentration did not change after application of PEEP, which otherwise could explain why ICP increased in both studies.

Suggestions based on comparison between the two studies, however, are not convincing because it is based on non-controlled conditions. Between the two studies several differences exist. In study 1 propofol-remifentanil was used, while propofol-fentanyl was used in study 2. The higher MABP and CPP in study 1 are reasonably explained by different principles for maintenance of anaesthesia. In contrast, the level of subdural ICP was lower in propofol-fentanyl-anaesthetized patients. The reason for this difference might be explained by the difference in MABP because a higher blood pressure elicits a vasoconstrictor effect, provided that cerebral autoregulation is intact.

The difference in JBP between the two studies also calls for considerations. One explanation is that all patients in study 1 received i.v. volume expanders (HAES 500 ml) before the measurements, while in study 2 only 4 of 12 patients received similar volume-expanding solutions. Using a 2×2 table and Fisher's exact test the difference was significant ($P<0.001$). Georgiadis et al. (2001) found a significant reduction in CPP after PEEP only in patients with low CVP, suggesting a deleterious effect of hypovolaemia during ventilation with PEEP. Interestingly, Doblar et al. (1981) found that volume loading just before the application of PEEP failed to show any protective action, causing a further increase in ICP.

Although the increase in ICP was significantly greater during $10\,cmH_2O$ PEEP compared with $5\,cmH_2O$ PEEP, conclusions regarding dose-dependent changes in subdural ICP as well as JBP are uncertain. Only a blinded, controlled crossover study might resolve this question.

The main finding in this study was that, in patients undergoing surgery for supratentorial tumours or aneurysm of the brain, applying low levels of PEEP resulted in an increase of ICP and JBP.

References

Caricato A, Conti G, Della Corte F et al (2005) Effects of PEEP on the intracranial system of patients with head injury and subarachnoid hemorrhage: the role of respiratory system compliance. J Trauma 58:571–576

Doblar DD, Santiago TV, Kahn AU (1981) The effect of positive end-expiratory pressure ventilation (PEEP) on cerebral blood flow and cerebrospinal fluid pressure in goats. Anesthesiology. 55:244–250

Frost EA (1977) Effects of positive end-expiratory pressure on intracranial pressure and compliance in brain-injured patients. J Neurosurg 47:195–200

Georgiadis MD, Schwarz S, Baumgartner RW et al (2001) Influence of positive end-expiratory pressure on intracranial pressure and cerebral perfusion pressure in patients with acute stroke. Stroke 32:2088–2092

Hedenstierna G, Rothen HU (2000) Atelectasis formation during anesthesia: causes and measures to prevent it. J Clin Monit Comput 16:329–335

Mascia L, Grasso S, Fiore T et al (2005) Cerebro-pulmonary interactions during the application of low levels of positive end-expiratory pressure. Intensive Care Med 31:373–379

McGuire G, Crossley D, Richards J (1997) Effects of varying levels of positive end-expiratory pressure on intracranial pressure and cerebral perfusion pressure. Crit Care Med 25:1059–1062

Shapiro HM, Marshall LF (1978) Intracranial pressure responses to PEEP in head-injured patients. J Trauma 18:254–256

Videtta W, Willarejo F, Cohen M et al (2002) Effects of positive end-expiratory pressure on intracranial pressure and cerebral perfusion pressure. Acta Neurochir Suppl 81:93–97

Chapter 19
Subdural Intracranial Pressure and Cerebral Haemodynamics During General Anaesthesia for Craniotomy in Patients with Cerebral Aneurysm

Alp Tankisi and Georg Emil Cold

Abstract

Patients with cerebral aneurisms are frequently presented to the neuro-anaesthesiologist, although the number is decreasing due to intravascular coiling. In the intensive care setting a significant correlation between ICP and Hunt & Hess gradation has been described in patients with subarachnoid haemorrhage. The relationship between H&H gradation and perioperative ICP is an important issue because measures to decrease ICP may prevent brain swelling and improve surgical access. It therefore seems reasonable to investigate this issue, taking both patient positioning and anaesthetic technique into consideration.

In this chapter two studies are presented. In the first study we investigated the subdural ICP and cerebral perfusion pressure in patients with cerebral aneurysm anaesthetized with either propofol-fentanyl or isoflurane-fentanyl. In the second study the effect of 10 degrees reverse Trendelenburg position on subdural ICP and cerebral perfusion pressure in patients subjected to craniotomy for cerebral aneurysm were investigated.

In a previous study no relationship was found between H&H gradation and perioperative ICP (Auer and Mokry 1990). In the intensive care setting, however, a significant correlation between ICP and H&H gradation has been described in patients with SAH (Hayashi et al. 1977; Hase et al. 1978; Hartmann 1980; Voldby and Enevoldsen 1982). The relationship between H&H gradation and perioperative ICP is an important issue because measures to decrease ICP may prevent brain swelling and improve surgical access. It therefore seems reasonable to re-investigate this issue. However, other questions arise, including comparison of the effects of volatile anaesthetics and intravenous anaesthetics, and the effect of rTp on ICP and CPP.

Two properties are common for inhalation anaesthetics: a dose-related decrease in $CMRO_2$ and a dose-related decrease in CVR. Intravenous anaesthetic agents have the same ability to reduce $CMRO_2$ but CVR is changed somewhat less. This will be discussed in depth later in this chapter. In addition to the anaesthetic technique used, patient position plays an important role. In supine-positioned patients subjected to craniotomy for cerebral tumours a significant decrease in ICP from 9.5 to 6.0 mmHg with unchanged CPP was observed after change in position to 10° rTp (Rolighed Larsen et al. 2002). Likewise, 10° rTp resulted in a significant decrease in subdural ICP averaging 3 mmHg from a median value of 10 mmHg in supine-positioned patients with cerebral tumours (Haure et al. 2003). In patients subjected to craniotomy in the prone position for occipital or fossa posterior tumours a significant decrease in subdural ICP from 21 to 15.6 mmHg and 18.3 to 14.2 mmHg was recorded, respectively (Tankisi et al. 2002). As a consequence of these studies, we found it of interest also to study the effect of rTp on ICP in patients with SAH.

This chapter is based on two studies, the second of which is based on data presented by Tankisi et al. in J Neurosurg Anesthesiol (2006) 18:11–17.

Study 1: Comparative Study of Subdural Intracranial Pressure and Cerebral Perfusion Pressure in Patients with Cerebral Aneurysm Anaesthetized with Either Propofol-Fentanyl or Isoflurane-Fentanyl

Aim Comparison of subdural ICP and CPP in patients with cerebral aneurysm anaesthetized with either propofol-fentanyl or isoflurane-fentanyl.

Method One hundred and ten patients with cerebral aneurysm, including 33 patients anaesthetized with isoflurane-fentanyl and 77 patients anaesthetized with propofol-fentanyl participated in the study. All patients with SAH were in treatment with nimodipine. Within 1 h of anaesthesia for craniotomy H&H gradation was performed. Before opening of dura subdural ICP and CPP were measured, and the degree of dural tension and cerebral swelling after opening of dura were estimated.

Statistical analysis Within groups the paired t-test was used for the analyses of normally distributed data. Between groups, analysis of variance was used. The chi-square test was used to estimate the difference in proportion. Mean±SD are indicated. $P<0.05$ was considered significant.

Results No significant differences as regards demographics, localization of the aneurysms or distributions of numbers of patients in the respective H&H groups were found between the two anaesthetic groups. The maintenance doses of anaesthetics are indicated in Table 19.1. The level of $PaCO_2$, PaO_2, rectal temperature, MABP and CPP did not differ between the two anaesthetic groups (Table 19.2). In H&H 0 and H&H I patients ICP was low, averaging 6.2 and

5.1 mmHg in the isoflurane group, and 3.8 and 3.9 mmHg in the propofol group, respectively. In H&H II and H&H III patients a gradual increase in subdural ICP was found in both groups, with subdural ICP in the H&H III averaging 18.3 mmHg in the isoflurane group against 17.2 mmHg in the propofol group. In the H&H III patients a significant decrease in CPP was also found in both anaesthetic groups. Compared with the isoflurane group, subdural ICP was lower in all H&H groups in propofol-fentanyl-anaesthetized patients, but the differences in subdural ICP in the respective H&H groups were not significant (Table 19.2). Neither did the degree of dural tension before opening of dura nor the degree of brain swelling after opening of the dura differ significantly between the two anaesthetic groups, but with increasing H&H classification the proportion between normal/increased tension and no swelling/swelling changed significantly (Table 19.3).

Table 19.1 Maintenance dosages of anaesthetics in the isoflurane-fentanyl group and the propofol-fentanyl group

Doses	Isoflurane-fentanyl	Propofol-fentanyl
Isoflurane (MAC)	1.0±0.2	0
Propofol (mg/kg/h)	0	9.0±1.7
Fentanyl (μg/kg/h)	2.2±0.5	2.3±0.6

Table 19.2 Number of patients and physiological variables in patients anaesthetized with isoflurane-fentanyl or propofol-fentanyl. The respective H&H gradations are indicated. Mean±SD are indicated

	H&H 0	H&H I	H&H II	H&H III
Isoflurane-fentanyl				
Number	6	7	12	8
Temperature (°C)	35.9±0.4	36.1±0.8	36.5±0.7	36.2±0.8
$PaCO_2$ (kPa)	4.6±0.5	4.3±0.6	4.1±0.8	4.4±0.6
PaO_2 (kPa)	22.0±6.0	24.0±6.0	27.0±10.0	22.0±10.0
MABP (mmHg)	88.0±12.0	77.0±10.0	80.0±6.0	78.0±10.0
ICP (mmHg)	6.2±4.9	5.1±3.5	9.6±3.2	18.3±4.4*,**
CPP (mmHg)	82.0±12.0	71.0±12.0	70.0±5.0	58.0±11.0**
Propofol-fentanyl				
Number	17	16	27	17
Temperature (°C)	35.9±0.6	36.6±0.8	36.4±0.6	36.7±0.9
$PaCO_2$ (kPa)	4.5±0.3	4.3±0.4	4.5±0.4	4.3±0.5
PaO_2 (kPa)	30.0±7.0	29.0±9.0	25.0±12.0	23.0±11.0
MABP (mmHg)	84.0±10.0	79.0±17.0	83.0±13.0	80.0±9.0
ICP (mmHg)	3.8±3.2	3.8±3.2	9.4±3.4*,**	17.2±4.6*,**
CPP (mmHg)	81.0±9.0	75.0±16.0	74.0±12.0	62.0±10.0*,**

*$P<0.05$ compared with the preceding H&H group
**$P<0.05$ compared with H&H 0

Table 19.3 Degree of dural tension and degree of brain swelling after opening of dura. Number of patients is indicated

	Isoflurane-fentanyl		Propofol-fentanyl	
Degree of dural tension	Normal tension	Increased tension	Normal tension	Increased tension
H&H 0	5	1	17	0
H&H I	6	1	15	1
H&H II	5	7	11	16*,**
H&H III	0	8**	0	17*,**
Degree of brain swelling	No swelling	Swelling present	No swelling	Swelling present
H&H 0	5	1	17	0
H&H I	5	2	15	1
H&H II	4	8	9	18*,**
H&H III	0	8**	0	17*,**

*$P<0.05$ compared with the preceding H&H grade
**$P<0.05$ compared with H&H 0

Conclusion Independent of anaesthetic agent (propofol contra isoflurane), subdural ICP increases with higher H&H gradation, but although the mean values of subdural ICP in all H&H groups were higher during isoflurane anaesthesia, these differences never reached significance.

Study 2: Effect of 10 Degrees Reverse Trendelenburg Position on Subdural Intracranial Pressure and Cerebral Perfusion Pressure in Patients Subjected to Craniotomy for Cerebral Aneurysm

Aims 1: To examine the effect of 10° rTp position on subdural ICP, CPP and dural tension during craniotomy in patients with cerebral aneurysm. 2: To analyse the relationship between subdural ICP in the neutral position and changes in subdural ICP (ΔICP) after change in position to 10° rTp in different H&H groups. 3: To investigate the relationship between preoperative H&H grade and ICP in the neutral position.

Method Twenty-eight patients with cerebral aneurysm were subjected to craniotomy in propofol-fentanyl ($n=15$) or propofol-remifentanil ($n=13$) maintenance anaesthesia, respectively. During anaesthesia the level of $PaCO_2$ was between 4.0 and 5.0 kPa, and PaO_2 was > 13 kPa. All patients were in treatment with oral nimodipine. The localization of the aneurysm was classified with preoperative four-vessel angiography. The localization was as follows: middle cerebral artery, 13 patients; anterior communicans artery, 7 patients; internal carotid artery, 6 patients; and posterior communicans artery, 2 patients. H&H grade was determined just before induction of anaesthesia. Twelve patients were classified as H&H 0, 8 patients as H&H I and 8 patients as H&H II. Intubated patients, patients with ventricular catheters and patients in treatment with mannitol were not included in the statistical analysis. These patients were classified separately as H&H III.

Catheters were inserted into the radial artery and into the jugular vein. After reference measurement of MABP, subdural ICP and JBP in the neutral position the operating table was adjusted to $10°$ rTp. All transducers were readjusted to the same level (point of the needle perforating the dura) and the measurements of MABP, subdural ICP and JBP were repeated after 1 min of stabilization. CPP was calculated as the difference between MABP and subdural ICP. Changes in subdural ICP (ΔICP) and changes in JBP (ΔJBP) were calculated as well. Tension of dura was estimated by the surgeon and graded as follows: low tension; normal tension; increased tension; and pronounced increased tension. These estimations were performed in the neutral position as well as in $10°$ rTp.

Statistical analysis Within groups the paired t-test was used for the analyses of normally distributed data. Between groups, analysis of variance was used. The chi-square test was used to estimate the difference in proportion. Mean±SD are indicated. $P<0.05$ was considered significant.

Results No significant differences between the anaesthetic groups with regards $PaCO_2$, PaO_2, subdural ICP, MABP, CPP, JBP, H&H classification, localization of aneurysms or demographic data were disclosed. Including all patients ($n=28$), $10°$ rTp was accompanied by a significant decrease in subdural ICP, MABP and JBP, whereas CPP remained unchanged (Table 19.4). In Table 19.5 the values of subdural ICP, MABP, CPP, JBP and ΔICP are related to the respective H&H groups. A progressive significant increase in subdural ICP was found with increasing H&H classification. Compared with H&H 0 (unruptured aneurysm), ΔICP was significantly higher in H&H II patients.

The relationship between subdural ICP in the neutral position and ΔICP was significant (ΔICP = 0.3661 ICP + 1.347; $r=0.627$, $P<0.001$). The relationship between ΔCPP and ΔICP was significant as well (ΔICP = 0.376 ΔCPP + 4.059; $r=0.596$; $P=0.001$). Change in position to $10°$ rTp was accompanied by a significant decrease in dural tension. The number of patients with increased tension of dura decreased from 10 to 4 patients. Additionally, a significant relationship between tension of dura and H&H grade was observed (Table 19.6).

Table 19.4 The effect of $10°$ rTp on MABP, subdural ICP, CPP, and JBP in 28 patients with cerebral aneurysm. Δ Values indicate change in pressure during rTp

Variable	Neutral position	$10°$ rTp	Δ Value
MABP (mmHg)	77.0±14.0	72.0±14.0*	4.6±3.4
ICP (mmHg)	6.6±4.6	2.8±3.6*	3.7±2.7
CPP (mmHg)	70.0±14.0	70.0±14.0	0.8±4.2
JBP (mmHg)	4.6±4.1	0.5±4.1*	4.2±1.6

*Significant change compared with neutral position

Table 19.5 Effect of 10° rTp on MABP, subdural ICP, CPP and JBP in different H&H gradations

H&H grade	Position	MABP (mmHg)	ICP (mmHg)	CPP (mmHg)	JBP (mmHg)	ΔICP (mmHg)
H&H 0	Neutral	75.0.±13.0	2.9±2.6	72.0±13.0	2.1±2.0	
(n=12)	10° rTp	70.0±14.0*	0.4±2.2*	70.0±14.0	−1.6±2.8*	2.5±1.4
H&H I	Neutral	81.0±14.0	6.8±3.3°	74.0±15.0	8.8±4.9°	
(n=8)	10° rTp	76.0±13.0*	2.9±2.4*	74.0±14.0	3.8±5.4*	3.9±2.6
H&H II	Neutral	78.0±17.0	11.9±2.0°#	66.0±17.0	4.5±2.4	
(n=16)	10° rTp	73.0±15.0*	6.3±3.3*°#	67.0±15.0	0.5±1.9*	5.5±3.4°
H&H I+II	Neutral	79.0±15.0	9.3±3.8°	70.0±16.0	6.9±4.4°	
(n=16)	10° rTp	75.0±14.0*	4.6±3.3*°	70.0±14.0	2.3±4.3*	4.7±3.0°
H&H III	Neutral	85.0±10.0	8.5±4.9	76.0±13.0	9.5±0.7	
(n=4)	10° rTp	77.0±9.0	3.7±5.1	73.0±13.0	3.0±1.4	4.7±1.3

*Significant difference from neutral position
°Significant difference from H&H 0
#H&H II data are significantly different from H&H I data

Table 19.6 Estimation of dural tension in the neutral position related to the H&H gradation. Number of patients is indicated. Pearson $\chi^2 = 15.750$, $P<0.003$

Tension of dura	H&H 0	H&H I	H&H II
Low or normal	1	2	0
Increased tension	10	4	1
Pronounced increased	1	2	7

Conclusion Subdural ICP in the neutral position is related to H&H gradation. Thus, the more severely injured patients with a high H&H gradation had a higher subdural ICP. Ten degrees rTp reduces subdural ICP, MABP and dural tension significantly, whereas CPP is unchanged.

Discussion

In study 1 it was documented that independent of anaesthetic agent (propofol contra isoflurane) subdural ICP increases with higher H&H gradation, but although the mean values of subdural ICP in all H&H groups were higher during isoflurane anaesthesia, these differences never reached significance.

Two properties are common for inhalation anaesthetics: a dose-related decrease in $CMRO_2$ and a dose-related decrease in CVR. As regards isoflurane experimental studies have demonstrated this (Cucchiara et al. 1974; Stullken et al. 1977; Newberg and Michenfelder 1983; Gelman et al. 1984; Todd and Drummond 1984). Comparative clinical studies in patients without cerebral lesions (Murphy et al. 1974; Algotsson et al. 1988; Olsen et al. 1994) and studies in patients with mass-expanding cerebral lesions (Eintrei et al. 1985; Madsen et al. 1987) have shown that the increase in CBF is dose dependent. Simultaneously, isoflurane induces a decrease in $CMRO_2$ (Murkin et al. 1986; Madsen et al. 1987; Algotsson et al. 1988; Olsen et al. 1994). The decrease in CVR is accompanied by an increase in CBF and CBV (Archer et al. 1987), an effect that increases ICP. Todd and Weeks (1996), however, made a comparative study of the effects of propofol, pentobarbital and isoflurane on CBF and CBV. They found that CBF in isoflurane-anaesthetized animals was 2.0–2.6 times greater than with propofol or pentobarbital. Nevertheless, although CBV was greater in the isoflurane group than in the propofol and pentobarbital groups, the magnitudes of the intergroup differences were much smaller (about 20%). In another experimental study, rabbits with brain tumour had a higher CBF and CBV when anaesthetized with isoflurane compared with propofol (Cenic et al. 2002). In comparison, in experimental studies, propofol is known to reduce both CBF and $CMRO_2$ (Werner et al. 1992). A dose-related decrease in CBF and $CMRO_2$ under conditions where blood pressure is maintained has been found (Ramani et al. 1992). However, in the same study a direct drug-related cerebral vasodilation cannot be excluded at excessive propofol concentrations. In dogs, a low and moderate dose of propofol decreases EEG activity and $CMRO_2$, and an associated decrease of CBF and CSF pressure were observed (Artru et al. 1992). Clinical studies support this. In other human studies propofol given as a bolus injection suppresses CBF and $CMRO_2$ (Stephan et al. 1987, 1988). Similar changes in CBF and $CMRO_2$ have been observed during continuous infusion with propofol (Vandesteene et al. 1988). Other clinical studies, including patients with cerebral tumours, indicate that subdural ICP is lower during propofol-fentanyl anaesthesia compared with isoflurane-fentanyl (Petersen et al. 2003). In children, however, a significant difference in subdural ICP between propofol and isoflurane anaesthesia was not found (Stilling et al. 2005).

Taking experimental and clinical evidence into consideration, all indicating that CBF and CBV are higher during isoflurane anaesthesia than during propofol anaesthesia, two conclusions concerning the effect of anaesthetic agents on ICP might be drawn from the first study:

1. The number of patients in the respective H&H groups was not sufficient. This combined with high standard deviations in the H&H groups makes statements concerning significant difference in subdural ICP invalid.
2. Although the mean values of subdural ICP were higher during isoflurane compared with propofol anaesthesia, the differences in the H&H II and III groups, where the highest levels of subdural ICP were recorded, only averaged 0.2 and 1.1 mmHg, indicating that this small difference hardly had clinical significance. In unruptured aneurysms, however, the difference was 2.4 mmHg, but the levels of subdural ICP in this group were far below the threshold for brain swelling of 10 and 13 mmHg, found in patients with cerebral aneurysm (Bundgaard et al. 1998) and patients with brain tumours (Rasmussen et al. 2004), respectively, and therefore also without

clinical significance as regards risk of cerebral swelling and impaired surgical access.

It is important to emphasize that the first study was not randomized. Thus, the clinical implication may be drawn with reservation. However, both experimental and human studies support the view that subdural ICP is higher during isoflurane compared with propofol anaesthesia. The first study does not deny this conclusion, but only a randomized study in children might settle this issue.

In a previous study no relationship was found between H&H gradation and perioperative ICP (Auer and Mokry 1990). In the intensive care setting, however, a significant correlation between ICP and H&H gradation has been described in patients with SAH (Hayashi et al. 1977; Hase et al. 1978; Hartmann 1980; Voldby and Enevoldsen 1982). This finding is in agreement with the result of the present study where a significant correlation between H&H gradation and ICP before and after tilting of the operating table was observed. The levels of ICP in H&H I and H&H II patients are identical with the values observed in awake patients where ICP in H&H I–II patients averaged 10.3 mmHg (Voldby and Enevoldsen 1982) or ranged between 10 and 13 mmHg (Hartmann 1982).

In the second study it was demonstrated that subdural ICP in the neutral position is related to H&H gradation. Thus, the more severely injured patients with a high H&H gradation had a higher subdural ICP. Furthermore, $10°$ rTp reduces subdural ICP, MABP and dural tension significantly, whereas CPP is unchanged.

Remifentanil and fentanyl have similar effects on cerebral haemodynamics, ICP and CO_2 reactivity (Guy et al. 1997; Ostapkovich et al. 1998; Balakrishnan et al. 2000). The present non-randomized study suggests that propofol-remifentanil and propofol-fentanyl have similar effects on MABP, ICP, ΔICP, CPP and JBP. These findings are in contrast to the study presented in Chapter 8, study 3, where subdural ICP and JBP were significantly lower in patients with supratentorial cerebral tumours during propofol-remifentanil compared with propofol-fentanyl anaesthesia. Only a randomized controlled study comparing subdural ICP and cerebral haemodynamics will settle this question, and seem justified.

Recently, we studied the effect of $10°$ rTp in patients with cerebral tumours in the supine and prone positions and found a significant decrease in subdural ICP as well as JBP (Rolighed Larsen et al. 2002; Tankisi et al. 2002; Haure et al. 2003). The results of the second study confirm these findings. In all H&H groups, expect H&H III, both subdural ICP and JBP decreased significantly. The lack of significant difference in the H&H III group is explained by the fact that only four patients were included.

In patients with head injury a positive correlation between the ICP level in the horizontal position and ΔICP during $30°$ head-up position has been disclosed (Feldman et al. 1992; Schneider et al. 1993). In the present study tilting of the operating table resulted in a significantly greater decrease in ICP in patients classified as H&H I–II compared with patients classified as unruptured aneurysm, and the correlation between ICP in the neutral position and ΔICP was positive and significant. These observations are in agreement with the ICP/volume concept, indicating that the decrease in ICP, effected by volume displacement, is reduced at low values of ICP, compared to the change in ICP observed during a high level of ICP (Langfitt et al. 1964). Difference in cerebral compliance between unruptured aneurysm patients and patients with SAH, however, may also explain the difference in ΔICP found in the present study.

In patients with head injury a decrease in mean ICP ranging from 4.5 to 11 mmHg with unchanged CPP during head-up position has been documented (Durward et al. 1983; Feldman et al. 1992; Schneider et al. 1993; Meixensberger et al. 1997; Moraine et al. 2000). An increase in ICP, however, secondary to a decrease in CPP has been described in patients with severe head injury. Thus, cerebral vasodilatation elicited by the autoregulatory mechanism might provoke an increase in ICP caused by a fall in CPP (Rosner and Coley 1986). In experimental studies (Hauerberg et al. 1993; Ma et al. 2000) as well as clinical studies (Voldby et al. 1985) of SAH cerebral autoregulation is disturbed. In the present study a significant relationship between the increase in CPP and decrease in ICP during rTp was found, suggesting that the autoregulatory mechanism influences the change in ICP, and that cerebral autoregulation, even in patients with ruptured aneurysm, predominantly was intact. Nevertheless, CPP did not differ between unruptured and ruptured aneurysm, and it is therefore unlikely that the level of CPP had any influence when ICP in unruptured and ruptured aneurysms was compared.

In a recent study, including 692 patients with cerebral tumour, cerebral swelling rarely occurred at subdural ICP < 5 mmHg (Rasmussen et al. 2004). Likewise, in patients with cerebral aneurysm cerebral swelling after opening of dura rarely occurred at subdural ICP < 7 mmHg, while cerebral swelling occurred with high probability at ICP $\geq$ 10 mmHg (Bundgaard et al. 1998). In the present study, the lowest ICP in H&H II patients was 9 mmHg, and 3 mmHg in H&H I patients. The highest ICP in patients without SAH was 6 mmHg. In all H&H groups 10° rTp significantly reduced ICP and dural tension. No cerebral swelling after dural incision occurred in patients (including all H&H 0 patients) with ICP $\leq$ 7 mmHg.

In awake patients without cerebral pathology ICP averages 11±2 mmHg (range 7–15 mmHg) (Albeck et al. 1991). In the present study the level of ICP in unruptured aneurysm, representing patients without intracranial mass-expanding lesion, averaged 2.9±2.6 mmHg. The difference in ICP level is supposed to be caused by propofol. In experimental studies (Ramani et al. 1992; Watts et al. 1998) and clinical studies (Stephan et al. 1987; Madsen 1991) reduces cerebral oxygen uptake and ICP. Furthermore, the low ICP may also be caused by hypocapnia (Petersen et al. 2003).

Lovell et al. (2000) examined changes in CBV before and after head elevation in awake and anaesthetized subjects. In awake subjects the decrease in CBV was more pronounced compared with subjects anaesthetized with propofol, probably because the CBV was already reduced by propofol anaesthesia. The ICP-reducing effect of head elevation was accompanied by a reduction in the cerebral venous blood volume and the capillary blood volume. In a recent study we found that the decrease in ICP was stable within 1 min after change in position, and the decrease in ICP was accompanied by a decrease in JBP (Haure et al. 2003). These findings indicate that the ICP-reducing effect of 10° rTp is secondary to mobilization of intracranial blood volume, but may also be caused by mobilization of intracranial CSF to the spinal segments.

References

Albeck MJ, Børgesen SE, Gjerris F et al (1991) Intracranial pressure and cerebrospinal fluid outflow conductance in healthy subjects. J Neurosurg 74:597–600

Algotsson L, Messeter K, Nordström CH et al (1988) Cerebral blood flow and oxygen consumption during isoflurane and halothane anaesthesia in man. Acta Anaestheiol Scand 32:15–20

Archer DP, Labrecque P, Tylor JL et al (1987) Cerebral blood volume is increased in dogs during administration of nitrous oxide or isoflurane. Anesthesiology 67:642–648

Artru AA, Shapira Y, Bowdle A (1992) Electroencephalogram, cerebral metabolism, and vascular responses to propofol anesthesia in dogs. J Neurosurg Anesthesiol 4:99–109

Auer LM, Mokry M (1990) Disturbed cerebrospinal fluid circulation after subarachnoid hemorrhage and acute aneurysm surgery. Neurosurgery 26:804–808

Balakrishnan G, Raudzens P, Samra SK et al (2000) A comparison of remifentanil and fentanyl in patients undergoing surgery for intracranial mass lesions. Anesth Analg 91:163–169

Bundgaard H, Landsfeldt U, Cold GE (1998) Subdural monitoring of ICP during craniotomy: thresholds of cerebral swelling/herniation. Acta Neurochir Suppl 71:276–278

Cenic A, Craen RA, Lee TY (2002) Cerebral blood volume and blood flow responses to hyperventilation in brain tumours during isoflurane or propofol anesthesia. Anesth Analg 94:661–666

Cucchiara RF, Theye RA, Michenfelder JD (1974) The effects of isoflurane on canine cerebral metabolism and blood flow. Anesthesiology 40:571–574

Durward QJ, Amacher AL, Del Maestro RF et al (1983) Cerebral and cardiovascular responses to changes in head elevation in patients with intracranial hypertension. J Neurosurg 59:938–944

Eintrei C, Leszniewski W, Carlsson C (1985) Local application of 133-Xenon for measurement of regional cerebral blood flow (rCBF) during halothane, enflurane and isoflurane anaesthesia in humans. Anesthesiology 63:391–394

Feldman Z, Kanter MJ, Robertson CS et al (1992) Effect of head elevation on intracranial pressure, cerebral perfusion pressure, and cerebral blood flow in head-injured patients. J Neurosurg 76:207–211

Gelman S, Fowler KC, Smith LR (1984) Regional blood flow during isoflurane and halothane anaesthesia. Anesth Analg 63:557–565

Guy J, Hindman BJ, Baker KZ et al (1997) Comparison of remifentanil and fentanyl in patients undergoing craniotomy for supratentorial space-occupying lesions. Anesthesiology 86:514–524

Hartmann A (1980) Continuous monitoring of CSF pressure in acute subarachnoid hemorrhage. In: Shulman K, Marmarau A, Miller JD, Becker DP, Hochwald GM, Brock M (eds) Intracranial pressure IV. Springer, Berlin, pp 220–228

Hase U, Reulen HJ, Fenske A et al (1978) Intracranial pressure and pressure volume relation in patients with subarachnoid haemorrhage (SAH). Acta Neurochir 44:69–80

Hauerberg J, Juhler M, Rasmussen G (1993) Cerebral blood flow autoregulation after experimental subarachnoid hemorrhage during hyperventilation in rats. J Neurosurg Anesthesiol 5:258–263

Haure P, Cold GE, Hansen TM et al (2003) The ICP-lowering effect of 10 degrees reverse Trendelenburg position during craniotomy is stable during a 10-minute period. J Neurosurg Anesthesiol 15:297–301

Hayashi M, Marukawa S, Fujii H et al (1977) Intracranial hypertension in patients with ruptured aneurysm. J Neurosurg 46:584–590

Langfitt TW, Weinstein JD, Kassell NF et al (1964) Transmission of increased intracranial pressure. I. Within the craniospinal axis. J Neurosurg 21:989–997

Lovell AT, Marshall AC, Elwell CE et al (2000) Changes in cerebral blood volume with changes in position in awake and anesthetized subjects. Anesth Analg 90:372–376

Ma X-D, Willumsen L, Hauerberg J et al (2000) Effects of graded hyperventilation on cerebral blood flow autoregulation in experimental subarachnoid hemorrhage. J Cereb Blood Flow Metab 20:718–725

Madsen JB (1991) Changes in CBF and $CMRO_2$ in patients undergoing craniotomy with propofol infusion. In: Prys-Roberts C (ed) Focus on infusion. Current Medical Literature pp 162–164

Madsen JB, Cold GE, Hansen ES et al (1987) The effect of isoflurane on cerebral blood flow and metabolism in humans during craniotomy for small supratentorial cerebral tumours. Anesthesiology 66:332–336

Meixensberger J, Baunach S, Amschler J et al (1997) Influence of body position on tissue-pO_2, cerebral perfusion pressure and intracranial pressure in patients with acute brain injury. Neurol Res 19:249–253

Moraine JJ, Berre J, Melot C (2000) Is cerebral perfusion pressure a major determinant of cerebral blood flow during head elevation in comatose patients with severe intracranial lesions? J Neurosurg 92:606–614

Murkin JM, Farrar JK, Tweed WA et al (1986) Cerebral blood flow, oxygen consumption and EEG during isoflurane anesthesia. Anest Analg 65:S107

Murphy FL, Kennell EM, Johnstone RE et al (1974) The effects of enflurane, isoflurane and halothane on cerebral blood flow and metabolism in man. Abstracts and scientific papers. Annual meeting of the Am Soc Anaesth, pp 61–62

Newberg LA, Michenfelder JD (1983) Cerebral protection by isoflurane during hypoxemia or ischemia. Anesthesiology 59:29–35

Olsen KS, Henriksen L, Owen-Falkenberg A et al (1994) Effect of 1 or 2 MAC isoflurane with or without ketanserin on cerebral blood flow autoregulation in man. Br J Anaesth 72:66–71

Ostapkovich ND, Baker KZ, Fogarty-Mack P et al (1998) Cerebral blood flow and CO_2 reactivity is similar during remifentanil/N_2O and fentanyl/N_2O anesthesia. Anesthesiology 89:358–363

Petersen KD, Landsfeldt U, Cold GE et al (2003) Intracranial pressure and cerebral hemodynamic in patients with cerebral tumours. A randomized prospective study of patients subjected to craniotomy in propofol-fentanyl, isoflurane-fentanyl, or sevoflurane-fentanyl anesthesia. Anesthesiology 98:329–336

Ramani R, Todd MM, Warner DS (1992) A dose-response study of the influence of propofol on cerebral blood flow, metabolism and the electroencephalogram in the rabbit. J Neurosurg Anesthesiol 4:110–119

Rasmussen M, Bundgaard H, Cold GE (2004) Craniotomy for supratentorial brain tumours: risk factors for brain swelling after opening of dura mater. J Neurosurg 101:621–626

Rolighed Larsen JK, Haure P, Col GE (2002) Reverse Trendelenburg position reduces intracranial pressure during craniotomy. J Neurosurg Anesthesiol 14:16–21

Rosner MJ, Coley IB (1986) Cerebral perfusion pressure, intracranial pressure, and head elevation. J Neurosurg 65:636–641

Schneider GH, von Helden GH, Franke R et al (1993) Influence of body position on jugular venous oxygen saturation, intracranial pressure and cerebral perfusion pressure. Acta Neurochir Suppl 59:107–112

Stephan H, Sonntag H, Schenk HD et al (1987) Effect of Disoprivan (propofol) on the circulation and oxygen consumption of the brain and CO_2 reactivity of brain vessels in the human. Anaesthesist 36:60–65

Stephan H, Sonntag H, Seyde WC et al (1988) Energie-und Aminosäurenstoffwechsel des Menschlichen Gehirns unter Desoprivan und verschiedenen paCO$_2$-Werten. Anaesthesist 37:297–304

Stilling M, Karatasi E, Rasmussen M et al (2005) Subdural intracranial pressure, cerebral perfusion pressure, and the degree of cerebral swelling in supra- and infratentorial space-occupying lesions in children. Acta Neurochir Suppl 95:133–136

Stullken AH, Milde JH, Michenfelder JD (1977) The nonlinear responses of cerebral metabolism to low concentrations of halothane, enflurane, isoflurane and thiopental. Anesthesiology 46:28–34

Tankisi A, Rolighed Larsen J, Rasmussen M et al (2002) The effects of 10 degrees reverse Trendelenburg position on ICP and CPP in prone positioned patients subjected to craniotomy for occipital or cerebellar tumours. Acta Neurochir 144:665–670

Tankisi A, Rasmussen M, Juul N et al (2006) The effects of 10° reverse Trendelenburg position on subdural intracranial pressure and cerebral perfusion pressure in patients subjected to craniotomy for cerebral aneurysm. J Neurosurg Anesthesiol 18:11–17

Todd MM, Drummond JC (1984) A comparison of the cerebrovascular and metabolic effects of halothane and isoflurane in the cat. Anesthesiology 60:276–282

Todd MM, Weeks J (1996) Comparative effects of propofol, pentobarbital, and isoflurane on cerebral blood flow and blood volume. J Neurosurg Anesthesiol 8:296–303

Vandesteene A, Trempont V, Engelman E et al (1988) Effect of propofol on cerebral blood flow and metabolism in man. Anaesthesia 43(suppl):42–43

Voldby B, Enevoldsen EM (1982) Intracranial pressure changes following aneurysm rupture. Part 1: clinical and angiographic correlations. J Neurosurg 56:186–196

Voldby B, Enevoldsen EM, Jensen FT (1985) Cerebrovascular reactivity in patients with ruptured intracranial aneurysms. J Neurosurg 62:59–67

Watts AD, Eliasziw M, Gelb AW (1998) Propofol and hyperventilation for the treatment of increased intracranial pressure in rabbits. Anesth Analg 87:564–568

Werner C, Hoffman WE, Kochs E et al (1992) The effects of propofol on cerebral blood flow in correlation to cerebral blood flow velocity in dogs. J Neurosurg Anesthesiol 4:41–46

Chapter 20
Subdural Intracranial Pressure in Children

Alp Tankisi, Etienne Karatasi and Georg Emil Cold

Abstract
Studies of ICP in adult supine-positioned patients with supratentorial tumours or prone-positioned patients with infratentorial tumours suggest a dependency of both tactile estimate of dural tension and the degree of brain swelling after opening of dura on subdural ICP monitored immediately before opening of dura. However, comparative studies of ICP and the degree of cerebral swelling during craniotomy for space-occupying lesions in children are not available. The pressure/volume relationship in children is different from that in adults because of the smaller intracranial volume and the compliancy of the cranial vault.

In this chapter data on children in supine and prone positions during surgery are discussed, the influence of the anaesthetic technique, either propofol-fentanyl or isoflurane-nitrous oxide 50%-fentanyl, is disclosed and the ICP-lowering effect of reverse Trendelenburg position are presented.

The pressure/volume relationship in children is different from adults because of the smaller intracranial volume and the compliancy of the cranial vault. As a consequence, the effects of anaesthetics on ICP may differ from that observed in adults. Likewise, the cerebral haemodynamic effect of change in position on ICP might differ from adults because cerebral as well as central circulation is age dependent.

Studies of ICP in adult supine-positioned patients with supratentorial tumours (Cold et al. 1996; Bundgaard et al. 1998; Rasmussen et al. 2004) or prone-positioned patients with infratentorial tumours (Jørgensen et al. 1999; Tankisi et al. 2002) suggest a dependency of both tactile estimate of dural tension and the degree of brain swelling after opening of dura on subdural ICP monitored immediately before opening of dura. However, comparative studies of ICP and the degree of cerebral swelling during craniotomy for space-occupying lesions in children are not available.

In this chapter two studies of subdural ICP in children will be presented. The first study was presented by Stilling et al. in Acta Neurochir Suppl (2005) 95:133–136; the second study has not been presented before.

Study 1: Subdural Intracranial Pressure, Cerebral Perfusion Pressure and Degree of Cerebral Swelling in Supra- and Infratentorial Space-Occupying Lesions in Children

Aim   To gather information on the degree of cerebral swelling, ICP and CPP in a group of children subjected to craniotomy.

Patients   Forty-eight children with space-occupying tumours were subjected either to isoflurane-nitrous oxide 50%-fentanyl ($n=22$) or propofol-fentanyl ($n=26$) anaesthesia, Twenty-five children were operated on supratentorially in the supine position, while 23 patients were operated on infratentorially in the prone position. Subdural ICP, CPP, estimation of dural tension and degree of cerebral swelling after opening of dura were monitored in accordance with the procedure described in detail in Chapter 3.

Statistical analysis   The data are presented as mean±SD. Intergroup differences were analysed with a one-way ANOVA model. The chi-square test was used for analyses of difference in distribution. *Post hoc* tests using Bonferroni corrections were performed. $P<0.05$ was considered significant.

Results   The age and weight of the children anaesthetized with isoflurane in the prone position were significantly lower than the propofol-anaesthetized children. No significant intergroup differences as regards tumour size, midline

Table 20.1   Demographic data, neuroradiological data and data related to anaesthesia. Mean±SD are indicated

	Isoflurane/ supine	Isoflurane/ prone	Propofol/ supine	Propofol/ prone
Number	14	8	11	15
Male/female	8/6	4/4	8/3	11/4
Age (years)	6.1±4.4	3.6±2.1	9.3±2.1*	8.3±4.3*
Weight (kg)	24.0±15.0	17.0±4.5	34.0±11.0*	29.0±11.0
Steroid therapy +/−	5.0/9.0	2.0/6.0	2.0/9.0	3.0/12.0
Neuroradiology				
Tumour area (cm^2)	10.4±10.0	9.5±4.7	10.4±9.7	9.4±8.5
Midline shift (mm)	0.7±2.7	1.0±1.9	1.4±3.2	3.3±6.4
Anaesthesia				
Propofol (mg/kg/h)	0	0	10.5±3.8	12.7±5.1
Fentanyl (µg/kg/h)	1.8±1.3	1.2±0.6	2.2±1.1	2.3±0.8
Isoflurane (% expiratory)	1.3±0.5	1.2±0.2	0	0

*$P<0.05$ significant difference from isoflurane prone position

shift, pathology, rectal temperature, mean blood pressure, PaO_2 and $PaCO_2$ were disclosed (Table 20.1). Subdural ICP in prone-positioned children averaged 16.9 mmHg against 9.0 mmHg in supine-positioned children ($P<0.001$). In prone-positioned patients the tension of dura and the degree of brain swelling were significantly more pronounced (Table 20.2). No significant difference as regard ICP was disclosed when isoflurane-nitrous oxide and propofol-fentanyl were compared. Mean blood pressure and CPP, however, were significantly lower in children anaesthetized with isoflurane-nitrous oxide than in the children anaesthetized with propofol. No significant difference between isoflurane-nitrous oxide- and propofol-fentanyl-anaesthetized children as regards tension of dura and the degree of brain swelling after opening of dura were disclosed (Tables 20.3 and 20.4).

Table 20.2 Data related to cerebral circulation, tension of dura and degree of cerebral swelling. Anaesthesia and positioning are indicated. Mean±SD are indicated

	Isoflurane	Propofol	Supine	Prone
$PaCO_2$ (kPa)	3.9±0.6	4.2±0.4	4.0±0.5	4.1±0.6
PaO_2 (kPa)	33.0±12.0	36.0±10.0	36.0±14.0	36.0±9.0
Temperature (°C)	36.8±0.9	36.4±0.7	36.3±0.0	36.4±0.7
ICP (mmHg)	12.5±9.1	13.0±7.6	9.0±6.9	16.9±7.6*
MABP (mmHg)	66.0±11.0	739.0±*	68.0±8.0	70.0±9.0
CPP (mmHg)	52.0±10.0	59.0±10.0*	59.0±10.0	52.0±11.0*
Tension of dura				
Normal	10	14	17	7
Increased	8	7	6	9
Pronounced increased	4	5	2	7
Degree of swelling				
No swelling	9	11	15	5
Moderate swelling	6	10	6	10
Pronounced swelling	7	5	4	8

*$P<0.05$ significant difference between isoflurane and propofol anaesthesia and supine and prone positioning

Table 20.3 Data related to cerebral circulation. Anaesthesia and positioning are indicated. Mean±SD are indicated

	Isoflurane/ supine	Isoflurane/ prone	Propofol/ supine	Propofol/ prone
$PaCO_2$ (kPa)	3.9±0.6	3.9±0.7	4.1±0.4	4.2±0.5
PaO_2 (kPa)	33.0±12.0	33.0±12.0	39.0±17.0	39.0±9.0
Temperature (°C)	36.7±0.9	36.9±1.1	36.1±0.9	36.0±0.6
ICP (mmHg)	9.5±6.8	17.6±10.8*#	8.3±7.3	16.5±5.7*
CPP (mmHg)	55.0±9.0	48.0±10.0	63.0±8.0	55.0±11.0*

*$P<0.05$ significant difference from propofol, supine position
#Significant difference from isoflurane, supine position

Table 20.4 Tension of dura and degree of cerebral swelling. Anaesthesia and position are indicated

	Isoflurane/ supine	Isoflurane/ prone	Propofol/ supine	Propofol/ prone
Tension of dura				
Normal	8	2	9	5
Increased	4	3	2	6
Pronounced increased	2	3	0	4
Degree of swelling				
No swelling	8	2	9	3
Moderate swelling	4	2	2	7
Pronounced swelling	2	4	1	4

Conclusion In children with space-occupying lesions subdural ICP is significantly higher and the degree of cerebral swelling after opening of dura significantly more pronounced in the prone-positioned compared with the supine-positioned children. In this study choice of anaesthesia did not significantly influence the level of ICP, but CPP was significantly lower in isoflurane-nitrous oxide-anaesthetized children.

Study 2: Effect of Reverse Trendelenburg Position on Subdural Intracranial Pressure in Children During Craniotomy

Aim To study the effects of 5° and 10° rTp in children subjected to craniotomy.

Method In 9 children, with cerebral tumour (n=8) or cerebral abscess (n=1), subdural ICP was measured in the neutral supine position, 5° rTp and 10° rTp.

Table 20.5 Subdural ICP and CPP during change in position from neutral to 5° rTp and 10° rTp

Patient number	Age (years)	ICP Neutral (mmHg)	5° rTp (mmHg)	10° rTp (mmHg)	CPP Neutral (mmHg)	5° rTp (mmHg)	10° rTp (mmHg)
1	2	2	1	1	54	59	51
2	2	9	7	6	52	51	52
3	8	2	0	−2	58	55	59
4	1	4	3	2	55	55	54
5	14	17	13	11	68	68	70
6	10	40	26	25	18	34	34
7	6	14	11	9	58	53	51
8	12	8	5	4	70	69	69
Median	7	8.5	6.0*	5.0*	56.5	55	53
Range	1–14	2–40	0–26	−2 to 25	18–70	34–69	34–70

*P<0.05 significant change compared with the preceding values

The time interval between each measurement was 1–2 min. Simultaneously, MABP was monitored and CPP was calculated as the difference between MABP and subdural ICP.

Statistical analysis Median and range were calculated. Wilcoxon's test was used to assess difference in values. $P<0.05$ was considered significant.

Results The median values decreased significantly between each change in position from neutral via 5° rTp to 10° rTp, the three values being 8.5, 6.0 and 5.0 mmHg. The changes in CPP were not significant (Table 20.5).

Conclusions In children with cerebral tumours, reverse Trendelenburg effectively reduces subdural ICP without significant change in CPP.

Discussion

In the first study it was demonstrated that subdural ICP and the degree of cerebral swelling after opening of dura were significantly more pronounced in children subjected to infratentorial surgery in the prone position, compared with children operated on in the supine position for supratentorial lesions. The difference in subdural ICP was not related to the level of $PaCO_2$, blood pressure or tumour size.

The volume of the infratentorial compartment is considerably smaller than the supratentorial compartment. As a consequence, space-occupying lesions in the posterior fossa might increase ICP more, compared with supratentorial space-occupying lesions of the same size. To our knowledge studies of ICP and CPP during infra- and supratentorial craniotomy are few. In adult patients with cerebral tumours subdural ICP was significantly higher in prone-positioned patients with infratentorial lesions (Tankisi et al. 2002) compared with supine-positioned patients with supratentorial lesions (Tankisi and Cold 2007), and a higher ICP in the prone position compared with the supine position has also been demonstrated in patients with severe head injury (Lee 1989). In the prone-positioned patients the head is rotated downwards in order to gain acceptable surgical access. As a consequence the pressure in the intracerebral venous system is increased, the reason being the hydrostatic difference between the central and the cerebral venous system. Moreover, in the adult patient with acute lung injury the prone position results in an increase in abdominal pressure (Hering et al. 2001), and in experimental studies it has been demonstrated that an increase in intraabdominal pressure during insufflation augments ICP (Halverson et al. 1998; Rosenthal et al. 1998).

In the adult patient with supratentorial cerebral tumours subdural ICP is significantly higher with isoflurane-propofol compared with propofol-fentanyl (Petersen et al. 2003). This finding is supported by studies in rabbits with brain tumour, indicating that CBF as well as CBV are significantly greater during isoflurane than with propofol anaesthesia (Cenic et al. 2002). To our knowledge comparative studies of ICP in isoflurane-fentanyl- compared with propofol-fentanyl-anaesthetized children are not available. A dose-related increase in ICP, however, has been demonstrated in children when isoflurane concentration was changed from 0.5 to 1.0 MAC, and in the same study ICP averaged 6 and 7 mm Hg, respectively (Sponheim et al. 2003). In contrast, increasing propofol infusion rates stabilize flow velocity at a low level in children (Karsli et al. 2002). Nitrous oxide also contributes to changes in ICP. Thus, addition of nitrous oxide to inhalation anaesthetics increases flow velocity in children (Sponheim et al. 2003) and increases ICP in patients with intracranial disorders (Henriksen et al. 1973). Other differences between the two anaesthetic regimes include preserved CO_2 reactivity in children during isoflurane and sevoflurane anaesthesia (Rowney et al. 2004), while the CO_2 reactivity is decreased during hypocapnic propofol anaesthesia (Leon and Bissonnette 1991). In the present study the mean values of subdural ICP were lower during propofol anaesthesia, compared with isoflurane anaesthesia, but the difference in pressures did not reach a significant level. This finding is surprising, the reasons being that the sample sizes were too small, combined with the small differences in subdural ICP and the relatively high SD. However, another reason might be that the pressure/volume relationship in children is different from adults because of the smaller intracranial volume and the compliancy of the cranial vault. Thus, changes in cerebral vascular resistance caused by anaesthetics might give rise to smaller changes in subdural ICP. Moreover, the present study was not controlled and randomized to the two anaesthetic procedures. Only a randomized controlled study might resolve this issue.

In many patients relatively low CPP values were observed in the present studies. In some patients the low CPP were related to the size of the space-occupying lesions. It is important, however, to emphasize that MABP is age and gender dependent, with relatively low values compared with adults (Jackson et al. 2007; Haque and Zaritsky 2007).

In the second study it was demonstrated that 5° and 10° rTp significantly reduced subdural ICP without significant change in CPP. These findings are in agreement with studies in adult patients with cerebral tumour in the supine (Haure et al. 2003, Tankisi and Cold 2007) and the prone positions (Tankisi et al. 2002), and in patients with cerebral aneurysm (Tankisi et al. 2006).

References

Bundgaard H, Landsfeldt U, Cold GE (1998) Subdural monitoring of ICP during craniotomy: thresholds of cerebral swelling/herniation. Acta Neurochir Suppl 71:276–278

Cenic A, Craen RA, Lee TY (2002) Cerebral blood volume and blood flow responses to hyperventilation in brain tumours during isoflurane or propofol anesthesia. Anesth Analg 94:661–666

Cold GE, Tange M, Jensen TM (1996) Subdural pressure measurement during craniotomy: correlation with tactile estimation of dural tension and brain herniation after opening of dura. Br J Neurosurg 10:69–75

Halverson A, Buchanan R, Jacobs L et al (1998) Evaluation of mechanism of increased intracranial pressure with insufflation. Surg Endosc 12:266–269

Haque IU, Zaritsky AL (2007) Analysis of the evidence for the lower limit of systolic and mean arterial pressure in children. Pediatr Crit Care Med 8:138–144

Haure P, Cold GE. Hansen TM (2003) The ICP-lowering effect of 10° reverse Trendelenburg position during craniotomy is stable during a 10-minute period. J Neurosurg Anesthesiol 15:297–301

Henriksen HT, Balslev Jørgensen P (1973) The effect of nitrous oxide on intracranial pressure in patients with intracranial disorders. Br J Anaesth 45:486–492

Hering R, Wrigge H, Vorwerk R et al (2001) The effect of prone positioning on intraabdominal pressure and cardiovascular and renal function in patients with acute lung injury. Anest Analg 92:1226–1231

Jackson LV, Thalange NK, Cole TJ (2007) Blood pressure centiles for Great Britain. Arch Dis Child 92:288–290

Jørgensen HA, Bundgaard H, Cold GE (1999) Subdural pressure measurement during posterior fossa surgery. Correlation studies of brain swelling/herniation and dural incision with measurement of subdural pressure and tactile estimation of dural tension. Br J Neurosurg 13:449–453

Karsli C, Luginbuehl I, Farrar M (2002) Propofol decreases cerebral blood flow velocity in anesthetized children. Can J Anaesth 49:830–834

Lee ST (1989) Intracranial pressure changes during positioning of patients with severe head injury. Heart Lung 18:411–414

Leon JE, Bissonnette B (1991) Cerebrovascular responses to carbon dioxide in children anaesthetized with halothane and isoflurane. Can J Anaesth 38:805–808

Petersen KD, Landsfeldt U, Cold GE et al (2003) Intracranial pressure and cerebral hemodynamic in patients with cerebral tumours. Anesthesiology 98:329–336

Rasmussen M, Bundgaard H, Cold GE (2004) Craniotomy for supratentorial brain tumours: risk factors for brain swelling after opening of dura. J Neurosurg 101:621–626

Rosenthal RJ, Friedman RL, Chidambaram A et al (1998) Effect of hyperventilation and hypoventilation on $PaCO_2$ and intracranial pressure during acute elevation of intraabdominal pressure with CO_2 pneumoperitoneum: large animal observations. J Am Coll Surg 187:32–38

Rowney DA, Fairgrieve R, Bissonnette B (2004) The effect of nitrous oxide on cerebral blood velocity in children anesthetized with sevoflurane. Anaesthesia 59:10–14

Sponheim S, Skraastad O, Helseth E et al (2003) Effects of 0.5 and 1.0 MAC isoflurane, sevoflurane and desflurane on intracranial and cerebral perfusion pressures in children. Acta Anaesthesiol Scand 47:932–938

Stilling M, Karatasi E, Rasmussen M (2005) Subdural intracranial pressure, cerebral perfusion pressure, and degree of cerebral swelling in supra- and infratentorial space-occupying lesions in children. Acta Neurochir Suppl 95:133–136

Tankisi A, Cold GE (2007) Optimal reverse Trendelenburg position in patients undergoing craniotomy for cerebral tumours. J Neurosurg 106:239–244

Tankisi A, Rolighed Larsen J, Rasmussen M et al (2002) The effect of 10 degrees reverse Trendelenburg position on ICP and CPP in prone positioned patients subjected to craniotomy for occipital or cerebellar tumours. Acta Neurochir 144:665–670

Tankisi A, Rasmussen M, Juul N et al (2006) The effects of 10° reverse Trendelenburg position on subdural intracranial pressure and cerebral perfusion pressure in patients subjected to craniotomy for cerebral aneurysm. J Neurosurg Anesthesiol 18:11–17

Chapter 21
Subdural Spinal Pressure During Surgery for Intradural Tumours and Surgery for Tethered Cord

Georg Emil Cold, Claus Mosdal and Niels Juul

Abstract

To our knowledge studies of subdural spinal pressure during spinal surgery have never been performed. Knowledge of the spinal subdural pressure could be of importance for the surgeon when resecting intradural tumour masses from the spine. Additionally it could be of interest for the team treating the patient with a spinal mass to gain knowledge of the pressure both cranial and caudal to the tumour.

In this chapter a study of the measurements of spinal subdural pressure was performed before opening of dura in patients subjected to spinal surgery for intradural tumour or tethered cord. Measurements were performed cranially and caudally to the tumour (if present) and the effect of hyperventilation and positive end-expiratory pressure on spinal subdural pressure studied.

To our knowledge studies of subdural spinal pressure during spinal surgery have never been performed. Knowledge of the spinal subdural pressure could be of importance for the surgeon when resecting intradural tumour masses from the spine. Additionally could it be of interest for the team treating the patient with a spinal mass to gain knowledge of the pressure both cranial and caudal to the tumour. In this study measurements of spinal subdural pressure (SSP) were performed before opening of dura in patients subjected to spinal surgery for intradural tumour or tethered cord.

Study Outline

Aims 1: To measure SSP and spinal perfusion pressure (SPP) in patients subjected to spinal surgery. 2: To study the effect of hyperventilation on SSP. 3: To study the effect of PEEP on SSP.

Method In 18 patients, 12 patients with spinal tumour and 6 patients with tethered cord, SSP and MABP were measured. SPP was calculated as the difference between MABP and SSP. Simultaneously, arterial blood was analysed for $PaCO_2$, PaO_2 and pH. The measurements were performed during general anaesthesia with the patient in the prone position. In 10 patients with spinal cord tumour SSP was measured cranially and caudally to the tumour. None of the patients had a complete block of CSF flow. The effect of 5 min hyperventilation on SSP and SPP were studied in 17 patients (12 patients with spinal tumour and 5 patients with tethered cord). In 11 patients with spinal tumour and 6 patients with tethered cord, 10 cm PEEP was applied for a period of 2 min.

Statistical analysis Medians and ranges are indicated. Wilcoxon's test was used for analysing intragroup differences, and the Mann-Whitney test was used for intergroup statistics. $P<0.05$ was considered significant.

Results In the neutral position of the operating table median SSP was 10 (4–17) mmHg in patients with spinal tumour and 8 (0–10) mmHg in patients with tethered cord. In 7 patients with spinal tumour, regional differences between cranial and caudal SSP were recorded with a difference in median of 5.5 (3–15) mmHg. A tendency was observed, indicating that the difference between pressures measured cranially and caudally to the tumour was positive when the tumour was placed cranially in the neuroaxis, and vice versa (Table 21.1). During hyperventilation $PaCO_2$ decreased from median 4.5 to 3.8 kPa. No significant change in SSP or SPP was observed (Table 21.2). In all groups, 10 cm PEEP increased SSP, and in the total number of patients PEEP increased SSP significantly from median 10 to 11 mmHg. Simultaneously, a significant decrease in SPP from median 57 to 52 mmHg was observed, $P<0.001$ (Table 21.3).

Table 21.1 Patients in whom SSP was measured cranially as well as caudally to the tumour. Tumour localization is indicated. Difference in SSP is calculated as the difference between SSP cranial and caudal to the tumour

Patient number	Tumour localization	Cranial spinal pressure (mmHg)	Caudal spinal pressure (mmHg)	Difference in pressure (mmHg)
1	C3–4	17	10	7
2	C6–7	9	12	−3
3	C7–T1	12	6	6
4	T3–4	9	4	5
5	T8	14	11	3
6	T10–11	15	8	7
7	T10	3	8	−5
8	T11–L1	2	6	−4
9	T12	4	19	−15
10	L2	9	15	−6
Median		9	9	5.5
Range		(2–17)	(4–19)	(−15 to 7)

Table 21.2 The effect of 5 min hyperventilation on $PaCO_2$, SSP and SPP in patients with spinal tumour and tethered cord. Median and range are indicated. Group 1: spinal tumour, SSP measured cranial to tumour (n=6). Group 2: spinal tumour, SSP measured caudal to tumour (n=6). Group 3: tethered cord (n=5). Group 4: tumour and tethered cord (n=17)

Group	$PaCO_2$ before (kPa)	$PaCO_2$ after (kPa)	SSP before (mmHg)	SSP after (mmHg)	SPP before (mmHg)	SPP after (mmHg)
1	4.6 (4.3–5.4)	3.9* (3.7–4.4)	6.0 (2.0–8.0)	4.0 (1.0–10.0)	68.5 (37.0–89.0)	69.0 (36.0–89.0.)
2	4.6 (4.2–5.4)	3.8* (3.5–4.4)	7.0 (4.0–21.0)	6.0 (3.0–19.0)	62.0 (54.0–86.0)	64.0 (50.0–84.0)
3	4.3 (4.1–4.7)	3.7* (3.5–4.0)	10.0 (0.0–12.0)	10.0 (−1.0 to 10.0)	50.0 (47.0–57.0)	54.0 (46.0–67.0)
4	4.5 (4.1–5.4)	3.8* (3.5–4.4)	8.0 (0.0–21.0)	7.0 (−1.0 to 19.0)	59.0 (37.0–89.0)	64.0 (36.0–89.0)

*P<0.05

Table 21.3 The effect of 10 cm PEEP on $PaCO_2$, SSP and SPP in patients with spinal tumour or tethered cord. The measurements are recorded immediately before and 2 min after 10 cmH_2O PEEP application. Median and range are indicated. Group 1: spinal tumour, SSP measured cranial to tumour (n=7). Group 2: spinal tumour, SSP measured caudal to tumour (n=4). Group 3: tethered cord (n=6). Group 4: tumour and tethered cord (n=17)

Group	$PaCO_2$ before PEEP (kPa)	$PaCO_2$ after PEEP (kPa)	SSP before PEEP (mmHg)	SSP after PEEP (mmHg)	SPP before PEEP (mmHg)	SPP after PEEP (mmHg)
1	4.4 (4.1–4.6)	4.40 (4.1–4.6)	10.0 (0.0–15.0)	11.0* (5.0–15.0)	59.0 (37.0–76.0)	58.0 (38.0–75.0)
2	4.3 (4.1–4.5)	4.30 (4.1–4.5)	14.0 (6.0–19.0)	15.5 (8.0–22.0)	61.5 (38.0–79.0)	58.0 (39.0–78.0)
3	4.4 (4.1–4.8)	4.45 (4.1–4.8)	8.5 (0.0–12.0)	10.0* (1.0–13.0)	51.0 (37.0–61.0)	49.0 (38.0–56.0)
4	4.4 (4.1–4.8)	4.40 (4.1–4.8)	10.0 (0.0–19.0)	11.0* (1.0–22.0)	57.0 (37.0–79.0)	52.0* (38.0–78.0)

*P<0.05

Conclusion During surgery SSP can be measured accurately. PEEP application significantly increases spinal pressure and reduces SPP. Hyperventilation decreases spinal pressure and increases SPP, but these changes are small. Regional differences in SSP were observed in patients with intradural spinal cord tumour.

Discussion

In the study on the effect of hyperventilation it was demonstrated that hyperventilation did not change SSP significantly. As the effect of hyperventilation is based on vasoconstriction, this finding must be related to experimental and clinical studies of spinal cord blood flow (SBF) and metabolism and its regulation, and the loss of an SSP-reducing effect might be discussed in relation to experimental and clinical data.

In the rat $CMRO_2$ averaged 3.5 ml/100 g/min in the grey matter and 1.0 ml/100 g/min in the white matter. These values are independent of spinal level (Hayashi 1984). With the hydrogen method SBF averages 64.5 and 20.4 ml/100 g/min in the rat grey and white matter, respectively. This difference corresponds to the increased density of the vascular bed in the grey matter (Jellinger 1974). While the blood flow in the white matter differs very little, the blood flow in the grey matter ranges from 39.6 to 79.4 ml. SBF, however, is independent of whether it is measured in the cervical, thoracic or lumbar segment (Hayashi 1984). Immediately after spinal cord injury a marked reduction of blood flow in the lesioned region occurs (Bingham et al. 1975; Kobrine et al. 1975; Griffiths 1976; Senter and Venes 1978; Fehlings et al. 1989; Tator and Fehlings 1991). Thoracic spinal cord ischaemia was induced by inflation of a balloon in aorta in cats. After spinal ischaemia regional SBF increased as much as 2 times the control values and decreased gradually thereafter. After 10 min of balloon occlusion, regional SBF returned to control value. After 30 min of occlusion hypoperfusion after recirculation correlated with irreversible amplitude changes in evoked spinal cord potential, and postischaemic paraparesis and pathological ischaemic changes in the spinal segments were recognized (Yamada et al. 1998).

In experimental studies autoregulation of SBF has been demonstrated (Flohr et al. 1971; Kindt 1971; Kindt et al. 1971; Kobrine and Doyle 1975; Kobrine et al. 1976a, b; Marcus et al. 1977; Hickey et al. 1986). Intact autoregulation has also been confirmed in human studies (Wullenweber 1967). In the monkey regional SBF remains constant in the normal range of MABP of 50 to 135 mmHg. Above MABP of 135 mmHg vasodilatation occurs, resulting in breakthrough of autoregulation (Kobrine et al. 1976b).

Spinal cord blood flow increases with hypercapnia and hypoxaemia, and it decreases with hypocapnia (Wullenweber 1967). When SBF and CBF are compared, the absolute change in SBF per unit CO_2 change is less than the change in CBF, but because SBF is lower the percentage changes in SBF and CBF are the same.

After reversible spinal cord ischaemia in the rat, marked hyperaemia was seen for the first 15 min, followed by hypoperfusion at 60 min. The CO_2 reactivity was completely absent at 60 min (Marsala et al. 1994).

In the present study, the loss of SSP-reducing effect was not related to autoregulatory mechanisms, because the period with hyperventilation was not accompanied by significant changes in blood pressure or SPP. Although it has been demonstrated that the CO_2 reactivity may be absent following trauma or ischaemia of the spinal cord, this explanation for the absent SSP-reducing effect seems unlikely because the tumour process in the majority of patients was localized to a few segments, leaving the intracranial as well as the functioning part of spinal cord compartments without pathological changes. In four patients a convincing ICP-reducing effect was found. ICP was unchanged in seven patients, while an increase in pressure was observed in three patients. This pattern was not related to the level of spinal pressure measured before hyperventilation, which otherwise might influence an expected SSP-reducing effect caused by the volume/pressure relationship. However, in contrast to the intracranial volume/pressure relationship, where a small reduction in volume elicits a considerably greater ICP reduction at high levels of ICP compared with low levels of ICP, experimental or clinical studies concerning the volume/pressure relationship in the spinal compartment are not available. However, it seems reasonable to hypothesize that the volume/pressure relationship obtained from spinal segments during operation, if present at all, is flat. The operative decompression of the spinal channel also is supposed to constrain any effect of volume-elicited pressure change. Furthermore, it is supposed that the high respirator peak and mean pressures during hyperventilation might impede venous return, increase intraabdominal pressure, dilate the epidural venous vessels and counteract any pressure-reducing effect of hyperventilation. Taking these factors into consideration, changes in spinal blood volume caused by hyperventilation-induced spinal vasoconstriction is not supposed to have a significant effect on SSP.

It has been demonstrated that the application of PEEP prevents the development of pulmonary atelectasis (Hedenstierna et al. 2000). As regards the effect of PEEP on the ICP, Mascia et al. (2005) elevated PEEP to 5 and 10 cmH_2O in patients with head injury, and showed that patients who achieved lung recruitment showed no increase in $PaCO_2$ and ICP remained stable. However, in non-recruiters alveolar hyperinflation occurred, and $PaCO_2$ increased with the consequence of an increase in ICP. These findings are in accordance with studies in patients with SAH (Caricato et al. 2005). McGuire et al. (1997) showed, in patients, that PEEP increased ICP when the applied PEEP was higher than the baseline ICP, but had less effect if the applied PEEP was lower than the ICP. In our study the baseline ICP was 5.7 and 5.1 mmHg in the two groups. So in the group where 10 cmH_2O PEEP was applied the PEEP was higher than the ICP and this may explain why the change in ICP in this group was more pronounced. Thus, it can be concluded that in the intensive care setting ICP is not affected by PEEP when a significant alveolar recruitment is achieved with PEEP, while patients who showed no increase in lung volumes had an increase in $PaCO_2$ resulting in a rise in CBF and an elevated ICP.

In the present study 10 cmH_2O PEEP application resulted in a significant increase in spinal pressure from 10 to 11 mmHg. The increase in SSP was not related to changes in $PaCO_2$, but a decrease in SPP averaging 5 mmHg was found when all studies were included. In cannot be excluded that autoregulatory vasodilatation occurred caused by the decrease in perfusion pressure, resulting in the detectable increase in SSP. Furthermore, it is supposed that the high respirator peak and mean pressures during PEEP application impedes venous return, increases intraabdominal pressure and dilates the epidural venous vessels, resulting in an increase in SSP.

References

Bingham WG, Goldman H, Friedman SJ et al (1975) Blood flow in normal and injured monkey spinal cord. J Neurosurg 43:162–171

Caricato A, Conti G, Della Corte F et al (2005) Effects of PEEP on the intracranial system of patients with head injury and subarachnoid hemorrhage: the role of respiratory system compliance. J Trauma 58:571–576

Fehlings MG, Tator CH, Linden RD (1989) The effect of nimodipine and dextran on axonal function and blood flow following experimental spinal cord injury. J Neurosurg 71:403–416

Flohr H, Pöll W, Brock M (1971) Regulation of spinal cord blood flow. In: Russell RWR (ed) Brain and blood flow. Pitman, London, pp 406–409

Griffiths IR (1976) Spinal cord blood flow after acute experimental cord injury in dogs. J Neurol Sci 27:247–259

Hayashi N (1984) Local spinal cord blood flow and oxygen metabolism. In: Davidoff RA (ed) Handbook of the spinal cord. Dekker, New York, pp 817–830

Hedenstierna G, Rothen HU (2000) Atelectasis formation during anesthesia: causes and measures to prevent it. J Clin Monit Comput 16:329–335

Hickey R, Albin MS, Bunegin L et al (1986) Autoregulation of spinal cord blood flow: Is the cord a microcosm of the brain? Stroke 17:1183–1189

Jellinger K (1974) Comparative studies of spinal cord vasculature. In: Cervos Nervarro J (ed) Pathology of cerebral microcirculation. de Gruyter, Berlin, pp 45–58

Kindt GW (1971) Autoregulation of spinal cord blood flow. Eur Neurol 6:19–23

Kindt GW, Ducker TB, Huddlestone J (1971) Regulation of spinal cord blood flow. In: Russell RWR (ed) Brain and blood flow. Pitman, London, pp 401–409

Kobrine AI, Doyle TF (1975) Physiology of spinal cord blood flow. In: Harper AM et al (eds) Blood flow and metabolism in the brain. Churchill Livingstone, Edinburgh, pp 4.16–4.19

Kobrine AI, Doyle TF, Martins AN (1975) Local spinal cord blood flow in experimental traumatic myelopathy. J Neurosurg 42:144–149

Kobrine AI, Doyle TF, Newby N et al (1976a) Preserved autoregulation in the rhesus spinal cord after high cervical cord section. J Neurosurg 44:425–428

Kobrine AI, Doyle TF, Rizzoli H (1976b) Spinal cord blood flow as affected by changes in systemic arterial blood pressure. J Neurosurg 44:12–15

Marcus ML, Heistad DD, Ehrhardt JC et al (1977) Regulation of total and regional spinal cord blood flow. Circ Res 41:128–134

Marsala M, Sorkin LS, Yaksh TL (1994) Transient spinal ischemia in rat: characterization of spinal cord blood flow, extracellular amino acid release, and concurrent histopathological damage. J Cereb Blood Flow Metab 14:604–614

Mascia L, Grasso S, Fiore T et al (2005) Cerebro-pulmonary interactions during the application of low levels of positive end-expiratory pressure. Intensive Care Med 31:373–379

McGuire G, Crossley D, Richards J (1997) Effects of varying levels of positive end-expiratory pressure on intracranial pressure and cerebral perfusion pressure. Crit Care Med 25:1059–1062

Senter HJ, Venes JL (1978) Altered blood flow and secondary injury in experimental spinal cord trauma. J Neurosurg 49:569–578

Tator CH, Fehlings MG (1991) Review of the secondary injury theory of acute spinal cord trauma with emphasis on vascular mechanisms. J Neurosurg 75:15–26

Wullenweber R (1967) First results of measurements of local spinal blood flow in man by means of heat clearance. In: Bain WH, Harper AM (eds) Blood flow through organs and tissues. Williams & Wilkins, Baltimore, pp 176–183

Yamada T, Morimoto T, Nakase H et al (1998) Spinal cord blood flow and pathophysiological changes after transient spinal cord ischemia in cats. Neurosurgery 42:626–634

Chapter 22
Studies of Jugular Pressure

Georg Emil Cold and Niels Juul

Abstract

It is well known that neck compression increases jugular venous pressure cranial to the compression and consequently ICP. Thus, the Queckenstedt manoeuvre, bilateral neck compression and coughing inevitably result in an increase in ICP. In contrast, clinical studies, including patients with space-occupying cerebral processes, have demonstrated that elevation of the head results in a decrease in ICP, while the head down position results in an increase in ICP. To what extent, however, rotation of the head results in changes in jugular venous pressure is sparsely investigated.

In this chapter the results of two studies of jugular pressure and the effect of neck movement, and the influence of the sitting position with either anti-G-suit or application of positive end-expiratory pressure are presented.

It is well known that neck compression increases jugular venous pressure to the compression, and consequently ICP. Thus, the Queckenstedt manoeuvre, bilateral neck compression and coughing inevitably result in an increase in ICP. In contrast, clinical studies, including patients with space-occupying cerebral processes, have demonstrated that elevation of the head results in a decrease in ICP (Hulme and Cooper 1976; Kenning et al. 1981; Ropper and Coley 1982; Goldberg et al. 1983; Rosner and Coley 1986; Feldman et al. 1992; Schneider et al. 1993; Yoshida et al. 1993), while the head down position results in an increase in ICP (Lee 1989; Mavrocordatos et al. 2000). A decrease in ICP is also observed during craniotomy when the position is changed from neutral to the rTp in patients with cerebral tumours (Rolighed Larsen 2002; Tankisi et al. 2002; Haure et al. 2003; Tankisi and Cold 2007) and patients with aneurysms (Tankisi et al. 2006). To what extent, however, rotation of the head results in changes in JBP is sparsely investigated.

Surgical assess for operation in the posterior fossa and control of haemorrhage are facilitated in the sitting position. Well-known risks of the sitting position include venous air embolism and postural hypotension. The risk of hypotension is decreased by assuring adequate intravascular volume before the change in position and by applying a pneumatic anti-G-suit to prevent peripheral pooling in the lower extremities. A pressure gradient of $5\,cmH_2O$ between the upper pole of the wound and the right atrium is sufficient to allow air to pass into the venous system (Albin et al. 1983). The risk of air embolism is supposed to be even greater if the pressure in the venous system is negative in comparison with atmospheric pressure (Engelhardt et al. 2006).

In this chapter the results of two studies of jugular pressure and the effect of neck movement and the influence of the sitting position with either anti-G-suit or application of PEEP are presented.

Study 1: Neck Compression and Jugular Bulb Pressure in Patients Subjected to Craniotomy

Aim   To study the influence of the degree of head rotation on JBP in patients subjected to craniotomy.

Patients and method   Thirteen patients subjected to elective craniotomy were included in the study. After induction of anaesthesia with propofol-fentanyl a jugular catheter was introduced percutaneously using the principles described in Chapter 3. Zero-point adjustment was performed with the transducer placed at the external auditory meatus. After 5 min of stabilization the JBP and MABP were measured over a period of 1 min with the head in the neutral position. Following this procedure the JBP and MABP were measured after change in head position according to the following procedure: (1) 1 min after 45° neck rotation to the ipsilateral side; (2) 1 min after maximal rotation of the head to the ipsilateral side of the catheter; (3) 1 min after 45° neck rotation to the contralateral side of the catheter; (4) 1 min after maximal rotation of the neck to the contralateral side of the catheter; and (5) after 10 s of bilateral neck compression. Before, between and after change in head position the bulb pressure was measured with the head in the neutral position. From the basal preoperative CT scans corrections caused by displacement of the tip of the catheter placed in the jugular bulb during the neck-rotation procedures were performed.

Statistical analysis   Median and ranges were calculated. For statistical analysis Wilcoxon's signed rank test and Pearson's product moment correlation were used. $P<0.01$ was considered significant.

Results   No significant differences in end-tidal CO_2 were disclosed during the procedures. MABP decreased from median 81 (66–120) mmHg to 64 (58–93) mmHg).

In Table 22.1 the corrected values of bulb pressures in 13 patients are indicated during the different procedures. During 45° neck rotation to the ipsilateral and the contralateral side of the catheter the bulb pressures were unchanged. Maximal rotation of the neck to the ipsilateral side resulted in an increase in bulb pressure from 10.0 to 15.0 mmHg on both sides ($P<0.01$). During bilateral neck compression the bulb pressure increased from 10 to 19 mmHg ($P<0.01$). As indicated the increase in bulb pressure is modest at 45° rotation, but increases considerably during maximal rotation and during bilateral neck compression (Table 22.1).

A positive significant correlation was found between body mass index (BMI) (weight (kg)/height (m^2)) of the patients and difference in bulb pressure measured before and after bilateral neck compression (difference in bulb pressure (mmHg) = $-7.43 + 0.633 \times$ BMI, $r = 0.664$, $P = 0.013$), and BMI and increase in bulb pressure during maximal ipsilateral neck rotation (difference in bulb pressure (mmHg) = $-13.1 + 0.820 \times$ BMI, $r = 0.724$, $P = 0.005$).

Conclusion The study demonstrates significant changes in bulb pressure caused by maximal neck rotation and neck compression; 45° rotation of the head, however, can safely be used during positioning of the head, as it hardly increases bulb pressure. A positive significant correlation between the BMI of the patients and the increase in bulb pressure during maximal ipsilateral rotation and during bilateral neck compression suggest that even 45° neck rotation might be critical in overweight patients.

Table 22.1 Change in JBP (mmHg) during rotation of the neck and bilateral neck compression

Patient number	Neutral position	45° rotation against catheter	Maximal rotation against catheter	45° rotation opposite to the catheter	Maximal rotation opposite to the catheter	Bilateral neck compression	Neutral position
1	10	10	10	10	10	15	10
2	11	12	16	14	16	21	12
3	9	10	11	10	13	17	9
4	5	5	28	6	26	28	5
5	13	13	16	13	16	16	12
6	14	14	14	13	13	19	14
7	10	10	15	9	16	20	9
8	7	7	15	8	13	19	8
9	17	20	26	19	27	27	16
10	12	12	14	12	15	15	12
11	3	4	11	4	10	12	4
12	7	8	13	9	14	16	6
13	9	12	17	11	18	22	10
Median	10	10	15*	10	15*	19*	10
Range	3–17	4–20	10–28	4–19	10–27	12–28	4–16

*$P<0.05$

Study 2: Studies of Jugular Bulb Pressure During Craniectomy in the Sitting Position

Aim To observe the changes in JBP when the position was changed from the supine to the sitting position, and to investigate the changes in bulb pressure after applying different combinations of anti-G-suit pressure, PEEP and applying superficial manual compression.

Patients and Method Eight adult patients with tumour in the posterior fossa, median age 44 years (range 16–61 years) underwent craniectomy in the sitting position. For anaesthesia propofol-fentanyl was used (Chapter 3). Intravenous fluid was administered in accordance with our standard (Chapter 3), but besides the standard treatment 500 ml 5% dextran in saline was given intravenously. An arterial line for measurement of MABP and a jugular bulb catheter were inserted. In the supine position, the middle axillary line was used as zero reference. In the sitting position both transducers were placed with the external auditory meatus as zero reference. A Doppler ultrasonic device for detection of air embolism was placed on the chest to the right of the sternum between the third and sixth intercostal space.

Bulb pressure and MABP were measured under the following conditions: (1) in the supine position; (2) after change to the sitting position with anti-G-suit pressure of 20 mmHg; (3) during application of PEEP (5, 10 and 15 cmH$_2$O) with anti-G-suit pressure of 20 mmHg; (4) during anti-G-suit pressures of 10, 20 and 30 mmHg; (5) during application of superficial manual neck compression for 30–60 s with anti-G-suit pressure of 20 mmHg, without PEEP and at PEEP of 5 and 10 cm H$_2$O. Between each measurement 3–4 min was used for stabilization.

Statistical analysis The results are presented as median and range. Wilcoxon's non-parametric rank sum test was used for intergroup analysis, and $P<0.05$ was considered significant.

Table 22.2 JBP (mmHg) in the supine and sitting position. Anti-G-suit pressure of 20 cmH$_2$O was applied during the study

Patient number	Supine position (mmHg)	Sitting position (mmHg)
1	15	−4
2	12	4
3	15	−6
4	1	−18
5	7	−4
6	4	−4
7	9	1
8	12	0
Median	11	−4*
Range	1–15	−18 to 1

*$P<0.05$

Results The medians and ranges of $PaCO_2$ and PaO_2 in the sitting position were 3.8 (3.7–4.5) kPa and 33 (23–48) kPa, respectively. In Table 22.2 the bulb pressures in the supine and the sitting position are indicated. In the supine position the median (range) were 11 (1–15) mmHg and in the sitting position −4 (−18 to 4) mmHg ($P<0.05$). The bulb pressures during PEEP application are indicated in Table 22.3. While the bulb pressures were unchanged at PEEP applications from zero to 10 cmH_2O, application of 15 cmH_2O was accompanied by a significant increase in bulb pressure from median values of −4 mmHg without PEEP to −1 mmHg during 15 cmH_2O PEEP ($P<0.05$). In Table 22.4 the effect of increasing anti-G-suit pressures from 10 to 20 to 30 mmHg on bulb pressure are indicated. No significant changes in bulb pressure occurred. In Table 22.5 the results of PEEP application combined with bilateral neck compression are indicated. Neck compression increased

Table 22.3 Jugular pressure in the sitting position without PEEP and after application of PEEP (5, 10 and 15 cmH_2O). Anti-G-suit pressure of 20 cmH_2O was applied during the study

Patient number	Zero PEEP	5 cmH_2O	10 cmH_2O	15 cmH_2O
1	−4	−3	−2	−1
2	4	4	4	4
3	−4	−6	−5	−5
4	−18	−16	−15	−12
5	−4	−3	−2	−1
6	−4	−3	−2	−1
7	1	2	1	5
8	0	1	2	2
Median	−4	−3	−2	−1*
Range	−18 to 4	−16 to 4	−15 to 4	−12 to 5

*$P<0.05$

Table 22.4 Jugular pressure in the sitting position during application of anti-G-suit (10, 20 and 30 cmH_2O). PEEP was not applied. No significant difference was found

Patient number	10 cmH_2O	20 cmH_2O	30 cmH_2O
1	−5	−4	−4
2	4	4	4
3	−7	−6	−6
4	−17	−16	−16
5	−5	−4	−3
6	−4	−4	−4
7	4	4	4
8	0	0	1
Median	−4	−4	−3
Range	−17 to 4	−16 to 4	−16 to 4

Table 22.5 Jugular pressure without and with PEEP application (5 and 10 cmH$_2$O), and with and without manual neck compression. Anti-G-suit pressure of 20 cmH$_2$O was applied during the study

Patient number	PEEP (cmH$_2$O)/Neck compression (yes/no)					
	Zero/No	Zero/Yes	5/No	5/Yes	10/No	10/Yes
1	−4	−4	−3	−3	−2	2
2	4	10	4	10	4	12
3	−6	−2	−6	−2	−5	2
4	−18	−15	−16	−12	−15	−11
5	−4	1	−3	2	−2	4
6	−4	8	−3	8	−2	10
7	1	10	2	9	1	10
8	0	3	1	3	2	4
Median	4	2*	−3	3*	−2	4*
Range	−18 to 4	−15 to 10	−16 to 4	−12 to 10	−15 to 4	−11 to 12

*$P<0.05$ from studies performed without neck compression

bulb pressure without PEEP application and during application of 5 and 10 cmH$_2$O PEEP ($P<0.05$).

Conclusion When the position of the patient is changed from supine to sitting the jugular pressure drops significantly from median 11 to −4 mmHg. The use of an anti-G-suit does not lead to any change in jugular pressure and the application of 15 cm PEEP leads to a significant but clinically unimportant drop in jugular pressure.

Discussion

One problem, which cannot be ignored when discussing the influence of head rotation on ICP, is zero point adjustment. Whether subdural or intraventricular pressure devices are used, rotation of the head might change the position of the intracranial part of the device in relation to the externally placed transducer. With the subdural screw, correction of zero point adjustment is fairly easy. With the intraventricular catheter, however, correction after head rotation is difficult, because the correct position of the tip of the ventricular catheter cannot be determined accurately. Adjustment for change in head position generally is performed with reference to the external auditory meatus, at the level of the foramen of Monro. Zero point adjustment based on this principle is acceptable during studies of the effect of head elevation or flexion, but during head rotation erroneous ICP values occur. The problem is illustrated in several studies (Hulme and Cooper 1976; William and Coyne 1993), where the increase in ICP during head rotation differed whether the head was rotated to the right or left side. The higher pressure associated with head rotation to the right side has been explained by differences in the anatomy of the two internal jugular veins, the right being generally larger in diameter than the left. Consequently, drainage via the right jugular vein is more efficient, and right rotation of the head compresses the venous drainage system more effectively and compromises the cerebral venous outflow (Watson 1974).

In studies of neurointensive patients (William and Coyne 1993; Mavrocordatos 2000) and neonates (Goldberg et al. 1983) rotation of the head is accompanied by an increase in ICP. In these studies the degree of rotation, however, is not described. To our knowledge pressure changes in the jugular bulb during head rotation procedures have not been studied. In the present study, well-defined degrees of head rotation (neutral position, 45° head rotation, maximal rotation) were investigated. By preoperative basal CT scans the sagittal displacement of the catheter was estimated with 45° rotation and maximal rotation of the head. We found that 45° head rotation did not increase bulb pressure, but a substantial increase was observed during maximal rotation. Our findings are in agreement with experimental studies of sagittal sinus pressure in the dog, indicating that the sinus pressure was dependent on simple hydrostatic mechanisms as long as the pressure was positive. At negative pressures, however, the collapsing nature of the jugular vein prevented the sinus pressure from decreasing to the same extent (Leighton and Winston 1994). Theoretically, unilateral hypoplasia of the jugular vein might influence the effect of head rotation and unilateral neck compression. Other factors include the length and circumference of the neck. In accordance with these considerations we found that pressure change even at 45° rotation differed from patient to patient, and a significant correlation was found between the BMI and the increase in bulb pressure observed during ipsilateral neck compression. These findings indirectly suggest that the degrees of adipositas also play a role during neck rotation, possibly because compression of the veins occurs more frequently in adipose patients.

In the present study the bulb pressure in the neutral position differed considerably with median 10 mmHg and range 3–17 mmHg. This variation was not correlated to age of the patients, respiratory peak pressure or different amounts of intravenous fluid administration, and all patients were in neutral supine position on the table. Considering the theoretical impact of increased bulb pressure on ICP, optimizing of the central haemodynamics by securing adequate blood pressure and cardiac output with a minimum of central venous pressure might be of importance. One possibility is to place the patients in 10° rTp as clinical studies during craniotomy indicate that within 1 min this position instantly reduces JBP and ICP without affecting CPP, and the pressures are stable for at least 10 min after change in position (Haure et al. 2003).

The present study confirms the usefulness of JBP measurement during craniotomy. The pressure measurements give valuable information concerning risk of increased ICP due to compromised venous outflow from the intracranial compartment, and blood samples from the jugular catheter together with samples from an arterial line give information concerning the risk of cerebral ischaemia when low values of jugular blood oxygen tension/oxygen saturation or high values of the $AVDO_2$ are detected. Furthermore, measurements of the relative CO_2 reactivity and cerebral autoregulation are possible.

In skilled hands, surgery in the sitting position is a safe procedure (Standefer et al. 1984; Matjasko et al. 1985). One complication that repeatedly has been studied is the occurrence of air embolism, and especially the occurrence of paradoxical air embolism, where air may pass through a persistent foramen ovale. Persistence of foramen ovale is considered a contraindication for surgery in the sitting position (Porter et al. 1999). The incidence of a persistent foramen ovale or a right-to-left shunt in patients scheduled for surgery in the sitting position varies between 0% and 29% (Black et al. 1990; Girard et al. 2003; Domainque 2005a). The occurrence of air embolism is dependent on the diagnostic facilities, being relatively low when it is based on end-tidal CO_2 monitoring, with the incidence ranging between 9.0% and 28% (Harrison et al. 2002; Bithal et al. 2004; Leslie et al. 2006). In one study, including 579 patients undergoing posterior fossa surgery in the sitting position, it was demonstrated that air embolism occurred more frequently in the sitting position (45% versus 12%), but neither morbidity nor mortality was attributed to venous air embolism (Black et al. 1988). In other studies, the incidence of venous air embolism varied between 31% and 50% (Matjasko et al. 1985; Sørensen et al. 1990; Domainque 2005a) being highest with transoesophageal echocardiography, which is considered as today's "gold standard" (Domainque 2005b), but contrast-enhanced transcranial Doppler ultrasonography is also highly sensitive (Stendel et al. 2000). In the present study of eight patients no signs of air embolism were detected by precordial Doppler and end-tidal CO_2 monitoring. The use of PEEP, however, is controversial because the release of PEEP may be accompanied by the occurrence of air embolism and especially paradoxical venous air embolism (Black et al. 1989; Schmitt and Hemmerling 2002) and because PEEP in experimental studies (Toung et al. 1988, 2000) and clinical studies (Iwabuchi et al. 1983) does not increase cerebral venous pressure, possibly because jugular venous collapse in the sitting position serves as a resistance in the transmission of central venous pressure to the cerebral venous compartment. We believe that the adjustment of bulb pressure monitoring with sufficient intravenous plasma expander before the change to the sitting position, combined with PEEP application, anti-G-suit facility and neck compression during critical periods of surgery might contribute to the absence of air in this study. Of great importance is also the surgical technique, the alertness of the anaesthesiologist and the communication between anaesthesiologist and surgeon. As demonstrated in a number of studies, air embolism occurs predominantly early in the surgical procedure (Standefer et al. 1984), especially during stripping of the muscles and fascia (Leivers et al. 1971), drilling of the skull (Ericsson et al. 1964) and closure of the fascia layer (O'Higgins 1970). Certainly, air embolism may also occur during opening of dura, sinus lesion and removal of tumour.

We assume the pressure in the jugular bulb in the sitting position equals venous pressure in the surgical field at the same sagittal level. This assumption might be erroneous, because the venous outflow and the venous pressure in the surgical field might be influenced by retractor pressure, surgical manipulation and the occurrence of space-occupying masses. During surgical dissection without PEEP or neck compression we observed that venous vessels were constricted, and we observed application of PEEP and neck compression was followed by dilation of the venous bed.

Our results indicate that change in position from the supine to the sitting position is accompanied by a decrease in bulb pressure, which generally is negative in the sitting position. In the sitting position great variation was observed between patients, with only two of eight patients having positive bulb pressure.

The level of bulb pressure after the change to the sitting position is not correlated with the bulb pressure in the supine position. Thus, in this study it was impossible to predict bulb pressure in the sitting position from bulb pressure in the supine position. The poor correlation between supine and sitting bulb pressures might be due to differences in cardiac performance, adjustment of peripheral resistance and the occurrence of collapse of the jugular bed during head elevation.

In the prevention of venous air embolism in the sitting position, manual neck compression (Michenfelder et al. 1969; Tausk and Miller 1983), inflation of a neck tourniquet or the use of a neck tie have been recommended (Hewer and Logue 1962; Buckland and Manners 1976; Sale 1984). In the present study, it was possible to increase the bulb pressure by 5 mmHg with superficial manual neck compression. In seven out of eight patients, positive bulb pressures were obtained by this manoeuvre. This finding is in accordance with Iwabuchi et al. (1983) who demonstrated that the confluence sinus pressure elevates by jugular compression.

References

Albin MS, Babinski MF, Gilbert J et al (1983) Venous air embolism is not restricted to neurosurgery. Anesthesiology 53:151

Bithal PK, Pandia MP, Dash HH et al (2004) Comparative incidence of venous air embolism and associated hypotension in adults and children operated for neurosurgery in the sitting position. Eur J Anaesthesiol 21:517–522

Black S, Ockert DB, Oliver WC et al (1988) Outcome following posterior fossa craniectomy in patients in the sitting or horizontal position. Anesthesiology 69:49–56

Black S, Cucchiara RF, Nishimura RA et al (1989) Parameters affecting occurrence of paradoxical air embolism. Anesthesiology 71:235–241

Black S, Muzzi DA, Nishimura RA et al (1990) Preoperative and intraoperative echocardiography to detect right-to-left shunt in patients undergoing neurosurgical procedures in the sitting position. Anesthesiology 72:436–438

Buckland EW, Manners JM (1976) Venous air embolism during neurosurgery. Anaesthesia 31:633–643

Domainque CM (2005a) Neurosurgery in the sitting position: a case series. Anaesth Intensive Care 33:332–335

Domainque CM (2005b) Anaesthesia for neurosurgery in the sitting position: a practical approach. Anaesth Intensive Care 33:323–331

Engelhardt M, Folkers W, Brenke C et al (2006) Neurosurgical operations with the patients in sitting position: analysis of risk factors using transcranial Doppler sonography. Br J Anaesth 96:467–472

Ericsson JA, Gottlieb JD, Sweet RB (1964) Closed chest massage in the treatment of venous air embolism. N Engl J Med 270:1353–1354

Feldman Z, Kanter M, Robertson CS et al (1992) Effect of head elevation in intracranial pressure, cerebral perfusion pressure, and cerebral blood flow in head-injured patients. J Neurosurg 76:207–211

Girard F, Ruel M, McKenty S et al (2003) Incidences of venous air embolism and patent foramen ovale among patients undergoing selective peripheral denervation in the sitting position. Neurosurgery 53:316–319

Goldberg RN, Joshi A, Moscoso P (1983) The effect of head position in intracranial pressure in the neonate. Crit Care Med 11:428–430

Harrison EA, Mackersie A, McEwan A (2002) The sitting position for neurosurgery in children: a review of 16 years' experience. Br J Anaesth 88:1–3

Haure P, Cold GE, Hansen TM et al (2003) The ICP-lowering effect of 10 degrees reverse Trendelenburg position during craniotomy is stable during a 10 minute period. J Neurosurg Anesthesiol 15:297–301

Hewer AJH, Loque V (1962) Methods of increasing the safety of neuroanaesthesia in the sitting position. Anaesthesia 17:476–482

Hulme A, Cooper R (1976) The effects of head position and jugular vein compression (JVC) on intracranial pressure (ICP). A clinical study. In: Beks JWF, Bosch DA, Brock M (eds) Intracranial pressure III. Springer, Berlin, pp 259–263

Iwabuchi T, Sobata E, Suzuki K et al (1983) Dural sinus pressure as related to neurosurgical positions. Neurosurgery 12:203–207

Kenning JA, Toutant SM, Sauders RL (1981) Upright patient positioning in the management of intracranial hypertension. Surg Neurol 15:148–152

Lee ST (1989) Intracranial pressure changes during positioning of patients with severe head injury. Heart Lung 32:1288–1291

Leighton SB, Winston K (1994) Cerebrospinal fluid pressure as a function of body position in dogs. Neurol Res 16:439–442

Leivers D, Spilsbury RA, Young JVI (1971) Air embolism during surgery in the sitting position. Br J Anaesth 43:84–90

Leslie K, Hui R, Kaye AH (2006) Venous air embolism and the sitting position: a case series. J Clin Neurosci 13:419–422

Matjasko J, Petrozza P, Cohen M et al (1985) Anesthesia and surgery in the seated position: analysis of 544 cases. Neurosurgery 17:695–702

Mavrocordatos P, Bissonnette B, Ravussin P (2000) Effects of neck position and head elevation on intracranial pressure in anaesthetized neurosurgical patients. J Neurosurg Anesthesiol 12:10–14

Michenfelder JD, Martins JT, Alterburg BM (1969) Air embolism during neurosurgery: an evaluation of right-arterial catheters for diagnosis and treatment. J Am Med Assoc 298:1353–1358

O'Higgins JW (1970) Air embolism during neurosurgery. Br J Anaesth 42:459–462

Porter JM, Pidgeon C, Cunningham AJ (1999) The sitting position in neurosurgery: a critical appraisal. Br J Anaesth 82:117–128

Rolighed Larsen J, Haure P, Cold GE (2002) Reverse Trendelenburg position reduces intracranial pressure during craniotomy. J Neurosurg Anesthesiol 14:16–21

Ropper MJ, Coley IB (1982) Cerebral perfusion pressure, intracranial pressure, and compliance. Neurology 32:1288–1291

Rosner MJ, Coley IB (1986) Cerebral perfusion pressure, intracranial pressure, and head elevation. J Neurosurg 65:636–641

Sale JP (1984) Prevention of air embolism during sitting neurosurgery. The use of inflatable venous neck tourniquet. Anaesthesia 39:795–799

Schmitt HJ, Hemmerling TM (2002) Venous air emboli occur during release of positive end expiratory pressure and repositioning after sitting surgery. Anesth Analg 94:400–403

Schneider F, Franke R, Lanksch WR et al (1993) Influence of body position and cerebral and cerebral perfusion pressure. Acta Neurochir 59:107–112

Sørensen J, Troelsen S, Kaalund J (1990) Changes in blood gases during venous air embolism. Eur J Anesthesiol 7:467–471

Standefer M, Bay JW, Trusso R (1984) G position in neurosurgery: a retrospective analysis of 488 cases. Neurosurgery 14:649–658

Stendel R, Gramm HJ, Schroeder K et al (2000) Transcranial Doppler ultrasonography as a screening technique for detection of a patent foramen ovale before surgery in the sitting position. Anesthesiology 93:971–975

Tankisi A, Cold GE (2007) Optimal reverse Trendelenburg position in patients undergoing craniotomy for cerebral tumours. J Neurosurg 106:239–244

Tankisi A, Rolighed Larsen J, Rasmussen M et al (2002) The effect of 10 degrees reverse Trendelenburg position on ICP and CPP in prone positioned patients subjected to craniotomy for occipital or cerebellar tumours. Acta Neurochir 144:665–670

Tankisi A, Rasmusssen M, Juul N (2006) The effects of 10 degrees reverse Trendelenburg position on subdural intracranial pressure and cerebral perfusion pressure in patients subjected to craniotomy for cerebral aneurysm. J Neurosurg Anesthesiol 18:11–17

Tausk HC, Miller R(1983) Anaesthesia for posterior fossa surgery in the sitting position. Bull N Y Acad Med 59:771–783

Toung TJ, Miyabe M, McShane AJ et al (1988) Effect of PEEP and jugular venous compression on canine cerebral blood flow and oxygen consumption in the head elevated position. Anesthesiology 68:53–58

Toung TJ, Aizawa H, Traystman RJ (2000) Effects of positive end-expiratory pressure ventilation on cerebral venous pressure with head elevation in dogs. J Appl Physiol 88:655–661

Watson G (1974) Effect of head rotation on jugular vein blood flow. Arch Dis Child 49:237–239

William A, Coyne SM (1993) Effects of neck position in intracranial pressure. Am J Crit Care 2:68–71

Yoshida A, Shima T, Okada Y et al (1993) Effects of postural changes on epidural pressure and cerebral perfusion pressure in patients with serious intracranial lesions. In: Avezaat CJJ, Eijndhoven JHM, Maas AIR, Tans JTJ (eds) Intracranial pressure VIII. Springer, Berlin, pp 433–436

Chapter 23
Differences in PCO_2, pH, Lactate, K^+ and Na^+ Between Arterial Blood and Jugular Bulb Blood in Patients Subjected to Craniotomy in Either Propofol-Fentanyl or Propofol-Remifentanil Anaesthesia

Georg Emil Cold and Niels Juul

Abstract
Studies of intensive care patients indicate that the arteriovenous difference (AVD) of PCO_2 in the systemic circulation increases during critical hypoperfusion. As regards the cerebral circulation, studies in pigs indicate that the AVD-PCO_2 increases with CBF reduction. In patients subjected to craniotomy for supratentorial cerebral tumours the AVD-PCO_2 or AVD-pH has not been studied. It has repeatedly been documented that low values of jugular bulb oxygen saturation (SjO_2) and high values of $AVDO_2$ occur during anaesthesia with propofol-fentanyl or propofol-alfentanil, and in a comparative study of propofol-fentanyl or propofol-remifentanil anaesthesia SjO_2 is even lower during the latter.

In this chapter, the results of a database study of AVD of physiological parameters are reported and discussed. We investigated the relationships between $AVDO_2$, AVD-PCO_2, AVD-pH, AVD of the electrolytes Na^+, K^+ and Ca^{++}, SjO_2, jugular oxygen content and jugular oxygen tension during maintenance anaesthesia with propofol-fentanyl and propofol-remifentanil.

Studies of intensive care patients indicate that the AVD of PCO_2 in the systemic circulation increases during critical hypoperfusion (Zhang and Vincent 1993; Mekontso-Dessap et al. 2002). As regards the cerebral circulation, studies in pigs indicate that the AVD-PCO_2 increases with CBF reduction (Rossi et al. 2002). In a case study, this finding has been documented in a patient with severe head injury (Chieregato et al. 1997) and in a series of 12 patients with severe cerebral damage, it was found that the relationship between the $AVDO_2$ and

AVD-PCO_2 was coupled, until severe cerebral ischaemia occurred, at which time the ratio of AVD-PCO_2 to $AVDO_2$ increases (Stocchetti et al. 2005).

In patients subjected to craniotomy for supratentorial cerebral tumours the AVD-PCO_2 or AVD-pH has not been studied. It has repeatedly been documented that low values of SjO_2/high values of $AVDO_2$ occur during anaesthesia with propofol-fentanyl (Jansen et al. 1999; Nandate et al. 2000; Petersen et al. 2003; Kuwano et al. 2004) or propofol-alfentanil (Moss et al. 1995), and in a comparative study of propofol-fentanyl or propofol-remifentanil anaesthesia SjO_2 is even lower during the latter (Schlünzen and Cold; Chapter 8). The threshold of SjO_2 at which cerebral ischaemia occurs, however, has not been defined. Until now, only $AVDO_2$ has been related to AVD-PCO_2, while the correlations between SjO_2, jugular venous oxygen tension (PvO_2) or cerebral venous oxygen content (O_2Ct) as dependent variables have not been studied. As cerebral ischaemia triggers ion dysfunction with movement of water and sodium into the cell, and lactate, potassium and calcium in the opposite direction (Stiefel et al. 2005), membrane failure of cerebral cells theoretically should be accompanied by an increase in the AVD of lactate, K^+ and Ca^{++} and a decrease in AVD-Na^+.

In this chapter, the results of a database study of AVD of physiological parameters are reported and discussed.

Study Outline

Aim   To investigate the relationships between $AVDO_2$, AVD-PCO_2, AVD-pH, AVD of the electrolytes Na^+, K^+ and Ca^{++}, SjO_2, jugular O_2Ct, and PvO_2 during maintenance anaesthesia with propofol-fentanyl and propofol-remifentanil.

Patients   In total 88 patients were included in the study, 38 patients were anaesthetized with propofol-fentanyl and 50 patients with propofol-remifentanil (see Chapter 3).

Method   During craniotomy, paired samples of arterial and jugular venous blood were analysed in 38 patients subjected to propofol-fentanyl and 50 patients subjected to propofol-remifentanil anaesthesia for supratentorial cerebral tumours. Immediately after induction of anaesthesia a jugular bulb catheter and an arterial line were inserted. At the time of opening of dura arterial and jugular blood were analysed for pH, PCO_2, PvO_2, SjO_2, PvO_2, jugular O_2Ct, lactate, K^+, Na^+ and Ca^{++}. The AVD of O_2, PCO_2, pH, lactate, K^+, Na^+ and Ca^{++} were calculated.

Statistical analysis   Sigma Stat and Sigma Plot programs were used for linear correlation, significance and power estimation. Data within anaesthetic groups were tested for normal distribution. Within groups the paired t-test or Wilcoxon's signed rank test were used. Between groups the normality test and equal variance test were applied. Intergroup analyses included one-way analysis of variance. Tukey's test was used for pair-wise multiple comparison procedures. The Kruskal-Wallis analysis of variance on ranks, and multiple comparisons versus control groups (Dunn's method) were used for statistical analysis when the normality test or equal variance test were not passed. The chi-square test was used for statistical analysis of proportions of observation within neuroradiological, histopathological findings and the degrees of dura tension and brain swelling. Medians (ranges) are indicated. $P<0.05$ was considered statistically significant.

Results of comparison between anaesthetic groups The demographic data (age, weight, height, sex), arterial Na^+, arterial K^+, arterial Ca^{++}, arterial lactate, $PaCO_2$, PaO_2 or rectal temperature were comparable (Table 23.1). The propofol maintenance dose was significantly lower in propofol-remifentanil-anaesthetized patients compared to patients anaesthetized with propofol-fentanyl (Table 23.1).

Table 23.1 Demographic, neuroradiological findings, data concerning maintenance doses of anaesthesia, data from arterial and jugular venous blood and data of MABP, subdural ICP and CPP are presented. Mean±SD are indicated

	Propofol-fentanyl	Propofol-remifentanil
Number	38	50
Men/women	29/21	25/13
Age (years)	53.00±9.0	53.00±11.0
Weight (kg)	72.00±16.0	71.00±13.0
Neuroradiological findings		
Maximal area of the tumour (cm^2)	14.00±11.0	13.00±8.2
Volume of the tumour (cm^3)	27.00±26.0	26.00±31.0
Midline shift (mm)	5.00±6.3	5.50±6.7
Data concerning anaesthesia		
Propofol maintenance dose (mg/h)	509.00±113.0	386.00±105.0*
Fentanyl maintenance dose (µg/h)	128.00±25.0	
Remifentanil maintenance dose (µg/h)		1.80±0.59
Data from arterial and venous samples		
Arterial Na$^+$ (mmol/L)	138.00±3.0	138.00±3.0
Arterial K$^+$ (mmol/L)	3.50±0.4	3.70±0.4
Arterial lactate (mmol/L)	1.17±0.53	1.18±0.7
Arterial Ca^{++}(mmol/L)	1.16±0.05	1.14±0.05
PaCO$_2$ (kPa)	4.70±0.3	4.50±0.3
PaO$_2$ (kPa)	20.00±6.5	24.00±5.7
AVDO$_2$ (mmol/L)	3.33±0.66	3.22±0.70
SjO$_2$ (%)	53.30±9.1	54.00±8.8
Temperature, MABP, subdural ICP and CPP		
Temperature (°C)	35.80±0.3	35.80±0.3
MABP (mmHg)	87.00±13.0	74.00±11.0*
Subdural ICP (mmHg)	8.70±5.7	7.70±5.7
CPP (mmHg)	78.00±15.0	66.00±13.0*

*$P<0.05$

The neuroradiological data, including midline shift, area and volume of the tumours did not differ significantly between propofol-fentanyl- and propofol-remifentanil-anaesthetized patients (Table 23.1). During propofol-fentanyl anaesthesia the mean±SD of MABP (87±13 mmHg) and CPP (78±15 mmHg) were significantly higher than the values obtained during propofol-remifentanil: MABP (74±11 mmHg) and CPP (66±13 mmHg). No significant difference was found as regards $AVDO_2$ or SjO_2.

Results of correlation studies with AVD-pH and AVD-PCO₂ as independent variables The highest values of correlation coefficients were found when the dependent variables were SjO_2 or $AVDO_2$ (Table 23.2). However, all correlations were highly significant with $P<0.001$ and powers of 1.000, or close to 1 (Table 23.3). The linear correlation of the relationship between propofol-

Table 23.2 Correlation coefficients between SjO_2, $AVDO_2$, PvO_2 and O_2Ct as abscissa, and the $AVD\text{-}PCO_2$ and AVD-pH as ordinate. The patients had supratentorial cerebral tumours and were anaesthetized with propofol-fentanyl or propofol-remifentanil

	Correlation coefficient (r) AVD-PCO₂ (kPa)	Correlation coefficient (r) AVD-pH
Propofol-fentanyl		
SjO₂ (%)	0.7970	0.7499
AVDO₂ (mmol/L)	0.8112	0.7463
(PvO₂) (kPa)	0.6672	0.6839
Jugular O₂Ct (mmol/L)	0.5517	0.4974
Propofol-remifentanil		
SjO₂ (%)	0.7943	0.7694
AVDO₂ (mmol/L)	0.7623	0.6373
PvO₂ (kPa)	0.6856	0.7035
Jugular O₂Ct (mmol/L)	0.5722	0.6867

Table 23.3 Power and statistical significance (P value) of the relationships between SjO_2, $AVDO_2$, PvO_2 and O_2Ct as abscissa, and the $AVD\text{-}PCO_2$ and AVD-pH as ordinate. The patients had supratentorial cerebral tumours and were anaesthetized with propofol-fentanyl or propofol-remifentanil

	AVD-PCO₂ (kPa)		AVD-pH	
	Power	P value	Power	P value
Propofol-fentanyl				
SjO₂ (%)	1.000	<0.001	1.000	<0.001
AVDO₂ (mmol/L)	1.000	<0.001	1.000	<0.001
PvO₂ (kPa)	0.997	<0.001	0.998	<0.001
Jugular O₂Ct (mmol/L)	0.952	<0.001	0.889	<0.001
Propofol-remifentanil				
SjO₂ (%)	1.000	<0.001	1.000	<0.001
AVDO₂ (mmol/L)	1.000	<0.001	1.000	<0.001
PvO₂ (kPa)	1.000	<0.001	1.000	<0.001
Jugular O₂Ct (mmol/L)	0.993	<0.001	1.000	<0.001

Table 23.4 Linear regressions of the relationships between SjO_2, $AVDO_2$, PvO_2 and O_2Ct as abscissa, and the $AVD\text{-}PCO_2$ and $AVD\text{-}pH$ as ordinate. The patients had supratentorial cerebral tumours and were anaesthetized with propofol-fentanyl or propofol-remifentanil

	Linear regression $AVD\text{-}PCO_2$ (kPa)	Linear regression $AVD\text{-}pH$
Propofol-fentanyl		
SjO_2 (%)	$AVD\text{-}PCO_2 = 2.9720 - 0.0270 \times SjO_2$	$AVD\text{-}pH = 0.1337 - 0.00109 \times SjO_2$
$AVDO_2$ (mmol/L)	$AVD\text{-}PCO_2 = 0.2774 + 0.3765 \times AVDO_2$	$AVD\text{-}pH = 0.0266 + 0.01478 \times AVDO_2$
PvO_2 (kPa)	$AVD\text{-}PCO_2 = 2.7910 - 0.3183 \times PvO_2$	$AVD\text{-}pH = 0.1310 - 0.01390 \times PvO_2$
Jugular O_2Ct (mmol/L)	$AVD\text{-}PCO_2 = 2.3210 - 0.2073 \times O_2Ct$	$AVD\text{-}pH = 0.1060 - 0.00798 \times O_2Ct$
Propofol-remifentanil		
SjO_2 (%)	$AVD\text{-}PCO_2 = 2.9150 - 0.0252 \times SjO_2$	$AVD\text{-}pH = 0.1473 - 0.00128 \times SjO_2$
$AVDO_2$ (mmol/L)	$AVD\text{-}PCO_2 = 0.5634 + 0.3072 \times AVDO_2$	$AVD\text{-}pH = 0.0349 + 0.01342 \times AVDO_2$
PvO_2 (kPa)	$AVD\text{-}PCO_2 = 2.8520 - 0.3386 \times PvO_2$	$AVD\text{-}pH = 0.1474 - 0.01800 \times PvO_2$
Jugular O_2Ct (mmol/L)	$AVD\text{-}PCO_2 = 2.4110 - 0.2342 \times O_2Ct$	$AVD\text{-}pH = 0.1321 - 0.01470 \times O_2Ct$

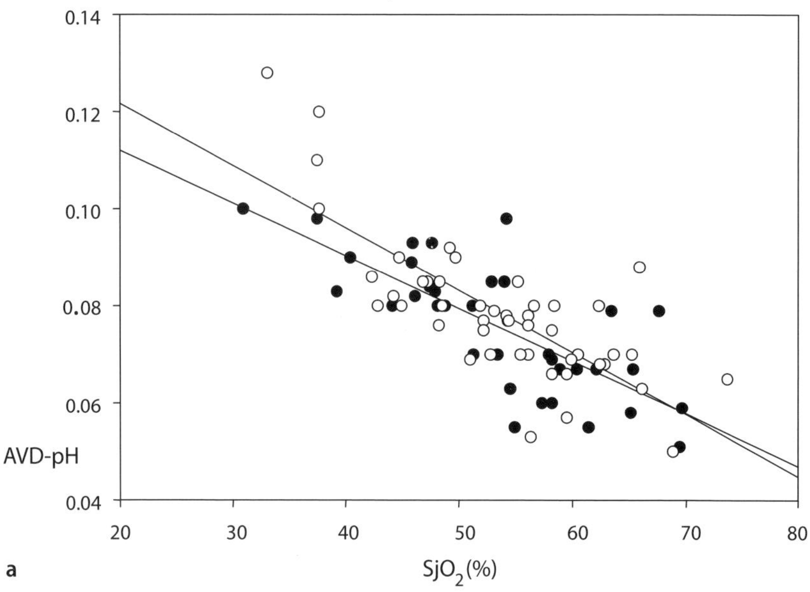

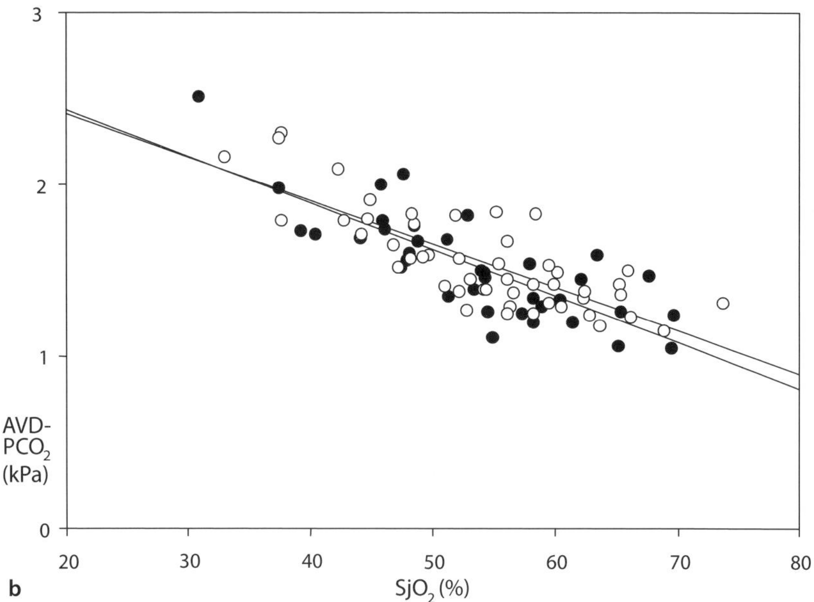

Fig. 23.1 Relationships between SjO$_2$ and AVD-pH (**a**), SjO$_2$ and AVD-PCO$_2$ (**b**), AVDO$_2$ and AVD-pH

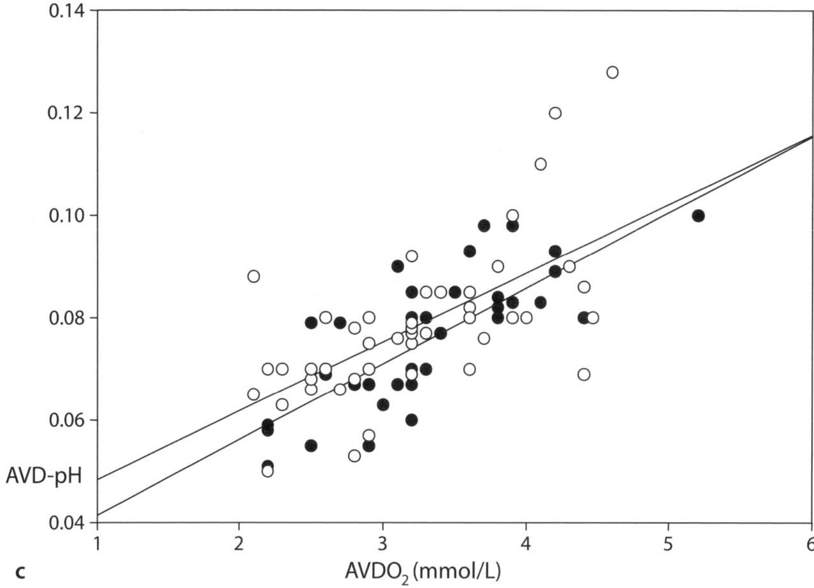

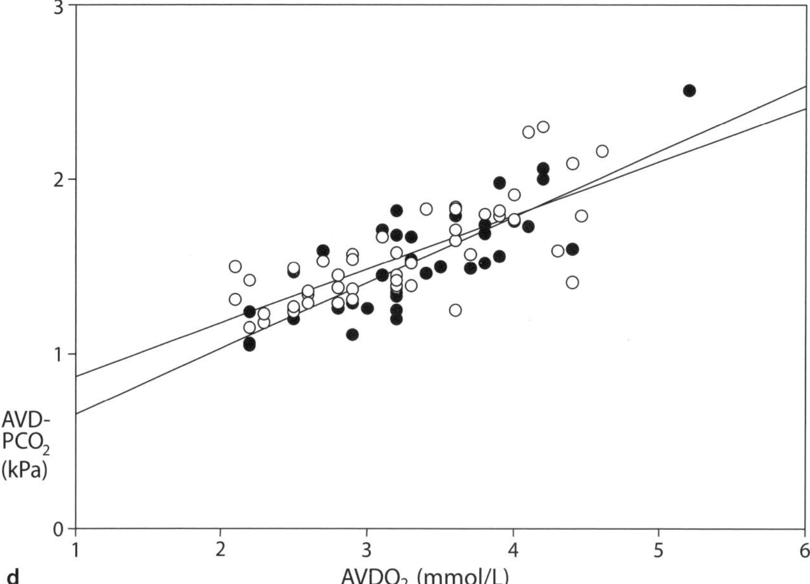

Fig. 23.1 *(continued)* (**c**) and $AVDO_2$ and $AVD\text{-}PCO_2$ (**d**) are indicated. Data were obtained during craniotomy in either propofol-fentanyl (*closed circle*) or propofol-remifentanil (*open circle*). The regression lines are indicated

fentanyl- and propofol-remifentanil-anaesthetized patients did not differ significantly (Table 23.4). The linear regressions between SjO_2 $AVDO_2$ as dependent variable and AVD-pH and AVD-PCO$_2$ as independent variable, respectively, are indicated in Fig. 23.1a–d.

Results of correlation studies with AVD of lactate, Na⁺, K⁺ and Ca⁺⁺ as independent variables

In Fig. 23.2a–d the correlations between SjO_2 as dependent variable and the AVD of lactate, Na⁺, K⁺ and Ca⁺⁺ as independent variables are indicated. All correlations were insignificant. In comparison with high values of SjO_2 low values were not associated with any significant changes in the AVD of lactate, Na⁺, K⁺ or Ca⁺⁺. As regards AVD-PCO$_2$ and AVD-pH, the correlation coefficients were highest for the relationships with SjO_2 or $AVDO_2$ as the dependent variable, followed by PvO_2 and O_2Ct, and the data concerning the correlations were close to the regression lines with both anaesthetic regimes, and without significant differences. Although high values of AVD-PCO$_2$ and AVD-pH were found at low SjO_2 and high $AVDO_2$ values, no signs of increased lactate, K⁺ or Ca⁺⁺ liberation from cerebral tissue suggesting impeding cerebral ischaemia were disclosed.

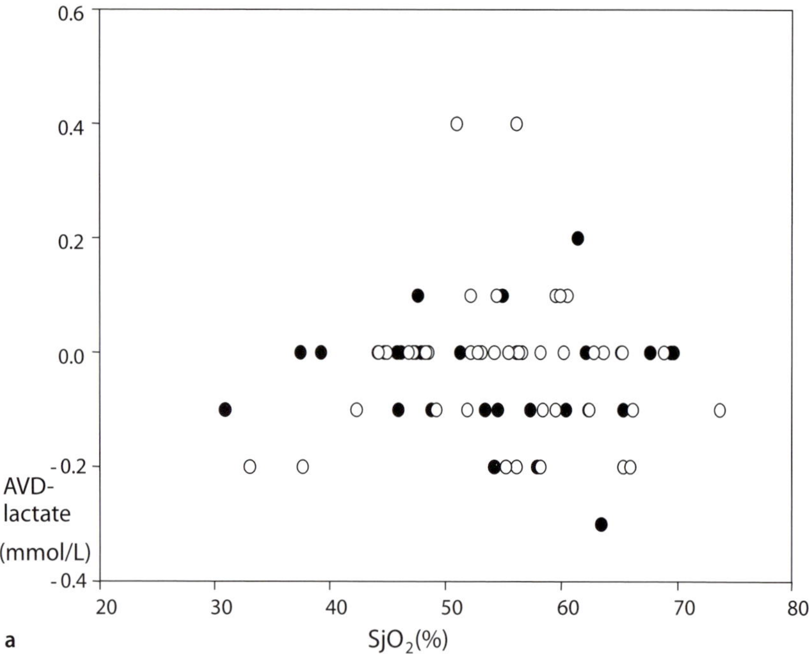

Fig. 23.2 Relationships between SjO_2 and AVD-lactate (**a**), SjO_2 and AVD-Na⁺

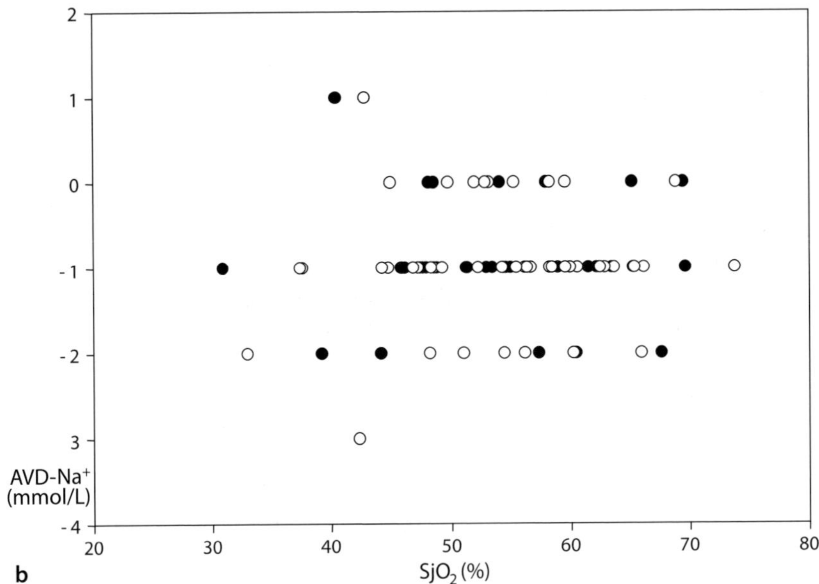

b

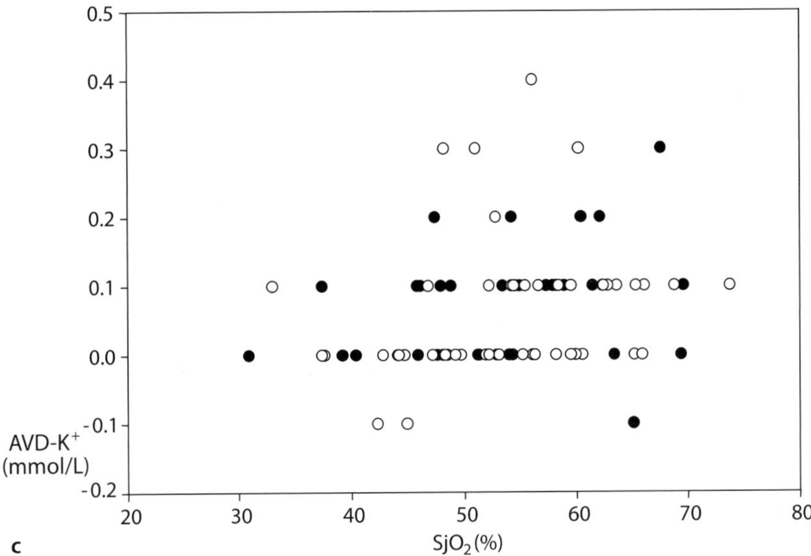

c

Fig. 23.2 *(continued)* (**b**), SjO$_2$ and AVD-K$^+$ (**c**) and SjO$_2$ and AVD-Ca^{++}

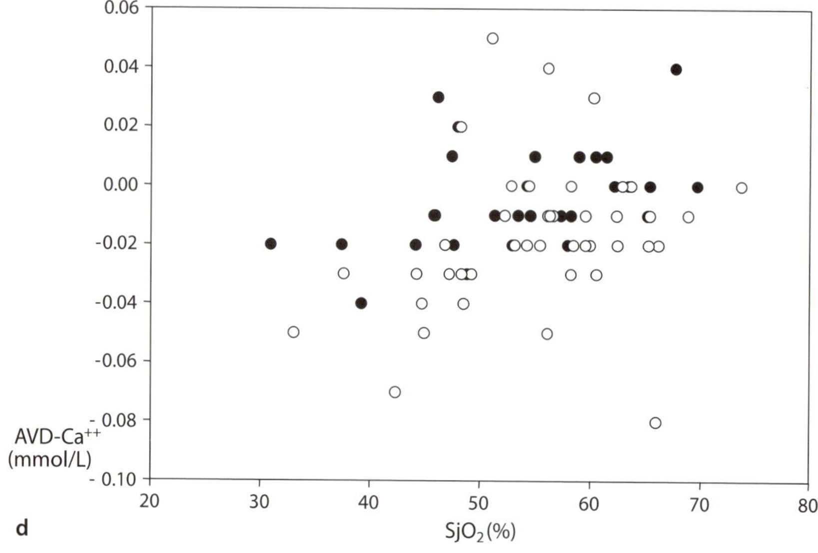

Fig. 23.2 *(continued)* (**d**) are indicated. Data were obtained during craniotomy in either propofol-fentanyl (*closed circle*) or propofol-remifentanil (*open circle*). No significant correlations were found

Conclusion Although an increase in AVD-pH and AVD-PCO₂ is found with low values of SjO₂ and high values of AVDO₂, it is not accompanied by significant changes in AVD-lactate, AVD-K+, AVD-Na⁺ or AVD-Ca⁺⁺ suggesting cerebral ischaemia.

Discussion

In the present study, patients scheduled for elective supratentorial tumour craniotomy were anaesthetized with either propofol-fentanyl or propofol-remifentanil. Blood from arterial and jugular venous catheters were analysed for oxygen tension, oxygen saturation, electrolytes (K⁺, Na⁺ and Ca⁺⁺) and lactate. The aims of the study were as follows: (1) to investigate the relationship between AVDO₂, SjO₂, PvO₂ or O₂Ct as dependent factor related to AVD-PCO₂ or AVD-pH; (2) to investigate whether the relationship between AVDO₂ with respect to SjO₂ and AVD-PCO₂ with respect to AVD-pH differed between propofol-fentanyl- and propofol-remifentanil-anaesthetized patients; and (3) to study the levels of AVD of lactate K⁺, Na⁺ and Ca⁺⁺ at low values of SjO₂ with respect to high values of AVDO₂.

The results of the study indicate that fairly good correlations were found between AVDO₂, SjO₂, PvO₂ or O₂Ct as dependent factor when related to

AVD-PCO_2 or AVD-pH as independent factors. The correlations between these factors were not significantly influenced by choice of anaesthesia, and low values of SjO_2 with respect to high values of $AVDO_2$ were not associated with signs of increased venous influx of lactate/Ca^{++}/Na^+ or venous efflux of K^+.

According to early clinical studies the lower limits of SjO_2 in conscious subjects without cerebral disease are 54.6% and 55.0% (Gibbs et al. 1942; Datsur et al. 1963). In a recent study, however, the lower limit of SjO_2 in patients without cerebral disease was 44.7% with confidence limits 36.5–53% (Chieregato et al. 2003). The authors suggest that contamination by extracerebral blood of the facial veins and the inferior petrosal sinuses is responsible for the higher values found in earlier studies. In accordance with a clinical study indicating that avoidance of extracerebral contamination is prevented when the tip of the catheter is placed within 2 cm of the base of the skull (Jakobsen and Enevoldsen 1989) we introduced the guide wire until resistance was obtained by the base of the skull, and introduced the jugular catheter with the guide wire in this position. Furthermore, we performed moderate neck compression cranial to the catheter to secure cranial direction of the catheter.

Experimental studies have shown that severe cerebral ischaemia is accompanied by flux of K^+ and lactate from the intracellular to the extracellular space, and movement of Na^+ in the opposite direction (Stiefel et al. 2005). Ca^{++} follows K^+, the result being an increased concentration in the extracellular space. In the present study we hypothesized that the AVD of K^+, Ca^{++} and lactate would increase and the AVD of Na+ decrease during cerebral ischaemia. $AVDO_2$, however, is dependent on CBF. If CBF is high, the $AVDO_2$ decreases, while $AVDO_2$ increases at low values of CBF. In several studies it has been observed that during propofol anaesthesia the reduction of CBF is larger than the reduction of $CMRO_2$, resulting in a decrease of the $CBF/CMRO_2$ ratio (Manohar 1986; Scheller et al. 1988, 1990; Mielck et al. 1999). Accordingly, relatively high values of $AVDO_2$ during both anaesthetic procedures were found in the present study, and the correlation between $AVDO_2$ and AVD-PCO_2 and AVD-pH was positive and highly significant, indicating prevention of efflux of CO_2 and H^+ caused by low CBF. During high $AVDO_2$/low SjO_2, however, the AVD of K^+, Ca^{++} and lactate did not increase, and the AVD-Na^+ did not fall, suggesting that cerebral ischaemia, giving rise to disturbed ion homeostasis and increased cerebral lactate efflux, did not occur. These findings support that, although high values of $AVDO_2$ were observed, the threshold of severe global cerebral ischaemia was not exceeded. However, as the AVD data are a global estimate, it does not exclude that regional ischaemia might occur.

References

Chieregato A, Zoppellari R, Targa L (1997) Cerebral arteriovenous PCO_2 difference and early global cerebral ischaemia in patients with severe head injury. J Neurosurg Anesthesiol 9:256–262

Chieregato A, Calzolari F, Trasforini G et al (2003) Normal jugular bulb oxygen saturation. J Neurol Neurosurg Psychiatry 74:784–786

Datsur DK, Lane MH, Hansen DB et al (1963) Effects of aging on cerebral circulation and metabolism in man. In: Birren JE, Butler RN, Greenhouse SW et al (eds) Human aging. A biological and behavioral study. US Government Printing Office, Washington, DC, pp 59–76

Gibbs EL, Lennox WG, Nims LF et al (1942) Arterial and cerebral venous blood. Arteriovenous differences in man. J Biol Chem 144:325–332

Jakobsen M, Enevoldsen E (1989) Retrograde catheterization of the right internal jugular vein for serial measurements of cerebral venous oxygen content. J Cereb Blood Flow Metab 9:717–720

Jansen GF, van Praagh BH, Kedaria MB et al (1999) Jugular bulb oxygen saturation during propofol and isoflurane/nitrous oxide anesthesia in patients undergoing brain tumour surgery. Anesth Analg 89:358–363

Kuwano Y, Kawaguchi M, Inoue S et al (2004) Jugular bulb oxygen saturation under propofol or sevoflurane/nitrous oxide anesthesia during deliberate mild hypothermia in neurosurgical patients. J Neurosurg Anesthesiol 16:6–10

Manohar M (1986) Regional brain blood flow and cerebral cortical O_2 consumption during sevoflurane anesthesia in healthy isocapnic swine. J Cardiovasc Pharmacol 8:1268–1275

Mekontso-Dessap A, Castclain V, Anguel N et al (2002) Combination of venoarterial PCO_2 difference with arterio-venous O_2 content difference to detect anaerobic metabolism in patients. Intensive Care Med 28:272–277

Mielck F, Stephan H, Weyland A et al (1999) Effects of one minimum alveolar anesthetic concentration sevoflurane on cerebral metabolism, blood flow, and CO_2 reactivity in cardiac patients. Anesth Analg 89:364–369

Moss E, Dearden NM, Berridge JC (1995) Effects of changes in mean arterial pressure on SjO_2 during cerebral aneurysm surgery. Br J Anaesth 75:527–530

Nandate K, Vuylsteke A, Ratsep I et al (2000) Effects of isoflurane, sevoflurane and propofol anaesthesia on jugular venous oxygen saturation in patients undergoing coronary artery by-pass surgery. Br J Anaesth 84:631–633

Petersen KD, Landsfeldt U, Cold GE et al (2003) Intracranial pressure and cerebral hemodynamic in patients with cerebral tumours. Anesthesiology 98:329–336

Rossi S, Colombo A, Magnoni S et al (2002) Cerebral veno-arterial pCO_2 difference as an estimator of uncompensated cerebral hypoperfusion. Acta Neurochir Suppl 81:201–204

Scheller MS, Tateichi A, Drummond JC et al (1988) The effects of sevoflurane on cerebral blood flow, cerebral metabolic rate of oxygen, intracranial pressure, and the electroencephalogram are similar to those of isoflurane in the rabbits. Anesthesiology 68:548–551

Scheller MS, Nakakimura K, Fleischer JE et al (1990) Cerebral effects of sevoflurane in the dog: comparison with isoflurane and enflurane. Br J Anaesth 65:388–392

Stiefel MF, Tomita Y, Marmarou A (2005) Secondary ischemia impairing the restoration of ion homeostasis following traumatic brain injury. J Neurosurg 103:707–714

Stocchetti N, Zanier ER, Nicolini R et al (2005) Oxygen and carbon dioxide in the cerebral circulation during progression of brain death. Anesthesiology 103:957–961

Zhang H, Vincent JL (1993) Ateriovenous differences of PCO_2 and pH are good indicators of critical hypoperfusion. Am Rev Respir Dis 148:867–871

Chapter 24
Limitations and Complications Connected with Monitoring of Subdural Intracranial Pressure and Insertion of Jugular Catheter

Georg Emil Cold and Niels Juul

Abstract

With any invasive monitoring procedure the risk of adverse events is present. The incidence of dural tears during opening of the surgical field has previously been reported in the literature. Predisposing factors for accidental dural tears occurring during supratentorial craniotomy have been reported. Predisposing factors included extracerebral pathology (meningioma), age of the patients, thickness of the cranial vault, the presence of hyperostosis frontalis and a frontal or pterional location. In elderly patients adhesions between the dura and the skull are increased, leaving dura more vulnerable during craniotomy. Moreover, with respect to the auxiliary surgical tools, the use of the drill was associated significantly with dural tears.

In this chapter the adverse effects of subdural monitoring are disclosed. In addition the potential dangers of jugular venous puncture and wound infection are discussed.

Since 1994 we have performed perioperative measurement of subdural ICP combined with arterial pressure, JBP and gas analysis in primarily elective patients subjected to craniotomy. ICP was measured with a 22G needle connected to a pressure transducer via a polyethylene catheter. Until May 2006 1,833 patients have been investigated, and in 989 patients insertion of a jugular bulb catheter was performed. The data have been collected in a database. The techniques used for subdural ICP measurement and insertion of a jugular bulb catheter are described in Chapter 3.

Study Outline

Aim In this study, the incidence of dural lesions, which in some cases may prevent subdural ICP measurement, the incidence of traumatic SAH due to needle insertion for ICP measurement, and the incidence of wound infection are analysed.

Method After removal of the skull the dura was inspected. If lesion of dura occurred it was registered. If a dural lesion greater than 2 cm was found subdural ICP measurement was omitted. After opening of dura the surface of the brain was inspected. Traumatic SAH was registered.

The occurrence of failed jugular catheter insertion and puncture of the internal carotid artery were registered as well. Via the records, skull wound infection was registered retrospectively for the year 2004. All patients were treated with i.v. cefuroxime (1.5 g for adults) administered shortly after induction of anaesthesia.

Table 24.1 Age of the patients related to number and percentage of patients with dural lesion where it was impossible to measure subdural ICP

Age (years)	Number of patients	Number of dural lesions	Percent of total
0–10	50	0	0.0
11–20	53	0	0.0
21–30	106	2	1.9
31–40	217	8	3.7
41–50	377	19	5.0
51–60	514	30	5.8
61–70	397	36	9.1
71–80	111	21	18.9
81–90	8	2	25.0
Total	1,833	117	6.4

Table 24.2 The incidence of failed subdural ICP monitoring due to large lesion of dura is indicated in different cerebral disorders. Patients undergoing supratentorial craniotomy are included

Pathology	Number	Percent	Total
SAH	19	8.4	225
Arteriovenous malformation	2	7.1	28
Head injury	0	0.0	15
Glioblastoma	21	4.5	467
Meningioma	40	11.6	345
Metastasis	20	7.3	275
Oligodendroglioma	7	6.3	111
Craniopharangioma	1	7.1	14
Glioma	6	7.0	86
Other tumours	1	6.1	21
Other disorders	0	0.0	63
Total	117	7.1	1,657

Results In 10 patients it was impossible to measure subdural ICP because of technical reasons (cable or transducer defect (n=4), bleeding (n=2) or unstable ICP (n=4)). In 293 patents (16%) dural lesion occurred, and in 117 patients (6.4%) ICP measurement was impossible because of dural lesion exceeding 2 cm. The occurrence of dural lesions increased with the age of the patients (Table 24.1) and in patients undergoing supratentorial craniotomy. Dural lesion was frequently found in patients with convexity meningioma and patients with cerebral aneurysm where the pterion approach was used (Table 24.2). In infratentorial surgery the incidence was highest in patients with angioma (9.8%) (Table 24.3). Traumatic SAH occurred in 16 patients (0.87%) (Table 24.4).

In 13 of 989 patients (1.3%) it was impossible to locate the jugular vein. Also, puncture of the carotid artery occurred in 12 cases (1.2%) and, in these

Table 24.3 The incidence of failed subdural ICP monitoring due to large lesion of dura is indicated in different cerebral disorders. Patients undergoing infratentorial craniectomy are included

Pathology	Number	Percent	Total
Angioma	4	9.8	41
Metastasis	4	5.8	69
Astrocytoma	1	6.7	15
Meningioma	2	8.0	25
Trigeminus	2	7.7	26
Total	13	7.4	176

Table 24.4 The occurrence of fresh traumatic SAH in 1,833 patients (10 male, 6 female), mean age 57.6 years (15–68 years)

	Number	Percent
Diagnosis		
Glioblastoma	6	
Oligodendroglioma	2	
Glioma	3	
Meningioma	1	
Astrocytoma	1	
Metastasis	1	
Ependynoma	1	
Intracerebral haematoma	1	
Total	16	0.87
Localization		
Frontal	4	
Parietal	2	
Temporal	7	
Occipital	3	
Total	16	0.87

cases, further attempts to insert a catheter were avoided. No further adverse events were reported as regards insertion of the jugular catheters. For a period of 12 months (year 2004) the incidence of wound infection was registered. During this period wound infections were not disclosed. In comparison, among the 143 patients subjected to acute craniotomy without ICP monitoring 4 patients (2.8%) suffered from deep skull wound infection.

Conclusion Perioperative subdural ICP measurement gives valuable information about ICP, and in addition information concerning the effects of ICP-reducing managements. Due to large dural lesions subdural ICP measurement could not be performed in 5.3% of patients. Traumatic SAH occurs rarely, and wound infections were not registered in the present study.

Discussion

The incidence of dural tears during opening in the present study is in accordance with the literature. Predisposing factors for accidental dural tears occurring during supratentorial craniotomy were studied by Engelhardt et al. (2005). They found an incidence of 26%. Predisposing factors included extracerebral pathology (meningioma), age of the patients, thickness of the cranial vault, the presence of hyperostosis frontalis and a frontal or pterional location. In elderly patients adhesions between the dura and the skull are increased, leaving dura more vulnerable during craniotomy. Moreover, with respect to the auxiliary surgical tools, the use of the drill was associated significantly with dural tears.

One reason for the relatively high incidence of lesion of dura in patients with meningioma is that meningioma generally is attached to dura, whereas meningioma without dural attachment is extremely rare (Zhang et al. 2007). Thus, in some meningioma opening of dura inevitably results in lesion of dura.

In the present study, the incidence of fresh SAH discovered after opening of dura was 0.87%. In all cases dura was intact after removal of the bone flap. The low incidence made estimation of risk factors futile. In three patients (0.17%) it was possible to locate the source of bleeding to cerebral veins, located just under the needle used for subdural ICP measurement. In the other cases the source of bleeding was undetectable. In these cases the source of bleeding might also be caused by incision of dura, and by the sewing of dura to the bone. If SAH was present some degree of brain swelling occurred, but in none of the cases did the presence of haemorrhage prevent the surgical procedure. Literature concerning the incidence of SAH after opening of dura is not available.

In order to avoid puncture of the carotid artery, catheterization of the jugular vein was performed with the head in the neutral position (Sulek et al. 1996) and with the patient positioned in 5–10° rTp. This position dilates the jugular vein (Clenaghan et al. 2006). Only the right jugular vein was used. Ultrasound guide in order to localize the jugular vein was not used in the present study, although the success rate is higher with this technique and complications are fewer (Hayashi and Amano 2002; Cajozza et al. 2004). Nevertheless, puncture of the carotid artery occurred in 12 patients (1.2%), and in 13 of 989 patients (1.3%) it was impossible to locate the jugular vein. Data concerning the incidence of carotid puncture are not available for jugular catheterization in the cranial direction. The incidence during central placement of jugular catheters varies between zero in children (Sheridan and Weber 2006) and 2.9% in critically ill patients (Schummer et al. 2007). Thus, the incidence in the present material seems acceptable. Infections localized to the jugular catheter were not observed, probably because the catheter was removed before extubation of the patients.

In the present study the incidence of wound infection was surprisingly low in the year 2004, and meningitis did not occur. One reason may be that the incidence was registered retrospectively. Moreover, in the present study, surgical site infections were not classified according to the guidelines of the Center for Disease Control (Barker 1994). An infection rate as high as 17.6% has been found (Idali et al. 2004). More seriously, postcraniotomy meningitis has been recorded in 5.5% of patients (Kourbeti et al. 2007). In a prospective study, where antibiotic prophylaxis was used, an incidence of 6.6% has been documented (Korinek et al. 2005). In the same study CSF leak, male gender, surgical diagnosis (glial tumours, meningioma, metastasis), early re-operation and surgical duration were independent risk factors, and it was documented that antibiotic prophylaxis decreased rates of infection significantly. That surgery for meningioma and metastasis is a risk factor for infection has also been documented in other studies (Blomstedt 1985; Tenney et al. 1985; Gaillard and Gilsbach 1991). Presence of diabetes mellitus, presence of foreign body and ICP monitoring were risk factors in a study by Erman et al. (2005), and the surgeon was found to be the most important risk factor influencing the infection rate (George et al. 1979; Blomstedt 1985). Taking the retrospective analysis of infection rate in the present study into consideration, it must be concluded that subdural ICP monitoring as such does not increase the rate of postcraniotomy infection.

References

Barker FG (1994) Efficacy of prophylactic antibiotics for craniotomy: a meta-analysis. Neurosurgery 35:484–490

Blomstedt GC (1985) Infections in neurosurgery: a retrospective study of 1143 patients and 1517 operations. Acta Neurchir 78:81–90

Cajozzo M, Quintini G, Cocchiera G et al (2004) Comparison of central venous catheterization with and without ultrasound guide. Transfus Apher Sci 31:199–202

Clenaghan S, McLaughlin RE, Martyn C et al (2006) Relationship between Trendelenburg tilt and internal jugular vein diameter. Emerg Med J 23:661

Engelhardt M, Uhlenbruch S. Christmann A et al (2005) Accidental dural tears occurring during supratentorial craniotomy. A prospective analysis of predisposing factors in 100 patients. Zentralbl Neurochir 66:70–74

Erman T, Demirhindi H, Göcer AI et al (2005) Risk factors for surgical site infections in neurosurgery patients with antibiotic prophylaxis. Surg Neurol 63:107–113

Gaillard T, Gilsbach JM (1991) Intra-operative antibiotic prophylaxis in neurosurgery. A prospective, randomised, controlled study on cefotiam. Acta Neurochir 113:103–109

George R, Leibrock L, Epstein M (1979) Long-term analysis of cerebrospinal fluid shunt infections. A 25-year experience. J Neurosurg 51:804–811

Hayashi H, Amano M (2002) Does ultrasound imaging before puncture facilitate internal jugular vein cannulation? Prospective randomized comparison with landmark-guided puncture in ventilated patients. J Cardiothorac Vasc Anesth 16:572–575

Idali B, Lahyat B, Khaleq K et al (2004) Postoperative infection following craniotomy in adults. J Med Mal 34:221–224

Korinek A-M, Golmard J-L, Elcheick A et al (2005) Risk factors for neurosurgical site infections after craniotomy: a critical reappraisal of antibiotic prophylaxis on 4578 patients. Br J Neurosurg 19:155–162

Kourbeti IS, Jacobs AV, Koslow M (2007) Risk factors associated with postcraniotomy meningitis. Neurosurgery 60:317–326

Schummer W, Schummer C, Rose N et al (2007) Mechanical complications and malpositions of central venous cannulation by experienced operators: a prospective study of 1794 catheterizations in critically ill patients. Intensive Care Med 33:1055–1059

Sheridan RL, Weber JM (2006) Mechanical and infectious complications of central venous cannulation in children: lessons learned from a 10-year experience placing more than 1000 catheters. J Burn Care Res 27:13–18

Sulek CA, Gravenstein N, Blackshear RH et al (1996) Head rotation during internal jugular vein cannulation and the risk of carotid artery puncture. Anesth Analg 82:125–128

Tenney JH, Vlahov D, Salcman M et al (1985) Wide variation in risk of wound infection following clan neurosurgery. Implications for perioperative antibiotic prophylaxis. J Neurosurg 62:243–247

Zhang J, Ling-Yi C, Meng B et al (2007) Meningioma without dural attachment: case report, classification, and review of the literature. Surg Neurol 67:535–539

Printing: Krips bv, Meppel, The Netherlands
Binding: Stürtz, Würzburg, Germany